PEPTIC ULCER DISEASE: BASIC AND CLINICAL ASPECTS

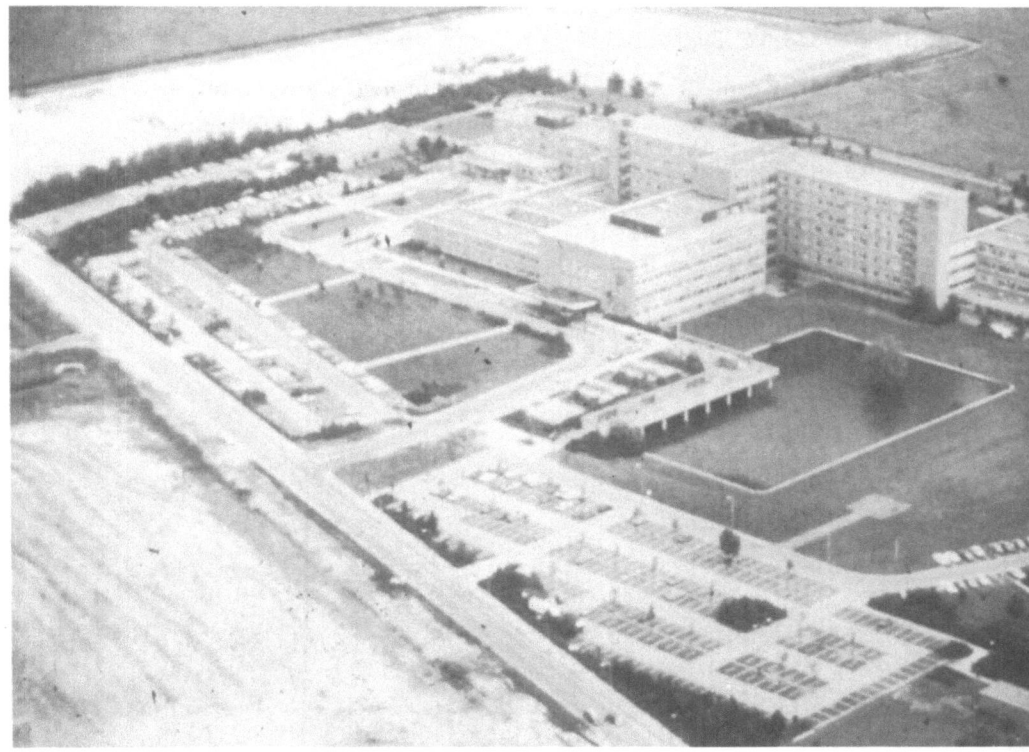

Air view photograph of the SOPHIA ZIEKENHUIS ZWOLLE, THE NETHERLANDS.
The SYMPOSIUM 'PEPTIC ULCER TODAY' was organized at the occasion of the
100th anniversary of the SOPHIA ZIEKENHUIS

DEVELOPMENTS IN GASTROENTEROLOGY

Pena, A.S., Weterman, I.T., Booth, C.C., Strober W., eds: Recent advances in Crohn's disease
ISBN 90 247 2475 9

Motta, P.M., Didio, L.J.A., eds: Basic and clinical hepatology
ISBN 90 247 2404 X

Rachmilewitz, D., ed.: Inflammatory bowel diseases
ISBN 90 247 2612 3

Fleischer, D., Jensen, D., Bright-Asare, P. eds: Therapeutic laser endoscopy in gastrointestinal disease
ISBN 0 89838 577 6

Borriello, S.P., ed: Antibiotic associated diarrhoea and colitis
ISBN 0 89838 623 3

Gips, Ch.H., Krom, R.A.F., eds: Progress in liver transplantation
ISBN 0 89838 726 4

Nelis, G.F., Boevé, J., Misiewicz, J.J., eds: Peptic ulcer disease: Basic and clinical aspects
ISBN 0 89838 759 0

PEPTIC ULCER DISEASE: BASIC AND CLINICAL ASPECTS

Proceedings of the Symposium Peptic Ulcer Today, 21–23 November 1984, at the Sophia Ziekenhuis, Zwolle, The Netherlands

edited by

G.F. NELIS
Department of Internal Medicine
Sophia Ziekenhuis
Zwolle, The Netherlands

J. BOEVÉ
Department of Surgery
Sophia Ziekenhuis
Zwolle, The Netherlands

J.J. MISIEWICZ
Department of Gastroenterology and Nutrition
Central Middlesex Hospital
London, United Kingdom

1985 **MARTINUS NIJHOFF PUBLISHERS**
a member of the KLUWER ACADEMIC PUBLISHERS GROUP
DORDRECHT / BOSTON / LANCASTER

Distributors

for the United States and Canada: Kluwer Academic Publishers, 190 Old Derby Street, Hingham, MA 02043, USA
for the UK and Ireland: Kluwer Academic Publishers, MTP Press Limited, Falcon House, Queen Square, Lancaster LA1 1RN, UK
for all other countries: Kluwer Academic Publishers Group, Distribution Center, P.O. Box 322, 3300 AH Dordrecht, The Netherlands

Library of Congress Cataloging in Publication Data

```
Symposium Peptic Ulcer Today (1984 : Sophia Ziekenhuis,
    Zwolle, Netherlands)
    Peptic ulcer disease.

    (Developments in gastroenterology)
    Symposium organized on the occasion of the 100th
anniversary of the Sophia Ziekenhuis, Zwolle, the
Netherlands.
    Includes bibliographies.
    1. Peptic ulcer--Congresses.  I. Nelis, G. F.
(G. Frits)  II. Boevé, J. (Jan)  III. Misiewicz, J. J.
IV. Sophia Ziekenhuis (Zwolle, Netherlands)  V. Title.
VI. Series. [DNLM: 1. Peptic Ulcer--congresses.
W1 DE997VYB / WI 350 S9897p 1984]
RC821.S925 1984      616.3'43       85-21457
```

ISBN-13:978-94-010-8730-8   e-ISBN-13:978-94-009-5034-4
DOI:10.1007/978-94-009-5034-4

Copyright

Preface

Despite a slow decrease in the incidence of peptic ulcer in the Western world during the past decade, general practitioners, physicians, gastroenterologists, and surgeons deal with patients suffering from peptic ulcer and its complications almost daily. It has been estimated that some 10% of the population in the Western world becomes afflicted by peptic ulcer at least once and many of them have chronic relapsing disease. This lays a heavy burden on the amount of money which is spent in general health care.

In recent years our understanding of peptic ulcer disease has increased tremendously, but considerable gaps in our knowledge remain. Originally the increase in our knowledge has been stimulated by the development of fibre-optic endoscopy in the sixties, and later by the development of new surgical techniques and drugs in the seventies.

New insights into the pathophysiology of the disease resulted from these developments and revived the scientific interest in peptic ulcer disease.

However, the field remains complicated and the studies are bedevilled by the large number of variables which can affect the results.

In the symposium 'PEPTIC ULCER TODAY' we have attempted to bring together recent knowledge on basic and clinical aspects of peptic ulcer disease.

The tremendous increase in the available data made it necessary to select only a limited number of issues to deal with. It is to be hoped that this presentation of the state of the art will provide insights into the basic and clinical aspects of peptic ulcer disease and will stimulate the search for answers to the many questions that are still open, to the benefit of our patients.

This symposium has been organized at the occasion of the 100th anniversary of the SOPHIA ZIEKENHUIS ZWOLLE, THE NETHERLANDS.

The organizers wish to thank in particular the Medical Staff of the SOPHIA ZIEKENHUIS whose Stichting Wetenschappelijk Werk Sophia Ziekenhuis (Founation for Scientific Work at the Sophia Ziekenhuis) provided a most generous grant which made the organization of this symposium possible. Also we wish to thank the Board of Directors of the STICHTING SOPHIA ZIEKENHUIS for their financial and technical support.

Zwolle, April 1985   Frits Nelis
                                                              Jan Boevé
                                                      George Misiewicz

Table of contents

Session III

Session IV

* Not read at the Symposium.

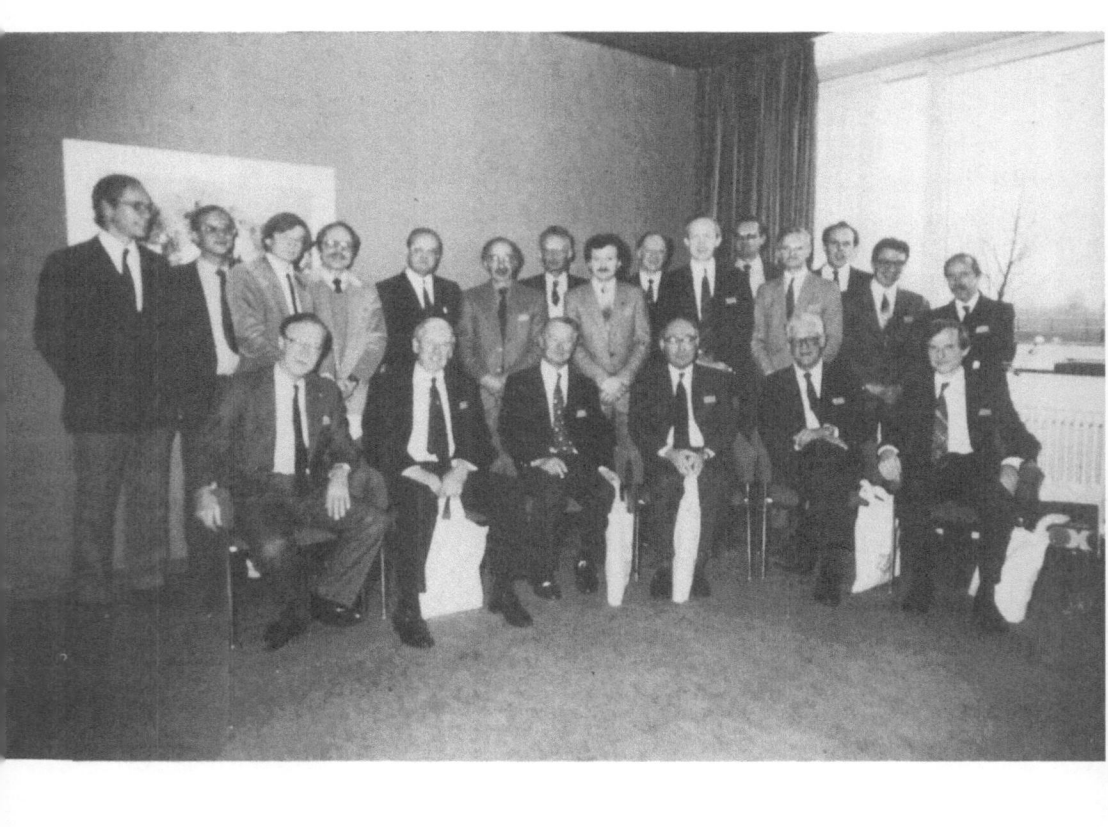

Contributors

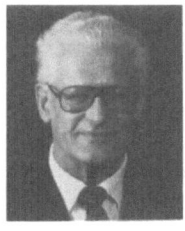

M. ALLGÖWER, M.D., M.D.(hon), F.A.C.S.(hon), F.R.C.S.(hon), Professor of Surgery.
Department of Surgery, Kantonsspital Basel, CH-4031, Switserland

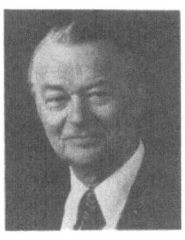

E. AMDRUP, M.D., Ph.D., Professor of Surgery.
Surgical Gastroenterological Department L.,
Århus Kommunehospital, 8000 Århus C, Denmark.

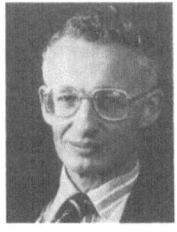

M. van BLANKENSTEIN, B.Sc., M.B., Lecturer in Medicine and Consultant Physician.
Department of Medicine II, Academisch Ziekenhuis Dijkzigt, Erasmus University, 3015 GD Rotterdam, The Netherlands.

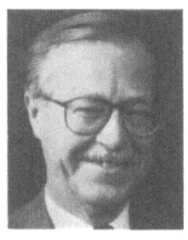

J. BOEVÉ, M.D., Consultant Surgeon.
Department of Surgery, Sophia Ziekenhuis, 8000 GK Zwolle, The Netherlands.

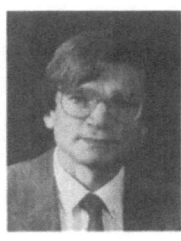

H.P.M. FESTEN, M.D., Lecturer in Medicine.
Department of Gastroenterology, University Hospital,
Free University, 1007 MB Amsterdam, The Nether-
lands.
Present post: Consultant Physician, Department of
Medicine, Groot Ziekengasthuis, 5211 NL 's-Hertogen-
bosch, The Netherlands.

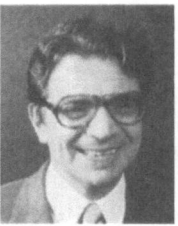

P.H. GUTH, M.D., Associate Professor of Medicine,
Consultant Physician, Assistant Chief of Gastro-
enterology.
Wadsworth Veteran Administration Medical Center,
Los Angeles, CA 90073, USA

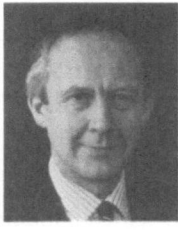

A.G. JOHNSON, M.D. Professor of Surgery and
Honorary Consultant Surgeon.
University Surgical Unit, Royal Hallamshire Hospital,
Sheffield S10 2JF, United Kingdom.

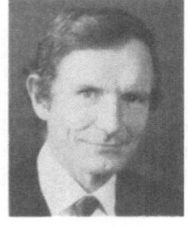

D. JOHNSTON, M.D., Professor of Surgery and
Honorary Consultant Surgeon.
University Department of Surgery, The General
Infirmary, Leeds LS1 3EX, United Kingdom.

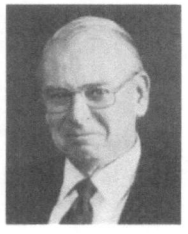

T. KENNEDY, M.D.(hon), Consultant Surgeon.
Department of Surgery, Royal Victoria Hospital,
Belfast BT12 6BA, Northern Ireland.

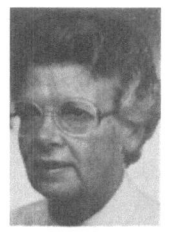

J. KREUNING, M.D., Associate Professor of Medicine, Consultant Gastroenterologist.
Department of Gastroenterology, State University, Academisch Ziekenhuis, 2333 AA Leiden, The Netherlands.

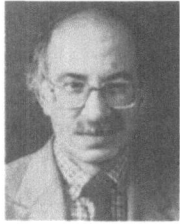

J.J. MISIEWICZ, B.Sc, M.B., F.R.C.P., Consultant Physician and Head of the Department.
Department of Gastroenterology & Nutrition, Central Middlesex Hospital, London NW10 7NS, United Kingdom.

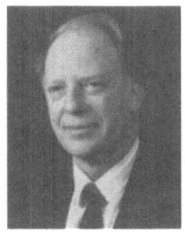

G.F. NELIS, M.D., Consultant Physician.
Department of Internal Medicine, Sophia Ziekenhuis, 8000 GK Zwolle, The Netherlands

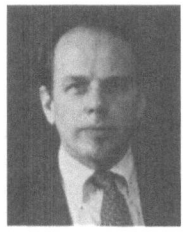

R.E. POUNDER, M.D., Senior Lecturer in Medicine and Honorary Consultant Physician.
University Department of Medicine, The Royal Free Hospital, London NW3 2QG, United Kingdom.

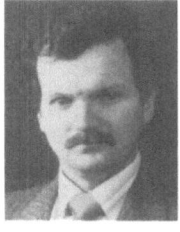

W.D.W. REES, M.D., M.R.C.P., Consultant Gastroenterologist.
Department of Medicine, University of Manchester, Hope Hospital, Salford M6 8HD, United Kingdom.

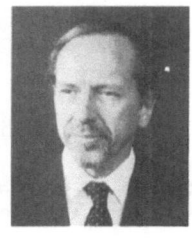

A. ROBERT, M.D., Ph.D.
Diabetes and GI Diseases Research, The Upjohn
Company, Kalamazoo, MI 490001, USA.

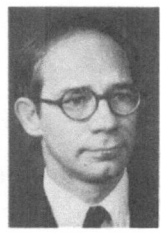

W. van ROOIJEN, B.Sc., Consultant Surgeon, Chairman of the surgical discussions.
Department of Surgery, Sophia Ziekenhuis, 8000 GK
Zwolle, The Netherlands.

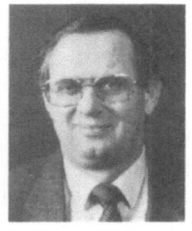

W. RÖSCH, M.D., Professor of Medicine, Chefarzt.
Medizinische Klinik, Krankenhaus Nordwest der Stiftung Hospital zum heiligen Geist, 6 Frankfurt am
Main 90, Federal Republic of Germany.

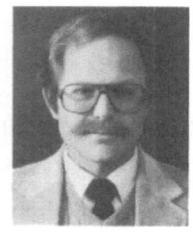

A.H. SOLL, M.D., Associate Professor of Medicine and
Key Investigator.
UCLA School of Medicine, Center for Ulcer Research
and Education, Los Angeles, CA 90073, USA.

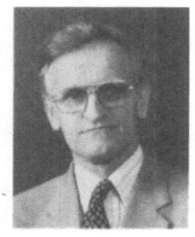

J. SPENCER, M.S., F.R.C.S., Senior Lecturer in
Surgery.
Department of Surgery, Royal Postgraduate Medical
School, Hammersmith Hospital, London W12 0HS,
United Kingdom.

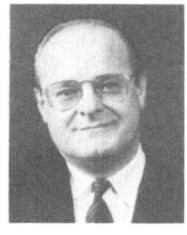

G.N.J. TIJTGAT, M.D., Professor of Gastroenterology. Department of Gastroenterology, University of Amsterdam, Academisch Medisch Centrum, 1105 AZ Amsterdam, The Netherlands.

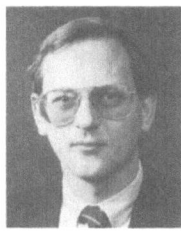

B.D. WESTERVELD, B.Sc., Consultant Physician, Chairman of the medical discussions. Department of Medicine, Sophia Ziekenhuis, 8000 GK Zwolle, The Netherlands.

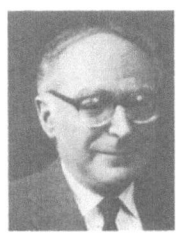

K.G. WORMSLEY, M.D., D.Sc., F.R.C.P., Reader in Medicine (hon), Consultant Physician. Department of Medicine, Ninewells Hospital, Dundee DD1 9SY, Scotland.

1. Introduction to the symposium

G.F. NELIS, M.D.

Department of Internal Medicine, Sophia Ziekenhuis, Zwolle, The Netherlands

Why does a general district hospital like the Sophia Ziekenhuis organize a three day symposium on PEPTIC ULCER TODAY on the occasion of its 100th anniversary?

Since the appointment in 1976 of mr D.W. Stol as a surgeon with a specific interest in gastroenterology and, perhaps, the appointment of a similar physician a few months later, an increasing interest in gastroenterology arose in this hospital. Apart from several regional meetings, this has led in the past to the organisation of two national symposia: on colorectal cancer and on proctology. Mr Stol originated from Dijkzigt University Hospital Rotterdam, which at the time was the prominent surgical gastroenterological clinic in The Netherlands under the guidance of the late professor H. Muller and professor H. van Houten. In his Rotterdam years mr Stol worked on the influence of suture material on abdominal wound healing, in which it was demonstated that Dexon® (polyglicolic acid) is superior to silk in promoting wound healing. At the end of his training period he worked together with professor J.L. Collis at the Queen Elizabeth Hospital, Birmingham, on the incidence of duodenogastric reflux in patients with symptoms of gastroesophageal reflux. Increased duodenogastric reflux was demonstrated by showing higher concentrations of fasting bile acids in gastric juice of the patients compared with healthy controls.

This work was extended at the Sophia Hospital Zwolle, at the request of the Union Européenne des Sociétées Nationales de Chirurgie, with a national survey of the surgical treatment of gastroesophageal reflux by Dutch surgeons.

Mr Stol left the Sophia Ziekenhuis in October 1983 to take up an insurance post and his place has been taken by mr W. van Rooijen, who also trained at the Rotterdam University Hospital and mainly worked on pancreatic surgery.

From the Department of Internal Medicine of the Sophia Ziekenhuis presentations have been given at national and international gastroenterological meetings and several publications appeared dealing with peptic ulcer and related subjects.

The first study started in 1977 and was inspired by Hall's observation of gynaecomastia and breast soreness during treatment with cimetidine, published in the New England Journal of Medicine, 1976;295:841. Using pituitary hormone profiles at − 5, 0, 10, 20 and 60 minutes following an intravenous bolus injection of hypothalamic releasing hormones (TRH 200 mcg and LHRH 150 mcg) before, during and after 4 week's standard cimetidine treatment (3x 200 mg at meals and 400 mg nocte) in duodenal ulcer patients, we demonstrated that oral cimetidine does not influence the response of prolactin, thyroid stimulating hormone, follicle stimulating hormone and luteinizing hormone. At the same time Van Thiel published observations on changes in LH-response to LHRH following cimetidine, which contrasted with our results, but his observations could not be confirmed in any study thereafter.

When ranitidine became available for clinical studies in 1979, we compared the response of serum prolactin concentration following intravenous bolus injections of cimetidine 200 mg and ranitidine 50 mg in equipotent dosages with respect to the inhibition of gastric acid secretion. A sharp rise in serum prolactin was observed following cimetidine, comparable to what had been described before by Carlson and Ippoliti, but no increase was observed after ranitidine. These results were significantly different at the $p < 0.01$ level. If the patients were divided into men, pre-menopausal and post-menopausal women, the results remained the same. Neither were the results influenced by the phase of the menstrual cycle in pre-menopausal women.

Meanwhile a controlled trial on the clinical efficacy of short and long-term treatment of duodenal ulcer with ranitidine 150 mg b.i.d. was started. Probably partly due to a remarkable compliance by the patients in this district, a very high healing rate was recorded after six weeks: 96% on ranitidine compared with 27% on placebo. On maintenance treatment with ranitidine 150 mg nocte for one year the relapse rate on placebo was 75% and on ranitidine 7%.

The study on the clinical use of ranitidine was extended to a placebo-controlled cross-over study of the clinical symptoms of gastroesophageal reflux, demonstrating a superior effect of ranitidine over placebo.

A side-step was a trial on the preparation for oral endoscopy. Confronted with the indignation of the nursing staff that we abandoned local throat anaesthesia and sedation, we compared three ways of patient preparation. It was shown that throat analgesia offered no benefit to either the patient, or the endoscopist and that sedation with diazepam 10 mg i.m. was unfavorable for patients and the endoscopist, resulting in significantly more retching and belching.

The latest study was done on a new compound inhibiting gastric acid secretion, RP 40749, which acts in the parietal cell at a level distal of cyclic AMP, probably by inhibition of the enzyme H^+-K^+-ATPase. We evaluated the efficacy of RP 40749 in the short-term treatment of duodenal ulcer. Complete ulcer healing was observed in 8 of 9 patients receiving RP 40749 100 mg nocte for 4 weeks and in all 9 patients receiving 150 mg nocte. The main part of this study was, however, to investigate the effect of RP 40749 on the gastrin content of the antral mucosa, basal and meal-stimulated serum gastrin and serum pepsinogen I. All these variables increased significantly after either dose of RP 40749. The magnitude of the meal-stimulated increase of serum gastrin did not change after RP 40749 treatment. From the increase in antral mucosa gastrin content it was concluded that the rise in serum gastrin was due to an increase in gastrin synthesis and not to merely enhanced release from gastrin stores. The only difference between the two doses of RP 40749 was a greater increase in serum pepsinogen I concentration on the higher dose of 150 mg.

From October 1983 we have enlarged our medical group with dr B.D. Westerveld, who trained at the Onze Lieve Vrouwe Gasthuis, Amsterdam and at the Free University Amsterdam. Together with the Department of Gastroenterology and the Institute of Human Genetics of the Free University he is working on pepsinogen I isozymogen determination in the human gastric mucosa, especially in the pre-malignant and malignant stomach. In these studies he demonstrated that the combination of a strong pepsinogen 5 isoprotein in the mucosa with a low serum pepsinogen I is highly suggestive of severe atrophic gastritis and/or gastric cancer. The sensitivity of the combined test, however, is too low to warrant its use for screening purposes.

At present research within the Department of Internal Medicine is being done on Campylobacter-like micro-organisms in the stomach and on prevention of stress ulcer bleeding.

4

List of publications on gastroenterological subjects from the Sophia Ziekenhuis Zwolle, The Netherlands

Department of Anaesthesia

Lip H. De dwarse en verticale incisie van de bovenbuik (Transverse and vertical abdominal incisions). MD Thesis, Rotterdam, 1981.

Department of Surgery

Boevé J. Acute afwijkingen aan de galwegen. Huisarts Wet 1962;5: 266 – 8.

Boevé J. Retroperitoneale tumoren en cysten. Ned T Geneesk 1976;111:15 – 20.

Stol DW. De invloed van hechtmateriaal op de wondgenezing (Influence of suture material on wound healing). MD Thesis, Rotterdam, 1978.

Stol DW, de Vries JE. Traitement des formes graves de l'oesophagite par reflux. In: 13ème Congrès Espagnol de Chirurgie, Barcelona, 1981:135 – 44.

Boevé J. Arterial obstruction as a complication of barium enema examination. Neth J Surg 1981;33:127 – 30.

Department of Medicine

Nelis GF, van de Meene JGC. The effect of oral cimetidine on the basal and stimulated values of prolactin, thyroid stimulating hormone, follicle stimulating hormone and luteinizing hormone. Postgrad Med J 1980;56:26 – 9.

Nelis GF, van de Meene JGC. The effect of oral cimetidine on the basal and stimulated values of PRL, TSH, FSH and LH. In: Torsoli A (Ed). Further experience with H2-receptor antagonists and progress in histamine research. Amsterdam: Excerpta Medica 1980:192 – 7.

Nelis GF, van de Meene JGC. Effetto della cimetidine somministrata per via orali sui valori basali e da stimolazione della prolatina, dell'ormone tireostimolante, dell'ormone follicolo-stimolante e dell'ormone luteinizzante. In: Torsoli A (Ed). Aggiornamento sugli antagonisti dei recettori H2 nelle malattie peptiche nelle ricerche sull'istamina. Amsterdam: Excerpta Medica 1980;204 – 10.

Nelis GF, van de Meene JGC. Effect of cimetidine on some hormones. In: Dresse A, Tijtgat GN (eds). Cimetidine, proceedings of the second national symposium Amsterdam: Excerpta Medica, 1980.

Nelis GF, van de Meene JGC. Comparative effect of cimetidine and ranitidine on prolactin secretion. Postgrad Med J 1980;56:478 – 80.

Nelis GF. Preparation for upper gastro-intestinal endoscopy; a controlled comparison of three regimens. Neth J Med 1981;23:191 – 2.

Nelis GF. Het effect van cimetidine en ranitidine op de plasma-prolactine concentratie. Ned T Geneesk 1980;124:2159A.

Nelis GF. Voorbereiding voor orale endoscopie; vergelijking van drie methoden. Ned T Geneesk 1980;124:2156A.

Nelis GF, van de Meene JGC. Comparative effect of intra-venous cimetidine and ranitidine on prolactin secretion. Hepatogastro-enterology Suppl 1980;256, E 32.4 A.

Nelis GF. Preparation for upper gastro-intestinal endoscopy; comparison of three regimes. IV. European Congress of Gastrointestinal Endoscopy, Georg Thieme Verlag, Stuttgart, 1980;11, E 3.1 A.

Nelis GF. Preparation for endoscopy. Lancet 1980;1:1750.

Nelis GF. Controlled trial with ranitidine in the treatment of peptic ulcer. Neth J Med 1981;24:224 – 8.

Nelis GF. De weg naar het coloncarcinoom. Mod Med 1982;6:1165 – 74.

Nelis GF. Behandeling van het ulcus pepticum met ranitidine; een dubbel-blind onderzoek (Treatment of peptic ulcer with ranitidine). Ned T Geneesk 1982;126:2320A.

Nelis GF. Controlled trial with ranitidine in the treatment of peptic ulcer. Scand J Gastroenterol 1982;17, suppl 78:92A.

Nelis GF. Experience with ranitidine in peptic ulceration and reflux oesophagitis. In: Tijtgat GN (Ed). Ranitidine, the selective new H2-receptor antagonist. Guildford: Theracom, 1982:25 – 32.

Nelis GF. Nitrofurantoin-induced pancreatitis. Gastroenterology 1983;84:1032 – 4.

Nelis GF. van Veen A. Deskundigen in discussie; ranitidine versus cimetidine. Mod Med 1984;8:455 – 6.

Nelis GF. RP 40749; results in treatment of duodenal ulcer. Lancet 1984;1:803.

Nelis GF, Lamers CBHW, Pals G. De invloed van RP 40749 op de basale en maaltijd-gestimuleerde waarden van serum-gastrine, serum pepsinogeen I en het gastrinegehalte van de antrummucosa. Ned T Geneesk 1985;129:330A.

6

Solleveldt HA, Nelis GF, Goossens JP. Vergelijking van cimetidine b.i.d. (800 mg) en q.i.d. (1000 mg) als acute behandeling van patienten met een benigne ulcus ventriculi. TGO/JDR 1985;10:540 – 3.

Nelis GF. Ranitidine in the management of gastro-oesophageal reflux disease. Neth J Med (in press).

Nelis GF, Lamers CBHW, Pals G. Influence of RP 40749 on basal and meal-stimulated serum gastrin, serum pepsinogen I and the gastrin content of the antral mucosa in duodenal ulcer patients. Dig Dis and Sci (in press).

Publications of consultants prior to their appointment to the Sophia Ziekenhuis

Department of Surgery

Boevé J. Enkele goedaardige gezwellen van de darm. Ned T Geneesk 1953;97:3240 – 4.

Stol DW, Murphy GM, Collis JL. Duodeno-gastric reflux and acid secretion in patients with symptomatic hiatal hernia. Scand J Gastroenterol 1974;9:97 – 101.

Van Rooyen W, van Blankenstein M, Eeftinck Schattenkerk M, de Vries JE, Obertop H, Bruining HA, van Houten H. Haemorrhage from the pancreatic duct; a rare form of upper gastrointestinal bleeding. Brit J Surg 1984;71:137 – 40.

Eeftinck Schattenkerk M, Obertop H, Bruining HA, van Rooyen W, van Houten H. Needle catheter jejunostomy for early postoperative feeding: Experience in 210 patients. Neth J Surg 1983;35:163 – 6.

Eeftinck Schattenkerk M, Obertop H. Bruining HA, van Rooyen W, van Houten H. Early postoperative enteral feeding by needle catheter jejunostomy after 100 oesophageal resections and reconstructions for cancer. Clin Nutr 1984;3:47 – 9.

Department of Internal Medicine

Pals G, Defize J. Meuwissen S, Westerveld BD, Verhoeven H, Ooms E, Kreuning J, Frants R, Eriksson AW. Pepsinogen I isoenzyme determination. Clinical significance? Gastroenterol 1981;80:1247A.

Westerveld BD, Pals G, Defize J, Ooms ECM, Kreuning J, van de Boomgaard DM, Frants RR, Eriksson AW, Meuwissen SGM.

Pepsinogeen I isoenzym bepaling en maagcarcinoom. Ned T Geneesk 1982;126:542A.

Eriksson AW, Meuwissen SGM, Kreuning J, Pronk J, Frants RR, Pena AS, Pals G, Defize J, *Westerveld BD*, Ooms ECM, Mullink H, Biemond J, van de Boomgaard DM. Pepsinogen in gastric mucosa and urine. Genetic and clinical implications. Am J Hum Genet 1982;34:66A.

Meuwissen SGM,. *Westerveld BD*, Nommensen FE, Starink TM, Ooms ECM, Coutinho RN. Anorectale chlamydiainfecties bij homosexuele mannen: klinische en differentieel-diagnostische aspecten. Ned T Geneesk 1983;127:812 – 6.

Westerveld BD, Hoitsma HWF, van Velzen D, Meuwissen SGM. Unusual confined perforation of a giant stomach ulcer into the liver with formation of a stomach tissue bridge. Acta Endosc 1983;13:29 – 32.

Eriksson AW, Frants RR, Pronk JC, Pals G, Defize J, *Westerveld BD*, Pena AS, Biemond I, Kreuning J, Meuwissen SGM. Genetics of urinary pepsinogen: A new multigene model. Am J Hum Genet 1983;35:184A.

Westerveld BD, Pals G, Defize J, Frants RR, Pronk JC, Kreuning J, Eriksson AW, Meuwissen SGM. A qualitative and quantitative study of pepsinogen I in (pre)malignant changes of the stomach. Proceedings of the 2nd European Conference on Clinical Oncology, Amsterdam, 1983.

Frants RR, Pronk JC, Pals G, Defize J, *Westerveld BD*, Meuwissen SGM, Kreuning J, Eriksson AW. Genetics of urinary pepsinogen: A new hypothesis. Am J Hum Genet 1984;65:385 – 90.

Defize J, Pals G, Frants RR, *Westerveld BD*, Meuwissen SGM, Eriksson AW. Pepsinogen synthesis and secretion in isolated gastric glands. J Clin Pathol 1984;37:531 – 36.

Westerveld BD, Pals G, Defize J, Frants RR, Pronk JC, Eriksson AW, Kreuning J, Meuwissen SGM. Kwalitatieve en kwantitative bepaling van pepsinogeen I en (pre)maligne afwijkingen van de maag. Ned T Geneesk 1984;128:1449A.

Frants RR, Pronk JC, Pals G, Defize J, *Westerveld BD*, Meuwissen SGM, Kreuning J, Eriksson AW. Pepsinogen and gastric cancer. Clin Genet 1984;26:240 – 41.

Lückens AEG, Thijs JC, *Westerveld BD*, Festen HPM, Meuwissen SGM. Is endoscopie van de proximale tractus digestivus op verzoek van de huisarts zinvol? Ned T Geneesk 1985;129:117 – 9.

8

Pals G, Biemond I, Defize J, *Westerveld BD*, Pronk JC, Meuwissen SGM, Eriksson AW. Pepsinogen I serum levels in relation to phenotypes. In: Kreuning J, Samloff IM, Rotter JI, Eriksson AW (Eds). Pepsinogen in Man: Clinical and Genetic Advances. Allan Liss, New York, 1985:91 – 100.

Defize J, Pals G, Frants RR, *Westerveld BD*, Meuwissen SGM, Eriksson AW. Pepsinogen synthesis and secretion in isolated gastric glands. In: Kreuning J, Samloff IM, Rotter JI, Eriksson AW (Eds). Pepsinogen in Man: Clinical and Genetic Advances. Allan Liss, New York, 1985:147 – 58.

Meuwissen SGM, Mullink H, Bosma A, Pals G, Defize J, Flipse M, *Westerveld BD*, Tas M, Brakke J, Kreuning J, Eriksson AW, Meyer CJML. Immunocytochemical localization of pepsinogen I and II in the human stomach. In: Kreuning J, Samloff IM, Rotter JI, Eriksson AW (Eds). Pepsinogen in Man Clinical and Genetic advances. Allan Liss, New York, 1985:185 – 98.

Westerveld BD, Pals G, Defize J, Pronk JC, Frants RR, Kreuning J, Eriksson AW, Meuwissen SGM. Qualitative and quantitative determination of pepsinogen I and (pre)malignant changes of the stomach. In: Kreuning J, Samloff IM, Rotter JI, Eriksson AW (Eds). Pepsinogen in Man: Clinical and Genetic Advances. Allan Liss, New York, 1985:201 – 12.

2. The epidemiology of peptic ulcer

G.F. NELIS, M.D.

Department of Medicine, Sophia Ziekenhuis, Zwolle, The Netherlands

"Peptic ulcer is a general public health problem throughout the world. Statistics from all sources indicate that 10% or more of the Western population may be afflicted by the disease at some time of their lives. Peptic ulcer also accounts for approximately 10% of all adult admissions to general medical and surgical hospitals and for an appreciable proportion of all new cases attending outpatient clinics." (from Langman[1]).

This means that peptic ulcer is an important economic problem for which 337 million guilders are spent every year in The Netherlands, 3224 million dollars in the USA, 1931 million marks in the Federal Republic of Germany and 480 million crowns in Sweden.[2,3] (Table I)

Table I. The cost of peptic ulcer in absolute values and (percentages of total costs).[2,3]

	USA 1977	Neth 1975	FRG 1976	Sweden 1975
Total expenses × 10^6	$3224	ƒ 337	DM 1931	SK 480
Direct expenses	149 (46)	71 (21)	585 (30)	106 (22)
drugs	13 (4)	3 (1)	49 (3)	15 (3)
admissions	107 (33)	61 (18)	453 (23)	72 (15)
others*	29 (9)	7 (2)	83 (4)	19 (4)
Indirect expenses	175 (54)	266 (79)	1346 (70)	374 (78)
loss of productivity	133 (41)		987 (51)	326 (68)
death	42 (13)		359 (19)	48 (10)

* includes fees and diagnostic procedures.

Considerable discrepancies appear to exist concerning the frequency with which peptic lesions of the stomach and duodenum afflict the general population. Clinical statistics underestimate the true incidence as only symptomatic ulcers are included. Given the low sensitivity of the history in peptic ulcer patients,[4] many ulcers will remain unrecognized in clinical studies. 'Typical' ulcer symptoms are only found in 26% of the patients with gastric ulcer under the age of 40 years and in 52% of the patients with duodenal ulcer in the same age group. In older people the history becomes even less reliable, reaching a nadir of 10% in patients over the age of 60 years with additional pathology. From the routine endoscopic follow-up in drug trials during the last decade, it has become apparent that many peptic ulcers are symptomless.

Necropsy studies are only reliable if not merely the presence, but also the absence of acute as well as chronic peptic lesions and scars have specifically been mentioned in the necropsy records, and only few such studies have been published.

Prevalence and incidence studies of uncomplicated and complicated peptic ulcer, investigating a localized population, or a random sample of that population, either during life, or at autopsy, are probably the best methods of studying peptic ulcer frequency.

Ulcer mortality

Peptic ulcer accounts for approximately 1% of all deaths in the general population. These figures, however, are mainly derived from death certificates, which are not necessarily reliable tools for epidemiological studies as shown by Steffelaar[5] for the Netherlands.

A sharp decline in mortality from peptic ulcer has been observed since the mid-sixties, possibly representing a decline in the incidence and prevalence of the disease. In the USA crude mortality rates from peptic ulcer dropped from 5.5/100,000 population in 1955 to 2.7/100,000 population in 1977, representing a decrease of 54%, whereas crude mortality rates from all causes dropped from 9500/100,000 population to 8800/100,000 population, representing a decrease of only 7%.[6,7] (Table II, fig. 1)

Table II. Death rates from peptic ulcer (USA)[6]

	1955	1977	Decrease 1955 – 1977
Crude mortality/100,000			
peptic ulcer	5.9	2.7	54%
all causes	9500	8800	7%

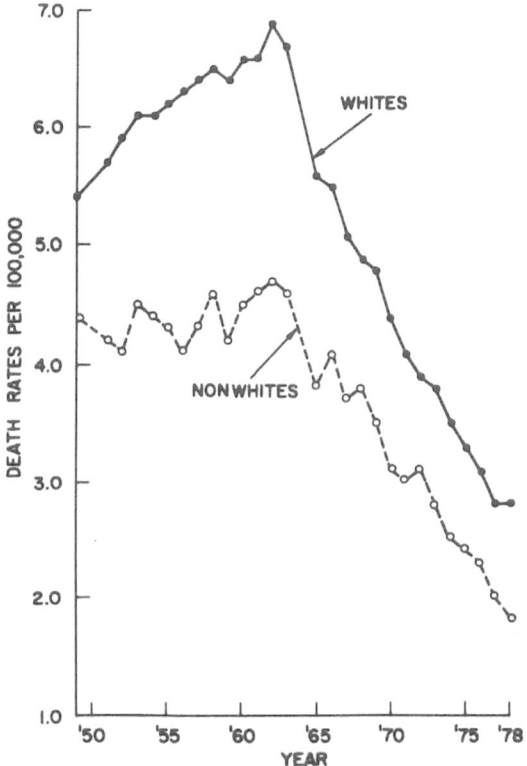

Figure 1. Death rates for peptic ulcer per 100,000 population in the USA, from 1949 to 1978. From: Kurata JH et al, 1982.[6]

Differentiation by sex shows a remarkable decrease of deaths from duodenal and gastric ulcer in males, but relatively stable rates in females: this has been observed in the USA, as well as in the United Kingdom and the Netherlands. Whereas in the past mortality rates for males were more than 4 times the mortality rate for females, in later years the male : female mortality ratio decreased to 2 : 1. (figs. 2 – 4)

Ulcer mortality varies greatly with age and is much more common in the elderly in the USA, the United Kingdom and the Netherlands.[7-10] (Table III, figs. 5 and 6)

In the past it has been suggested that ulcer mortality tended to occur more frequently during spring and autumn,[11] but a recent longitudi-

12

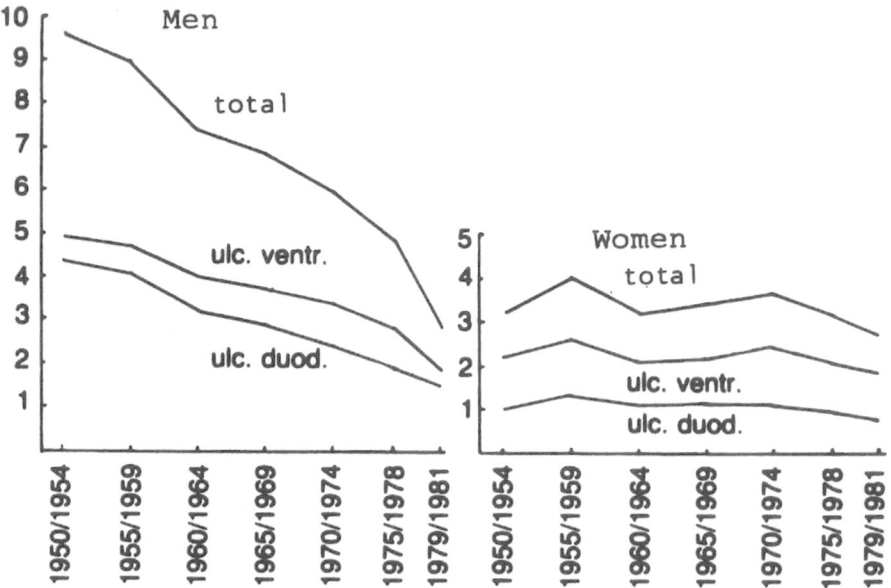

Figure 2. Age-adjusted death rates for gastric ulcer and duodenal ulcer by sex per 100,000 population in the Netherlands, from 1950/54 to 1979/81. From: Hoogendoorn D, 1984.[10]

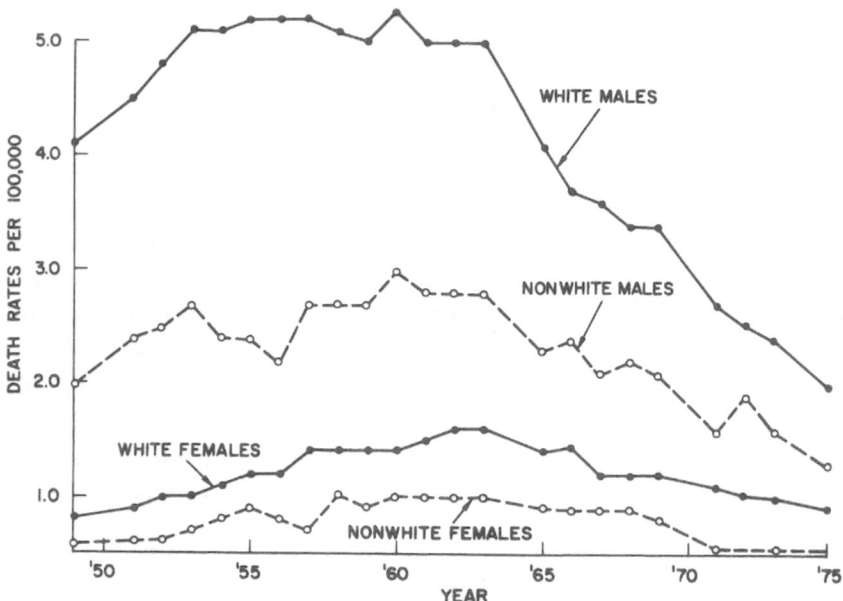

Figure 3. Death rates for duodenal ulcer by sex and race per 100,000 population in the USA, from 1949 to 1975. From: Kurata JH et al, 1982.[6]

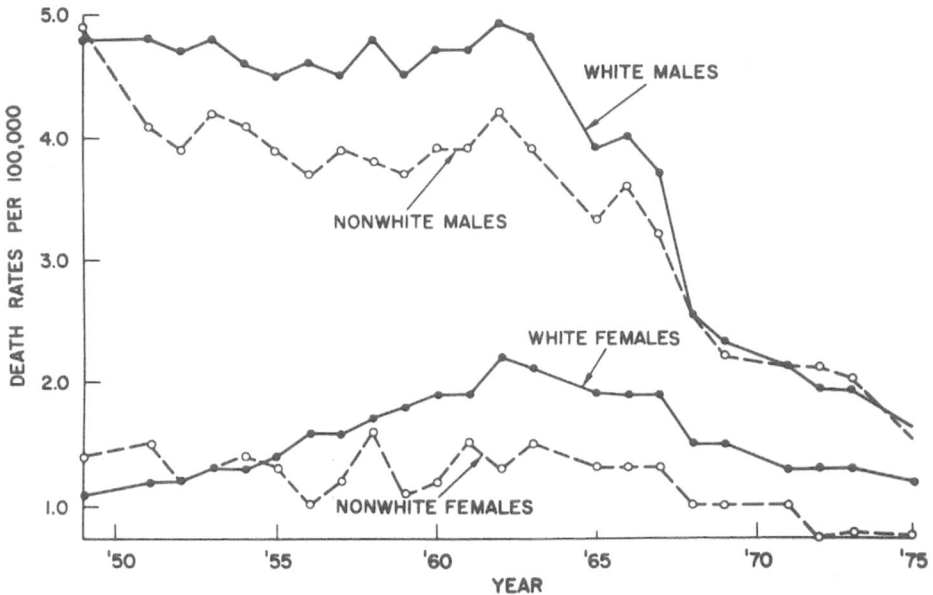

Figure 4. Death rates for gastric ulcer by sex and race per 100,000 population in the USA, from 1949 to 1975. From: Kurata JH et al, 1982.[6]

Table III. Age-specific death rates from peptic ulcer in England and Wales, per year, per 10^6 population. Years of survey: 1973 – 1977. From: Coggon et al.[9]

Age (yr)	25 –	35 –	45 –	55 –	65 –	75 +
Gastric ulcer						
men	1.9	5.6	22	72	202	573
women	0.8	3.0	10	31	100	416
Duodenal ulcer						
men	2.2	9.5	34	85	235	586
women	0.5	2.1	12	24	68	240
Total mortality	5.4	20.2	78	212	605	1815

14

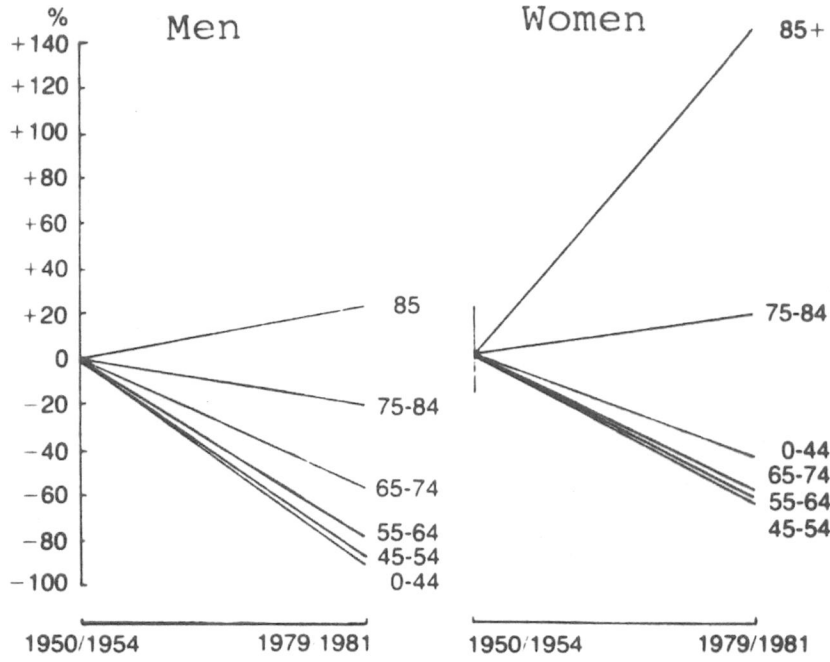

Figure 5. Death rates for peptic ulcer by age in the Netherlands, 1979/81 compared with 1950/54. From: Hoogendoorn D, 1984.[10]

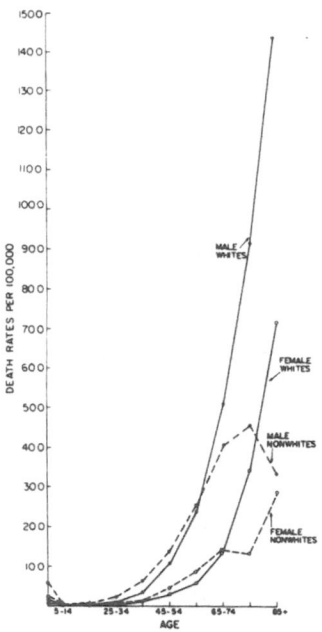

Figure 6. Death rates for peptic ulcer by age, sex and race per 100,000 population in the USA, 1963. From: Kurata JH et al, 1982.[6]

nal study from the USA has clearly shown that ulcer deaths are most common in the winter and least common in the summer months,[12] in accordance with the pattern of death in the general population.

As peptic ulcer displays only a low mortality rate but has a relatively high morbidity rate, studies of incidence and prevalence are probably more important.

Incidence and prevalence

Necropsy studies from the third to fifth decade of this century have demonstrated that a high percentage of males and females coming to autopsy have evidence of past or present peptic lesions. In the Swedish necropsy study by Falconer,[13] covering the period of 1930 – 1941 18.1% of 4553 males and 17.9% of 4747 females showed evidence of peptic ulcer, past or present. In the Leeds study by Watkinson,[14] covering the period of 1930 – 1949 the percentages were 20.5 for males and 11.0 for females and in the Rotterdam study by Levij and De la Fuente,[15] covering the period of 1940 – 1959 they were 27.3 and 17.2% respectively. (Table IV)

Table IV. Lifetime prevalence of peptic ulcer from necropsy studies.[13–15]

Author	Period	Men	Women
Falconer[13]	1930 – 41	18.1%	17.9%
Watkinson[14]	1930 – 49	20.5%	11.0%
Levij[15]	1940 – 59	29.2%	17.8%

The frequency of chronic lesions showed a regular increase with advancing age in females in the Rotterdam as well as in the Stockholm series, with a peak in the age frequency curves in males between 40 and 60 years of age. This would be consistent with a cohort phenomenon of certain population groups as suggested by Levij[15] and Susser and Stein.[16]

Prevalence is usually indicated as one-year prevalence, but this can also be done as point prevalence, or lifetime prevalence. In an endoscopic survey of 3458 healthy controls Ihamaki et al[17] in Finland found a point prevalence of active ulcer of 1.68% and deduced from ulcer scars and operations a lifetime prevalence of 5.88%, which is likely to be an underestimate of real lifetime prevalence, as the average age of his study population was only 46 years. The survey among Massachusetts physicians reporting a lifetime prevalence of 9%, is open to the same criticism, as the average age in this study was 50 years. In those above the age of 45, the prevalence rose sharply to 12.5%.[18]

The annual incidence of gastric and duodenal ulcer varies with geographical location and with the population studied. The overall annual incidence rates for new cases of peptic ulcer were 1.8/1000 population in a Danish survey,[19] 2.9/1000 population in the USA[20] and 6.0/1000 population in males and 1.6/1000 population in females in a rural area of South-West Scotland.[21]

In Denmark and the USA a linear relationship was found between incidence and increasing age, while in the United Kingdom peptic ulcer was less frequent in the older age groups than at middle age, both in rural areas and in urban conurbations.[19-24] (Tables V and VI)

Table V. Age-specific incidence rates of duodenal ulcer per 1000 population.

Reference	Men			Women			1960	1970
	19*	21	23**	19*	21	23**	22	22
Age (yr)								
20 –	0.9	5.8	2.1	0.2	1.2	0.5	1.6	0.7
30 –	1.3	8.2	2.5	0.5	3.2	0.7	4.6	1.5
40 –	2.2	10.0	2.3	1.3	2.7	0.8	5.6	2.7
50 –	3.0	15.5	2.3	1.4	3.2	0.6	7.8	3.0
60 –	3.2	8.7	2.0	1.4	1.7	0.4	7.5	3.7
70 +	3.7	2.8		2.1	1.4			

* only new cases; cases of recurrent ulcer excluded.
** adapted from 10 year periods starting at age 15.

Table VI. Age-specific incidence rates of gastric ulcer per 1000 population.

Reference	Men		Women		1960	1970
	19*	23**	19*	23**	22	22
Age (yr)						
20 –	0.1	0.2	0.1	0.1	1.1	0.1
30 –	0.2	0.4	0.1	0.2	1.2	0.1
40 –	0.4	0.6	0.3	0.3	2.1	0.4
50 –	0.7	0.7	0.6	0.3	3.1	1.2
60 –	1.1	0.5	0.7	0.3	3.4	1.6
70 +	1.2		1.0			

* only new cases; cases of recurrent ulcer excluded.
** adapted from 10 year periods starting at age 15; body of stomach only.

There are marked geographical differences in incidence and prevalence in different areas of the world and within single countries. Incidence and prevalence rates are higher in the West than in underdeveloped countries. However, peptic ulcer by no means coincides with a high standard of living, as duodenal ulcer is common among the rice-eating population of India, in Ethiopia, at the Nile-Congo watershed and in West-Africa.[1] Even within countries great variations in incidence and prevalence are present. This applies to duodenal, but not to gastric ulcer according to the data of Brown et al.[25] (Table VII)

Table VII. Admission rates for peptic ulcer in the United Kingdom per 1000 population, 1967.[25]

	England		Scotland
	South	North	
Gastric ulcer			
perforaterd	4 – 8	3 – 10	7
total	40 – 65	47 – 59	57
Duodenal ulcer			
perforated	7 – 14	22 – 31	45
total	84 – 93	140 – 226	294

Urban : rural ratio's have been studied extensively in a rural area in South-West Scotland by Litton and Murdoch[21] and show marked differences for gastric and duodenal ulcer. For duodenal ulcer a ratio of 2.43 was given for males and 2.03 for females, for gastric ulcer a ratio of 2.82 was given for males and 2.13 for females.

The incidence rates for duodenal ulcer are closely related to socioeconomic class for which no plausible explanation exists. These discrepancies have been noted in York and in Scotland.[21,23] (Table VIII)

Table VIII. Observed and expected rates for peptic ulcer by socio-economic class, South-West Scotland, 1957 – 59.[21]

	Socio-economic class				
	1	2	3	4	5
Gastric ulcer					
observed	0	11	12	13	28
expected	2	11	30	14	7
Duodenal ulcer					
observed	13	41	125	136	158
expected	14	80	218	108	52

Time trends

Hospital admission rates changed dramatically during the past few decades. In the nineteenth century gastric ulcer was predominantly seen in young women and duodenal ulcer was exceedingly rare. In the first half of the twentieth century there was a progressive decline in the frequency of gastric ulcer combined with an enormous increase in the frequency of duodenal ulcer, which ran parallel with an increase in the male : female ratio from 0.2 in 1867 to 1.4 in 1924. Mortality from gastric ulcer perforation changed towards the older age groups. In 1867 57% of the deaths from perforated ulcer were in persons under the age of 35 years compared to 12% in 1924.[1]

Changes in hospital admission rates have been reported from the USA, the United Kingdom, the Federal Republic of Germany and the Netherlands.[6-10,26-27]. This decline was clearly apparent before the introduction of highly effective drugs for the treatment of gastric and duodenal ulcer. Possible causes for this decline in admission rates include changes in peptic ulcer incidence, changes in the severity of the disease, changes in diagnostic or coding practices, changes in effectiveness of treatment or changes in criteria for hospitalization.

Overall hospitalization rates show a steady decrease for duodenal ulcer in all series; for gastric ulcer hospitalization rates are decreasing to a lesser extent in the United Kingdom, the Netherlands and the Federal Republic of Germany and are practically stable in the USA. The decrease is more pronounced in males than in females. Age-specific admission rates show decreases to a greater extent in the young, while the decrease in the elderly is less obvious and the rate is slightly increasing in elderly women in some series.[9,10]

In Coggon's series male admission rates fell steadily by more than 50% for gastric ulcer throughout the study period of 1957 – 1977. In contrast, the rate for duodenal ulcer remained stable till 1968 and then dropped sharply by 45%. For women a gradual decrease of 30 – 40% was observed in both duodenal and gastric ulcer, evenly distributed over the total study period. In the USA out-patient consultations for duodenal ulcer decreased from 13.7 per 1000 person-years in 1967 to 4.1 per 1000 person-years in 1973, representing an annual change of – 1.67/year. Consultations for gastric ulcer decreased only by – 0.25/year, being 4.6/1000 person-years in 1967 and 2.2/1000 person-years in 1973.[28] Mendeloff observed a 50% decrease in the out-patient episodes of duodenal ulcer in the

1960 – 1972 period in the US Army.[29]

Hospital admission rates do not necessarily represent incidence rates. It follows from Kurata's series[8] that criteria for hospitalization can have profound influences on hospital admission rates, as stable and low admission rates were found for gastric and duodenal ulcer throughout the study period of 1970 – 1980 among members of a health maintenance organization (HMO), while levels were rapidly declining for non-HMO members. As the total number of patients with haemorrhage and perforation were the same in both groups, HMO-members are not a healthier population, because the complication rate is comparable, nor do they represent an undertreated group because mortality rates are the same for HMO-members and non-HMO-members. In accordance with these suggestions is the fact that out-patient episodes for all causes were more frequent among HMO-members. Another study showing stable rates for the incidence of new cases of peptic ulcer was performed in Copenhagen County.[19]

Langman[30] emphasizes the fact that ulcer perforations are mandatory causes of admission and therefore probably more reliable in determining incidence and prevalence rates. In the USA and Denmark the number of admissions for perforated gastric and duodenal ulcer have been stable throughout the study period of 1970 – 1980, but age-specific rates have not been given in these series.[6,8,19] Smith reported a decrease in the number of perforated duodenal ulcers from 183 in 1966 – 1970 to 117 in 1971 – 1975 operated upon in five Seattle-area hospitals, but changes in referral patterns or changes in the adherent population could affect the results of this study.[31] The most recent data reported by Watkins from the United Kingdom show a decreased rate for perforated gastric and duodenal ulcers in males, stable rates for perforated gastric ulcer in females and nearly doubled rates for perforated duodenal ulcer in females, on comparison of 1977 – 1982 to 1965 – 1970.[32] (Table IX)

Table IX. Perforated peptic ulcer per 100,000 population per year.[32]

	1965 – 1970		1977 – 1982	
	men	women	men	women
Gastric ulcer	2.3	0.5	0.7	0.5
Duodenal ulcer	11.0	2.3	8.3	4.4
Total	13.3	2.8	9.0	4.9

20

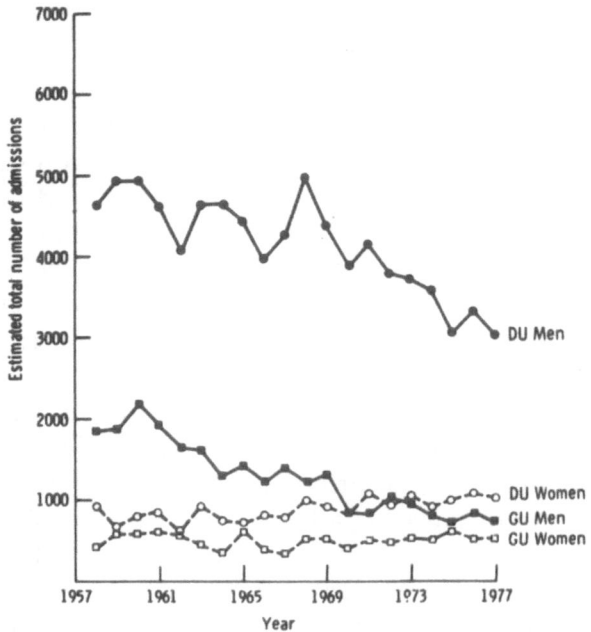

Figure 7. Number of hospital admissions for perforated duodenal and gastric ulcer in men and women in England and Wales, from 1958 to 1972. From: Coggon D, et al, 1981.[9]

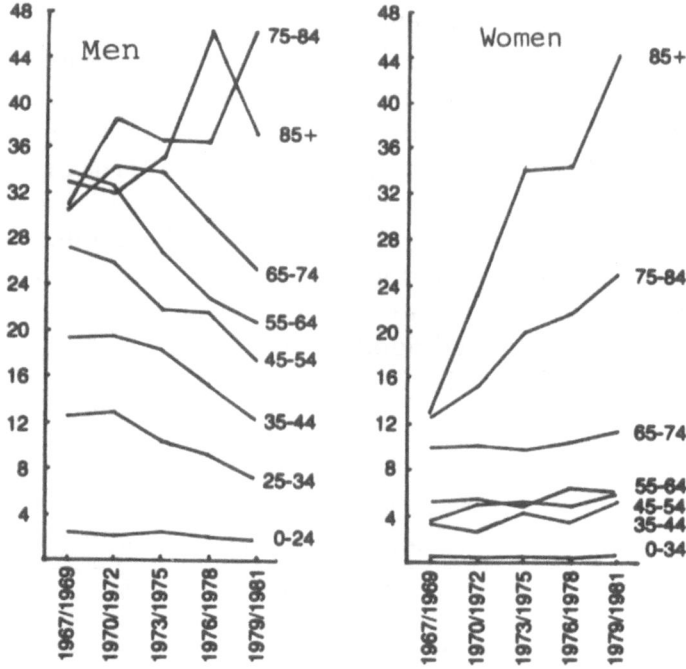

Figure 8. Hospital admission rates for perforated peptic ulcer by sex and age in the Netherlands, from 1967/69 to 1979/81. From: Hoogendoorn D, 1984.[10]

In the United Kingdom and the Netherlands overall changes in the number of ulcer perforation have been observed.[9,10,25,32] (figs 7 and 8) Perforated gastric ulcer has become virtually absent in the young and perforated duodenal ulcer decreased by approximately 40% in younger males and females and by 20 – 30% in elderly males. However, in the elderly woman rates of perforated gastric ulcer remained stable, but duodenal perforations sharply increased.

In summary, hospital admission rates and death rates due to perforated and non-perforated peptic ulcer are declining rapidly throughout the Western world, except in elderly women. This could support the hypothesis of either a change in the incidence of peptic ulcer in many parts of the world or a change in the clinical attributes of the disease.

Although perforation rates started to decline several years before the introduction of histamine H_2-receptor antagonists, the decline seems to be more rapid thereafter. The same pattern has been shown for total operation rates.[33]

Associated factors

Geographical location, age, sex and socio-economic class have been dealt with above. For genetic influences the reader is referred to the contribution by Kreuning[34] in this volume. The varying incidence of peptic ulcers during different decades and in various areas of the world indicate that environmental factors are important, especially diet, smoking and anti-inflammatory drugs.

Diet

High incidence rates of peptic ulcer are found in India among the rice-eating population and low incidence rates among the wheat-eating population. These differences could be due to the different fibre content of the diet in these populations, but this is not confirmed by controlled data.[35,36] On the other hand, a recent endoscopically-controlled study demonstrated that patients on high-fibre diets experienced fewer recurrences of peptic ulcer.[37] But the number of patients in this study is small and it is hard to extrapolate the results to epidemiological data.

A study of the influences of different types of beverages on ulcer incidence showed a positive correlation for coffee and cola-type soft drinks and a negative correlation for milk, between consumption patterns and the later development of peptic ulcer. No influence was apparent for tea, or moderate amounts of alcohol (Table X).

Table X. Incidence rates for peptic ulcer per 1000 former college students, by previous habits of beverage consumption.[38]

	Yes	No
Previous use		
coffee	31.7	17.7
tea	20.9	21.3
soft drinks	22.0	14.9
alcohol	9.9	10.6
milk	15.4	30.3

Smoking

Smoking correlates with the incidence rate of and the mortality rate from peptic ulcer. Retrospective studies support a significant increase of ulcer prevalence among smokers, compared with non-smokers, which was more pronounced in men than in women.[39-42] To prevent bias due to the relation of smoking and socio-economic class, Paffenbarger studied prospectively former college students and demonstrated a positive correlation between smoking and the risk of developing peptic ulcer later in life.[38] An even more homogenous socio-economic group of Massachusetts physicians was studied by Monson, with comparable results and also suggesting an increased probability of developing an ulcer if smoking started early in life.[18] Ulcers heal more slowly in smokers, on placebo, or on active treatment[43-46] and have a significantly higher symptomatic and asymptomatic relapse rate on placebo, or on maintenance treatment with cimetidine.[47] (Table XI)

Non-smokers receiving placebo had an even lower recurrence rate (21%) than smokers receiving maintenance treatment with cimetidine (34%), although this remarkable difference did not reach statistical significance at the 5% level.

The mechanisms by which smoking decreases ulcer healing and increases relapse rates is not evident. Suggested mechanisms include a direct stimulatory effect of nicotine on gastric acid secretion, an augmented acid load to the duodenum by an accelerated rate of gastric emptying,[48] decreased acid neutralizing capacity of the duodenal contents by inhibition of pancreatic bicarbonate secretion[45,50] or interference with the pharmacological effect of histamine H_2-receptor antagonists.[51]

Table XI. The effect of smoking on ulcer recurrence rate.[47]

	Non-smokers		Smokers	
	plac	cimet	plac	cimet
Recurrence rate % at 1 year				
symptomatic	13	4	51	22
asymptomatic	8	14	21	12
Total	21	18	72	34

Anti-inflammatory drugs

Case-control studies have suggested a relationship between aspirin-consumption and an increased risk of peptic ulcer.[52–54] Although in the majority of these patients the ulcer will have resulted from aspirin consumption, it can not be excluded that the patients have taken aspirin because they experienced epigastric pain from a pre-existing peptic ulcer. Thompson found among 21 women over the age of 60 admitted with perforated duodenal ulcer 8 current users of indomethacin, while there were no women taking indomethacin among 222 females over 60 years of age admitted for cholesytectomy.[55]

In combining incidences of perforated, or non-perforated peptic ulcer a systematic bias could be present in drug consumption data, which has indeed been shown to be present by using medication with paracetamol as positive control.[1,56]

The most suggestive study is by the Aspirin Myocardial Infarction Study Group in which patients randomly assigned to aspirin 1 g daily had a sixfold increase in ulcer incidence compared with those on placebo.[57]

Evidence suggesting a relationship between treatment with corticosteroids and peptic ulcer is even more difficult to evaluate, partly because several trials were conducted in diseases known to have a high prevalence of peptic ulcer, such as hepatic cirrhosis. Although Conn and Blitzer in their classic study denied the relationship between peptic ulcer and corticosteroids in moderate doses and for a moderate length of time, Messer et al demonstrated a relative risk of 2.3 in 3064 steroid-treated patients compared with 2897 controls.[58,59]

At present, circumstantial evidence suggests a relationship between peptic ulcer and the use of aspirin and corticosteroids. In future only those studies should be accepted whose methodological design corresponds to the ideas outlined by Kurata et al.[60]

Acknowledgements

Figures 1, 3, 4 and 6 have been reproduced by permission of JH Kurata, PhD, and the editor of Gastroenterology. Figures 2, 5 and 8 have been reproduced by permission of D Hoogendoorn, MD, and the editor of the Nederlands Tijdschrift voor Geneeskunde. Figure 7 has been reproduced by permission of prof. MJS Langman, MD FRCP, and the editor of The Lancet.

References

1. Langman MJS. The epidemiology of chronic digestive disease. Chapter 2, Peptic ulcer. London: Edward Arnold, 1979:9–39.
2. Bodemar G, Gotthard R, Ström M, et al. Socioeconomic aspects of treatment with cimetidine in peptic ulcer disease. In: Torsloli A, Luchelli PE, Brimblecombe RW (Eds). H_2-antagonists. Amsterdam, Oxford, Princeton: Excerpta Medica 1980:59–67.
3. Sonnenberg A, Fritch A, Sierp D, Bapst L, Horisberger B. Was kostet ein Ulcus. In: Blum AL, Siewert JR (Eds). Ulcus Therapie. Berlin, Springer Verlag 1982:138–50.
4. Hess H, Würsch TG, Killer-Walser R, et al. How often does peptic ulcer produce 'typical' ulcer symptoms? Acta Hepatogastroenterol (Stuttg.) 1980;27: 57–61.
5. Steffelaar JW. Analyse van een doorlopende reeks obducties: een bijdrage aan de kwaliteitsverbering van het medisch handelen. Ned T Geneesk 1979; 123:1898–1905.
6. Elashoff JD, Grossman MI. Trends in hospital admission and death rates for peptic ulcer in the United States from 1970 to 1978. Gastroenterology 1980;78:280–85
7. Kurata JH, Haile BM. Racial difference in peptic ulcer disease: fact or myth? Gastroenterology 1982;83:166–72.
8. Kurata JH, Honda GD, Frankl H. Hospitalization and mortality rates for peptic ulcers: a comparison of a large HMO and US data. Gastroenterology 1982;83:1008–16.
9. Coggon D, Lambert P, Langman MJS. 20 Years of hospital admissions for peptic ulcer in England and Wales. Lancet 1981;1:1302–4.
10. Hoogendoorn D. Opmerkelijke verschuivingen in het epidemiologische patroon van het ulcus pepticum. Ned T Geneesk 1984;128:484–91.
11. Ivy AC. The problem of peptic ulcer. JAMA 1946;132:1053–59.

12. Kurata JH, Haile BM. Epidemiology of peptic ulcer disease. In: Isenberg JI, Johansson C (Eds). Peptic ulcer disease. Clinics in gastroenterology, volume 13/2. London, Philadelphia, Toronto: WB Saunders Company, 1984:289–307.
13. Falconer B. Über die peptischen Laesionen. Jena: Fischer Verlag, 1943.
14. Watkinson G. The incidence of chronic peptic ulcer found at necropsy. Gut 1960;1:14–30.
15. Levij IS, de la Fuente AA. A post-mortem study of gastric and duodenal peptic lesions. Gut 1963;4:349–59.
16. Susser S, Stein Z. Civilisation and peptic ulcer. Lancet 1962;1:115.
17. Ihamaki T, Varis K, Siurala M. Morphological, functional and immunological state of the gastric mucosa in gastric carcinoma families. Comparison with a computer-matched family sample. Scand J of Gastroenterol 1979;14:801–12.
18. Monson RR, MacMahon B. Peptic ulcer in Massachusetts physicians. N Engl J Med 1969;281:11–15.
19. Bonnevie O. Peptic ulcer in Denmark. Scand J Gastroenterol (suppl 63) 1980;15:163–74.
20. National Center for Health Statistics. Prevalence of selected chronic digestive conditions, United States. 1975. Data from the National Health Interview Survey. Vital and Health Statistics. US Department of Health, Education and Welfare, Publication Number (PHS) 1979:79–1558.
21. Litton A, Murdoch WR. Peptic ulcer in South West Scotland. Gut 1963;4:360.
22. Almy TP. Prevalence and significance of digestive disease. Gastroenterology 1975;68:1351–71.
23. Pulvertaft CN. Peptic ulcer in town and country. Brit J Prev Soc Med 1959;13:131–8.
24. Pulvertaft CN. Comments on the incidence and natural history of gastric and duodenal ulcer. Postgrad Med J 1968;44:597–602.
25. Brown RC, Langman MJS, Lambert PM. Hospital admission for peptic ulcer during 1958–1972. Br Med J 1976;1:35–7.
26. Daten des Gesundheitswesens, Ausgabe 1977. Bonn: Bundesminister für Jugend, Familien und Gesundheit.
27. Fritsch A, Sonnenberg A, Erckenbrecht J. Epidemiologie der Ulkuskrankheit in der Bundesrepublik Deutschland 1952–1978. Z Gastroenterol 1981;19:493.
28. Vogt TM, Johnson RE. Recent changes in the incidence of duodenal and gastric ulcer. Am J Epidemiol 1980;111:713–20.
29. Mendeloff AI. What has been happening to duodenal ulcer? Gastroenterology 1974;67:1020–2.
30. Langman MJS. The tide of peptic ulcer. Scand J Gastroenterol 1980;15 (suppl 63):149–56.
31. Smith MP. Decline in duodenal ulcer surgery. JAMA 1977;237:987–88.
32. Watkins RM, Dennison AR, Collin J. What has happened to perforated peptic ulcer? Br J Surg 1984;71:774–6.
33. Fineberg HV, Pearlman LA. Surgical treatment of peptic ulcer in the United States. Trends before and after the introduction of cimetidine. Lancet 1981;1:1305–7.
34. Kreuning J. Genetic aspects of peptic ulcer. In: Nelis GF, Boevé, Misiewicz JJ (Eds). Peptic ulcer today. Dordrecht: Martinus Nijhoff Publishers, 1985:173–81.
35. Malhotra SL. The role of saliva in the aetiology of peptic ulcer. Br Med J 1965;1:1220–22.
36. Malhotra SL. A comparison of unrefined wheat and rice diets in the management of duodenal ulcer. Postgrad Med J 1978;54:6–9.

37. Rydning A, Berstad A, Aadland E, Odegaard B. Prophylactic effect of dietary fibre in duodenal ulcer disease. Lancet 1982;2:736–9.
38. Paffenbarger RS, Wing AL, Hyde RT. Chronic disease in former college students. AM J Epidemiol 1974;100:307–15.
39. Harrison A, Elashoff J, Grossman MI. Cigarette smoking and ulcer disease. In: The Surgeon General's Report on Smoking and Health. US Department of Health, Education and Welfare, Public Health Service 1979:9–21.
40. Friedman GD, Siegelaub AB, Seltzer CC. Cigarettes, alcohol, coffee and peptic ulcer. N Eng J Med 1974;290:469–73.
41. Petitti DB, Friedman GD, Kahn W. Peptic ulcer disease and the tar and nicotine yield of currently smoked cigarettes. J Chron Dis 1982;35:503–7.
42. Pfeiffer CJ, Fodor J, Geizerova H. An epidemiologic study of the relationships of peptic ulcer disease in 50–54 year old, urban males with physical health and smoking factors. J Chron Dis 1973;26:291–302.
43. Doll R, Jones F, Pygott F. Effect of smoking on the production and maintenance of gastric and duodenal ulcers. Lancet 1958;1:657–62.
44. Doll R, Peto R. Mortality in relation to smoking: 20 years' observation on male British doctors. Br Med J 1976;2:1525–36.
45. Gugler R, Rohner HG, Kratochvil P, et al. Effect of smoking on duodenal ulcer healing with cimetidine and oxmetidine. Gut 1982;23:866–71.
46. Korman MG, Hansky J, Eaves ER, Schmidt GT. Influence of cigarette smoking on healing and relapse in duodenal ulcer disease. Gastroenterology 1983;85:871–4.
47. Sontag S, Grahm DY, Belsito A, et al. Cimetidine, cigarette smoking and recurrence of duodenal ulcer. N Eng J Med 1984;311:68993.
48. Grimes DS, Goddard J. Effect of cigarette smoking on gastric emptying. Br Med J 1978;2:460–1.
49. Brown P. The influence of smoking on pancreatic function in man. Med J Aust 1976;2:290–3.
50. Murthy S, Dinoso V, Clearfield H, Chey W. Simultaneous measurement of basal pancreatic, gastric acid secretion, plasma gastrin, and secretin during smoking. Gastroenterology 1977;73:758–61.
51. Boyd EJS, Wilson JA, Wormsley KG. Smoking impairs therapeutic gastric inhibition. Lancet 1983;1:95–7.
52. Billington BP. The Australian gastric ulcer change: interstate variations. Australasian Ann Med 1963;12:153–9.
53. Billington BP. Observations from New South Wales on the changing incidence of gastric ulcer in Australia. Gut 1965;6:121–33.
54. Levy M. Aspirin use in patients with major upper gastrointestinal bleeding and peptic ulcer disease. N Engl J Med 1974;290:1158–62.
55. Thompson MR. Indomethacin and perforated duodenal ulcer. Br Med J 1980;280:448.
56. Coggon D, Langman MJS, Spiegelhalter D. Aspirin, paracetamol and haematemesis and melaena. Gut 1982;23:340.
57. Aspirin Myocardial Infarction Study Group. A randomized, controlled trial of aspirin in persons recovered from myocardial infarction. JAMA 1980;243:661–9.
58. Conn HO, Blitzer BI, Medical progress: non-association of adrenocorticosteroid therapy and peptic ulcer. N Engl J Med 1976;294:473.
59. Messer J, Reitman D, Sacks HS, Smith H, Chalmers TC. Association of adrenocorticosteroid therapy and peptic ulcer disease. N Engl J Med 1983;309:21–4.

60. Kurata JH, Elashoff JD, Grossman MI. Inadequacy of the literature on the relationship between drugs, ulcers and gastrointestinal bleeding. Gastro-enterology 1982;83:373 – 6.

3. Regulation of acid secretion: receptors, antagonists, and interactions

A.H. SOLL, M.D.

Center for Ulcer Research and Education, Department of Medicine, UCLA School of Medicine and Medical Research Services, Wadsworth VA Hospital Center, Los Angeles, USA

Introduction

The secretion of gastric acid is a property preserved in all species higher in the phylogenetic tree than the hagfish. The advantages to the species offered by gastric acid are improved digestion, sterilization of gastric contents before transport into the small intestine and elimination of certain pathogenic microorganisms such as salmonella. However, to individuals suffering from acid-peptic disease, gastric acid is an essential permissive factor for ulcer formation. In some patients, acid hypersecretion is a primary factor. Inhibition of acid secretion is the major modality for therapeutic intervention in these disorders.

The complex physiology of acid secretion

Unravelling the potentional pathogenic role of gastric acid in peptic ulcer and the mode of action of the modalities used to treat these disorders requires knowledge of the mechanisms regulating the secretory process. Gaining such knowledge has been slow because the regulation of acid secretion is exceedingly complex, with redundant stimulatory and inhibitory control pathways. Three major pathways deliver the chemical messenger that regulate acid secretion: neurocrine (neurotransmitters released from postganglionic nerves innervating the fundic mucosa); endocrine (hormones such as gastrin delivered by blood); and paracrine (transmitters that diffuse across the intercellular compartment from local tissue stores). All three of these pathways are physiologically important.[1,2] Several chemical transmitters are produced in fundic mucosal cells, including histamine, somatostatin, glucagon, and prostaglandins. These agents are candidates for local regulation of secretory function, but thus paracrine regulation remains difficult to study. In fact, despite the close association of histamine and acid secretion, the role of histamine in the regulation of acid secretion was hotly debated[3,4] until Black and coworkers introduced the histamine H_2-receptor antagonists blocked not only the action of histamine on acid secretion, but also stimulation by food, gastrin, and vagal stimuli thereby establishing that histamine played an essential role in the regulation of acid secretion.[5,6,7]

The interdependence between pathways regulating acid secretion

An additional layer of complexity of the mechanisms regulating acid secretion results from an interdependence that exists between the three pathways in their effects. This interdependence is clearly evident in the ability of specific histamine H_2-receptor antagonists and muscarinic receptor antagonists to inhibit basal acid secretion and the response to most stimuli. For example, the cephalic phase of acid secretion (that occurs with the smell, sight or thought of food) that is mediated by vagal delivery of acetylcholine to the fundic micosa is blocked by histamine H_2-receptor antagonists, indicating a dependence upon endogenous histamine. Although the release of gastrin with a protein meal appears to largely account for the acid secretory response, both histamine H_2-receptor antagonists and anticholinergic agents inhibit this gastric phase, indicating dependency upon input from the neurocrine and paracrine pathways. Basal acid secretion is inhibited by both anticholinergic agents and histamine H_2-receptor antagonists, suggesting that the 'resting' parietal cell receives both cholinergic and histamine input. The three pathways stimulating acid secretion are markedly interdependent.

Hypothesis for regulatory interdependency

The mechanisms underlying this interplay between the various pathways regulating acid secretion are poorly understood. A basic question that remains unresolved is the identity of the target cell(s) within the fundic mucosa mediating gastrin and acetylcholine effects on acid secretion. Code (1965), building upon earlier observations by Mac-

Intosh, hypothesized that histamine was the final chemostimulator at the parietal cell; receptors for gastrin and acetylcholine resided on the histamine cell and served to release histamine, which alone acted on parietal cell receptors. This hypothesis gained support from the findings that gastrin and acetylcholine influenced histamine formation in the rat gastric mucosa and by the demonstration thatmine H_2-receptor antagonists blocked the acid secretion response to all stimuli. However, this model did not account for the ability of anticholinergic agents to block histamine action and the interdependency between cholinergic pathways and gastrin. These factors led the late Morton I Grossman[6] to hypothesize that the parietal cell has separate specific receptors for histamine, gastrin and acetylcholine, with the interdependency between the pathways reflecting interaction at the parietal cell itself. The controversy thus centered about whether gastric secretagogues stimulated acid secretion by acting in parallel on the parietal cell, or in series with their final effects being mediated by release of histamine. It is also possible that the neurocrine, endocrine, and paracrine pathways influence the release of chemotransmitters other than histamine, which in turn mediate or modulate the secretory response.

Rationale for a reductionist approach

Two steps necessary to unravel the mode of direct action and interaction between the pathways are localization of the receptors mediating the actions of histamine, cholinergic agents and gastrin within the fundic mucosa and elucidation of the points of intersection between these pathways. Studies in intact mucosa are complicated by the heterogeneous cell population in the fundic mucosa and the presence of acetylcholine and histamine in the mucosa in the vicinity of the parietal cell. Cell separation techniques provide one approach to elucidating the receptors regulating acid secretory function. With isolation by enzyme treatment, the parietal cell can be removed from these background influences, thus allowing the effects of individual agents to be studied alone or in combination. The remainder of this review focuses on studies with isolated canine fundic cells aimed at elucidating the receptor interactions mediating acid secretion.

Separation of mucosal cells

Cells are dispersed from the fundic mucosa by treatment with enzymes. A variety of specific approaches have been developed, including rabbit gastric glands prepared with crude collagenase,[8] parietal cells dispersed from canine,[9] rat,[10,11] guinea pig,[12,13] or amphibian[14] gastric mucosa using sequential treatment with collagenase and EDTA or pronase. Several procedures have been used to enrich parietal cells, including velocity separation at either unit gravity or in an elutriator rotor and density gradient separation.[15,16]

Studies of parietal cell function

With dispersion, parietal cells lose their polar orientation as a component of an epithelium, and thus H^+-ions secreted at the apical surface are neutralized by the concomitant secretion of bicarbonate ions. Indirect indices provide evidence of functional responses. With stimulation, isolated parietal cells undergo a morphologic transformation similar to that observed *in vivo*;[8-15] tubulovesicles which fill the cytoplasm in the basal state transform into secretory canaliculi. Since the secretion of acid is a highly energy-dependent process, oxygen consumption and glucose oxidation both provide a reflection of the overall degree of cell activation. The accumulation of weak bases, such as ^{14}C-aminopyrine (AP), provides indirect evidence for the secretion of acid by isolated parietal cells.[17,18] AP, with its pKa of 5.0, is largely unionized at cytoplasmic pH and freely diffuses across plasma membranes. Once AP has entered an acidic compartment, such as the tubulo-vesicles and secretory canaliculi of the stimulated parietal cell, it becomes ionized and is thus locked in by the surrounding plasma membranes. (fig. 1) Using fluorescent microscopy, another weak base, acridine orange, has been shown to accumulate within vesicles of stimulated rabbit gastric glands.[17] It is important to emphasize that AP accumulation provides an index of the quantity of acid sequestered by parietal cells, rather than of the actual rate of acid secreted.

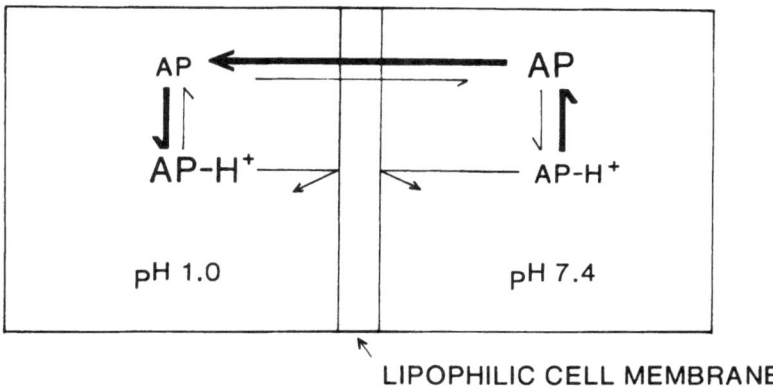

^{14}C-AMINOPYRINE ACCUMULATION

AP ← AP

AP-H$^+$ — AP-H$^+$

pH 1.0   pH 7.4

LIPOPHILIC CELL MEMBRANE

AMINOPYRINE, A WEAK BASE, pK$_a$ 5.0, PASSIVELY DIFFUSES ACROSS LIPOPHILIC MEMBRANES WHEN IN THE NON-IONIZED STATE. IT THUS BECOMES TRAPPED IN THE ACIDIC CANALICULUS.

Figure 1. The principle of ^{14}C-aminopyrine accumulation in parietal cells.

Regulation of parietal cell function

Histamine, gastrin and cholinergic agents each stimulate oxygen consumption, AP accumulation, and glucose oxidation by canine parietal cells.[9,15] Histamine and cholinergic agents have been shown to stimulate parietal cell function in rabbit gastric glands,[8,19] and parietal cells dispersed from the rat,[11,20] guinea pig[12] and frog.[14]

Histamine H$_2$-receptors

Several studies lead to the conclusion that histamine action on dispersed parietal cells is mediated by an histamine H$_2$-receptor. Histamine H$_2$-receptor antagonists competitively inhibit histamine

34

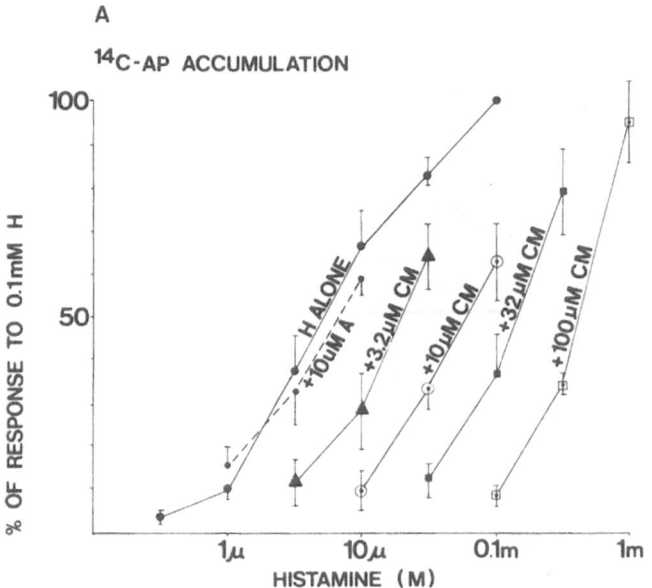

Figure 2. Competitive inhibition of histamine-stimulated ^{14}C-aminopyrine accumulation into parietal cells by cimetidine. Canine parietal cells were stimulated by the indicated concentrations of histamine in the presence of the 4 indicated concentrations of cimetidine.[18]

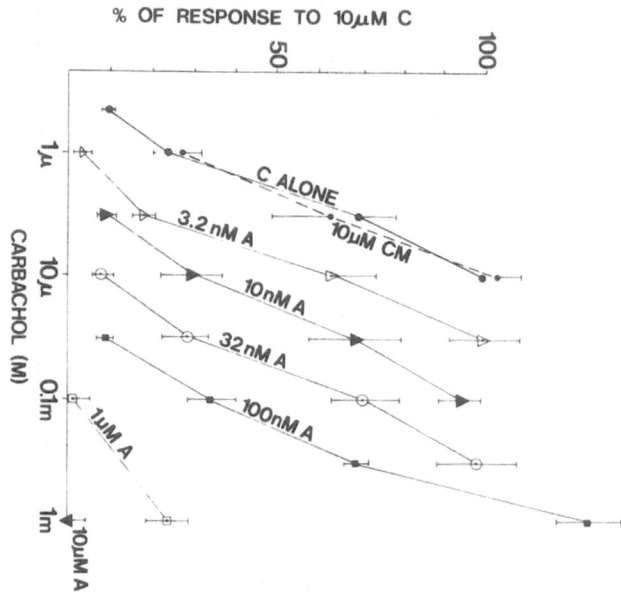

Figure 3. Competitive inhibition of cholinergic-stimulated ^{14}C-aminopyrine accumulation into parietal cells by atropine. Canine parietal cells were stimulated by the indicated concentrations of carbachol in the presence of the 4 indicated concentrations of atropine.[18]

stimulation of oxygen consumption and AP accumulation by rabbit gastric glands[19,21] and isolated canine, guinea pig, and rat parietal cells.[9,12,20] For example, cimetidine in increasing concentrations produced a progressive parallel shift of the dose-response for histamine stimulation of AP accumulation in canine parietal cells.[18] (fig. 2) The dissociation constant calculated from these data using a Schild plot is 1 μM and thus similar to those found in guinea pig atrium and rat uterus. Anticholinergic agents in concentrations that markedly inhibit the response to cholinomimetics, fail to shift the dose-response to histamine.

Muscarinic receptors

Muscarinic antagonists competively inhibit cholinergic stimulation of oxygen consumption and AP accumulation.[9,11,12,21] Atropine at concentrations between 3.2 nM and 100 nM produced a progressive, parallel rightward shift of the dose-response for carbachol stimulation of AP accumulation by isolated canine parietal cells, whereas cimetidine (10 μM) did not alter this dose-response relation.[18] (fig. 3) The dissociation constant determined for atropine was 1 nM[11,18] a value typical of muscarinic receptors in other tissues. Thus the isolated parietal cell after enzyme dispersion retains pharmacologically typical muscarinic and histamine H_2-receptors.

Gastrin receptors

The presence of gastrin receptors on the parietal cell remains controversial. With isolated canine parietal cells, gastrin produced a small, but definite increase in both oxygen consumption[9] and AP accumulation.[18] These responses were not blocked by either histamine H_2-receptor antagonists or anticholinergic agents, indicating interaction at a separate receptor site. This gastrin effect was found in elutriator fractions enriched in parietal cells, but depleted in histamine cells, thus making it unlikely that gastrin action was mediated by release of histamine. Direct effects of gastrin on parietal cells isolated from species other than dog are less dramatic. Pentagastrin did not stimulate oxygen consumption by parietal cells isolated from amphibian mucosa,[14] and only about one-third of parietal cell preparations from guinea pig responded to gastrin.[12] Gastrin has only a

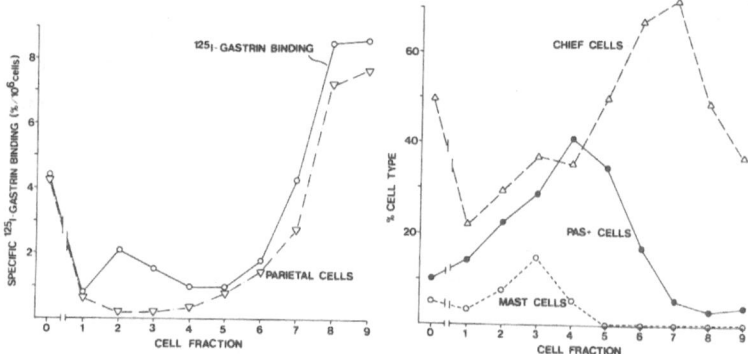

Figure 4. The binding of ^{125}I-[Leu^{15}]-G17 to cell fractions separated by elutriation. Fractions of increasing size were collected using a Beckman elutriator rotor. Parietal, cheif, and mucous cells were identified on cytocentrifuge slides stained with periodic acid Schiff. In the left panel, ^{125}I-[Leu^{15}]-G17 binding in fmol/10^6 cells and the percentage content of parietal cells, mucous cells (PAS +) and mast cells, the latter stained with toluidine blue.[16]

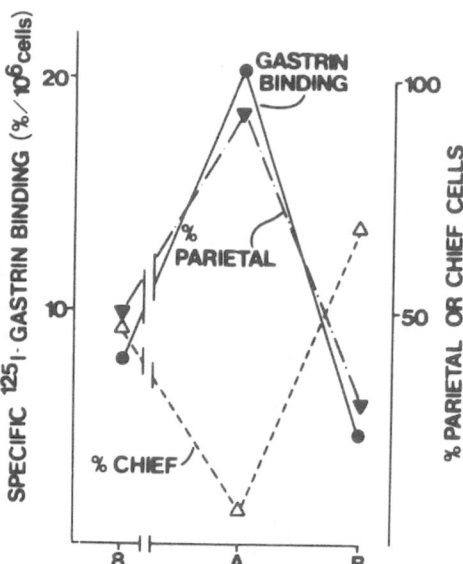

Figure 5. Binding of ^{125}I-[Leu^{15}]-G17 to highly enriched parietal and chief cells. The elutriator fraction enriched in parietal cells was further separated using a step density gradient of albumin and Ficoll. The binding of ^{125}I-[Leu^{15}]-G17 to these fractions was correlated with the content of parietal and not of chief cells. Modified from.[16]

small direct effect stimulating rabbit parietal cells.[22] However, in the presence of isobutyl methyl xanthine (IMX), gastrin did produce an incremental increase in AP accumulation that was largely inhibited by cimetidine.[22,23] The mechanisms accounting for these observations remain uncertain, but gastrin has been reported to release histamine from rabbit gastric glands, as discussed later.

The strongest evidence for the existence of a specific gastrin receptor on canine parietal cells comes from studies using a biologically active ^{125}I-[Leu^{15}]-G17 as a probe for the gastrin receptor.[16] ^{125}I-[Leu^{15}]-G17 has been used to study the gastrin receptor in a crude homogenate of rat fundic mucosa.[24] In our studies of the gastrin receptor on parietal cells, we also found it necessary to use [Leu^{15}]-gastrin for iodination, since oxidative damage presumably of methionine in the 15 position of native gastrin rendered specific receptor interactions inconsistent. In fractions containing 50 – 70% parietal cells 8 – 12% of the ^{125}I-[Leu^{15}]-G17 bound per million cells, with about 85% of the binding being specific as determined by the difference of binding in the presence and absence of excess unlabelled gastrin. At 37°C, binding was rapid and reversible. In cell separation studies using the elutriator rotor, ^{125}I-[Leu^{15}]-G17 binding correlated with the distribution of parietal cells, indicating that parietal cells accounted for the majority of the gastrin binding to canine fundic mucosal cells. (fig. 4) Step density gradients were performed on the parietal cell enriched elutriator fractions to provide enriched of greater than 85% parietal or chief cells respectively; ^{125}I-[Leu^{15}]-G17 binding correlated positively with the parietal cell content ($r = 0.96$) and negatively with the chief cell content ($r = -0.97$) of these fractions. (fig. 5) These data leave little question that the parietal cell, and probably not the chief cell, has a specific gastrin receptor. However, in the elutriator separation, there was indication of gastrin binding to one of more additional cell types that present in the small cell elutriator fractions (SCEF), as discussed subsequently. Gastrin binding was found to correlate with gastrin stimulation of parietal cell function.[16] Proglumide inhibited gastrin binding and the inhibition of binding was proportional with inhibition of gastrin stimulation of parietal cell function.

Potentiating interactions between secretagogues

Muscarinic and histamine H_2-receptor antagonists were specific for the actions on the isolated parietal cell function of carbachol and histamine, respectively. These findings are thus at odds with the *in vivo* observations that these inhibitors block all forms of acid secretion. This apparent contradiction may reflect the existence of potentiating interactions between secretagogues at the parietal cell itself. Data obtained with studies of both oxygen consumption[25] and AP accumulation[26] indicate that potentiating interactions occur between histamine and gastrin and histamine and carbachol, but not between carbachol and gastrin, in that the responses to these former two combinations are significantly greater than the sum of the individual responses. A three-way interaction, in addition, may exist between histamine, carbachol, and gastrin.[26] Interactions between cholinergic agents and histamine[7] and possibly between gastrin and histamine[22] have been found in rabbit gastric glands. In the presence of these potentiating interactions, the actions of cimetidine and atropine display an apparent nonspecific reminiscent of that found *in vivo.* thus, for example, when gastrin action on isolated parietal cells was enhanced by potentiating interaction with histamine, cimetidine caused an apparent inhibition of the response to gastrin, which presumably reflected withdrawal of histamine's enhancement of gastrin's action.[25,26]

Activation of parietal cell function

The parietal cell is activated by both calcium- and cyclic AMP-dependent mechanisms. These secondary signals are specific for acetylcholine and histamine, respectively, thus providing further support for the view that these transmitters act directly on parietal cell receptors.

Parietal cell activation by cyclic AMP

Histamine stimulated cyclic adenosine monophosphate (AMP) production by isolated canine fundic cells and this effect correlated with parietal cell content of fractions separation by elutriation.[28,29] In contrast, prostaglandin (PG) E$_2$ in micromolar concentrations also stimulated cyclic AMP production, but this effect was more pronounced in nonparietal cell fractions. Stimulation of parietal cells by histamine, but not by carbachol or gastrin, was linked to enhanced production of cyclic AMP. PGs in nanomolar concentrations did molulate parietal cell function; PGE$_2$ and PGI$_2$ selectively inhibited histamine-stimulated [^{14}C]-aminopyrine accumulation and interfered with the cellular accumulation of cyclic AMP. Prostaglandins did not block the response to gastrin of acetylcholine when these agents were studied as single agents. However, when the response to gastrin or acetylcholine was enhanced by histamine, PGE$_2$ and PGI$_2$ blocked the response to the extent of removing the component reflecting histamine enhancement.[30] This conclusion regarding blockade of histamine enhancement by PGs was underlined by the observation that PGs did not inhibit cholinergic or gastrin potentiation by dibutyryl cyclic AMP. Prostaglandins appear to inhibit histamine at a proximal step in action, presumably receptor activation of adenylate cyclase.

Parietal cell activation by calcium-dependent mechanisms

In many cell types, increases in cytosol calcium appear to mediate cell activation by chemical transmitters. Such increases in cytosol calcium can be achieved by either enhanced influx of extracellular calcium or mobilization of intracellular calcium. Cholinergic stimulation of parietal cell function appears coupled to enhanced influx of extracellular calcium. The experiments supporting this conclusion include a dependency of cholinergic stimulation on extracellular calcium.[23] Furthermore, lanthanum, which blocks calcium fluxes across plasma membranes, also caused marked impairment of cholinergic action.[31] Lastly, carbachol stimulation is associated with enhanced ^{45}Ca^{++} influx into parietal cells, which, in turn, is closely correlated with cholinergic stimulation of oxygen consumption and AP accumulation.[31] In contrast to these findings, histamine stimulation of parietal cell function was only modestly impaired by removal of extracellular calcium and was not blocked by lanthanum nor associated with enhanced influx of ^{45}Ca^{++}. Gastrin action showed an intermediate dependency upon the concentration of extracellular calcium, and treatment with lanthanum caused modest impairment of gastrin responsiveness. However, stimulation by gastrin was not

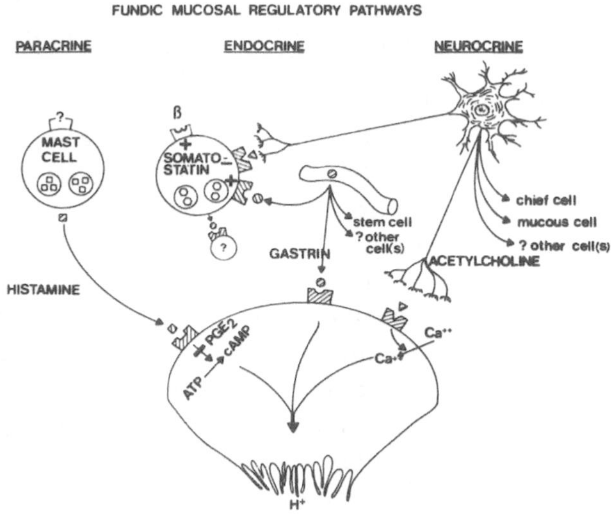

FUNDIC MUCOSAL REGULATORY PATHWAYS

Figure 6. Fundic mucosal regulatory pathways. Depicted is a model outlining a present view of the receptors and pathways regulating parietal cell function. Histamine, gastrin, and acetylcholine act in parallel on specific receptors on the parietal cell, with their actions amplified by potentiating interactions. Gastrin, delivered by capillaries, also acts directly on receptors on the somatostatin cell to activate an inhibitory pathway. Gastrin receptors are probably also present on the stem cell and possibly on other cell types. Histamine is delivered from mast cells locating in the lamina propria; receptors regulating mast cell histamine formation and release remain uncertain. Acetylcholine is delivered by postganglionic nerves to muscarinic receptors on parietal cells, but also to muscarinic receptors on the somatostatin cell that attenuate somatostatin release, and thus dampens the inhibitory pathway mediated by somatostatin. This 'double negative' effect of acetylcholine at the somatostatin cell – inhibition of an inhibitor – serves to enhance the acid secretory response. Muscarinic receptors on other cell types may also modulate the acid secretory response and many factors may influence acetylcholine delivery, but these elements remain to be elucidated.

found to be associated with enhanced calcium influx, and although gastrin action may be linked to the mobilization of intracellular calcium, studies available with cells preloaded with $^{45}Ca^{++}$ failed to confirm this gastrin effect on calcium flux.[31] Preliminary studies using Quin2 as a fluorescent probe for cytosolic $[Ca^{++}]$ indicated that both gastrin and carbachol induced increases in cytosolic calcium.[32]

Parietal cell vs nonparietal cell receptors

Studies with isolated canine parietal cells support the hypothesis that histamine, gastrin, and acetylcholine modulate acid secretion by directly interacting with receptors on the parietal cell. (fig. 6) Furthermore, potentiating interactions may be an important mechanism underlying the interdependency between secretagogues *in vivo*. Histamine activation of parietal cell function is linked to enhanced formation of cyclic AMP. Stimulation of parietal cell function by cholinergic agents and gastrin are linked to increases in cytosolic calcium that appear, in the case of cholinergic agents, to represent enhanced influx of extracellular calcium. These findings provide a basis for understanding the mechanisms of action of the modalities used to treat peptic ulcer disease, as noted below.

This discussion has not thus far considered the possibility that cholinergic and gastrin receptors may exist on other cells within the mucosa that also participate in the regulation of secretory function. These other cells with a potential regulatory role are endocrine, paracrine or even neurocrine cells that release transmitters such as histamine or somatostatin. Thus, integration between the pathways regulating acid secretion may occur by mechanisms in addition to potentiating interactions between secretagogues at the parietal cell itself. The next section will review recent studies with canine fundic mucosal cells indicating that receptors for gastrin and acetylcholine exist on cells other than parietal cells.

Nonparietal gastrin and acetylcholine receptors

^{125}I-[Leu^{15}]-G17 binding to elutriator (velocity) separated fractions, specific gastrin binding was found to a small cell(s), in addition to parietal cells.[16] (fig. 4) These small cell elutriator fractions had a heterogenous cell population including histamine cells, endocrine cells containing somatostatin and glucagon, and endocrine-like cells marked by the presence of serotonin and DOPA decarboxylase. To determine if ^{125}I-[Leu^{15}]-G17 binding was localized to a specific cell type, density separation of this small cell elutriator fraction was performed using a linear gradient formed with albumin and Ficoll.[33] In this density separation, a positive correlation was found between ^{125}I-[Leu^{15}]-G17 binding and the distribution of cells containing somatostatin-like immunoreactivity (SLI). Since the presence of specific receptors means little without testing functional responses, techniques were sought for determining if gastrin altered release of SLI from canine fundic endocrine cells. For these studies, the small cell elutriator fraction was placed in short term culture in full growth medium on a bed of type 1 collagen.[34] The presence of gastrin receptors on SLI cells was confirmed by finding that gastrin stimulated the release of SLI from these cultures.

Epinephrine and dibutyryl cyclic AMP also stimulated SLI release and marked potentiation was found between gastrin and both epinephrine and dibutyryl cyclic AMP. The beta-adrenergic antagonist propranolol, but not alpha-adrenergic receptor antagonists, competitively inhibited this epinephrine response.[35] Cholecystokinin was also found to be more effective than gastrin as a stimulant of SLI release,[36] whereas both peptides were equally effective stimulating parietal cell function.[16] Of interest, muscarinic receptors also regulated SLI cell function, but cholinergic agents inhibited – rather than stimulated – SLI release.[35] This cholinergic effect was surmountably blocked by atropine; the dissociation constant was o.4 nM, consistent with interaction at a typical muscarinic receptor. These data indicate that the fundic somatostatin cell is directly stimulated by gastrin, CCK, and epinephrine and inhibited by muscarinic agents. The greater ability of CCK than gastrin to release somatostatin may be a factor in the poor effectiveness of CCK as a gastrin acid secretagogue in dog.

Histamine cells in the canine fundic mucosa

Another potential target for gastrin and cholinergic regulation is the fundic mucosal histamine cell. Despite the central role for histamine in the regulation of gastric acid secretion, knowledge remains quite incomplete regarding the stores of histamine within the gastric mucosa and the regulation of histamine formation and release. In studies with canine fundic mucosal cells, histamine-containing cells were enriched using elutriation followed by density gradient separation. Morphologically typical mast cells appeared to fully account for the histamine content of these dispersed canine fundic cells.[37] To determine the factors regulating histamine release, this small cell elutriator fraction was placed in overnight suspension culture and factors regulating histamine release then characterized. These mast cells retained their histamine content and released histamine in response to the calcium ionophore A23187 and to antibody to IgE, which presumably crosslinks surface receptors saturated with IgE. However, despite these indications of cell viability and responsiveness, neither acetylcholine nor gastrin released histamine from these dispersed cells. The conclusion that these histamine cells lack gastrin[33] and muscarinic (unpublished observations) receptors was supported by direct binding with ^{125}I-[Leu^{15}]-G17 and [^{3}H]-quinuclindinyl benzylate respectively; neither of these receptors were present in density gradient fractions maximally enriched in mast cell content. The absence of gastrin and muscarinic receptors on canine fundic mast cells contrasted with their presence on fundic mucosal somatostatin cells, as discussed above. Since gastrin and acetylcholine receptors survived dispersion and separation of somatostatin cells, it seems unlikely that the rigors of cell separation accounted for the absence of receptors on mast cells, although it is possible that receptors on specific cells may display selective sensitivity to certain treatments.

Considerable evidence indicates that the cellular stores of histamine in the fundic mucosa vary among species. In contrast to the presence of histamine in mast cells in the dog (*vide supra*), in the rat fundic mucosa, histamine is also present in endocrine-like cells.[38] Techniques similar to those applied in the dog (enzyme dispersion, sequential velocity and linear density separation) were also used to enrich histamine cells from the rat fundic mucosa; histamine was found in a light cell fraction that possessed high activities of histidine decarboxylase (the histamine-forming enzyme) and DOPA decarboxylase.[39] In man present studies indicated that histamine is present only in mast cells.[40] The implication of these findings is that the factors regulating histamine formation and release may vary as a function of the cell type storing histamine. For example, histamine formation is induced in the rat fundic mucosa by gastrin and food,[41,42] but there is no indication of a similar effect in man or dog.[40] Even with these indications that gastrin influences histamine formation and possibly release in the rat there is no proof in the rat that gastrin stimulation of acid secretion is mediated by release of histamine.[4]

As a further caveat to this complex story, gastrin and acetylcholine have been found to release histamine from rabbit gastric glands[43] and from amphibian gastric mucosa.[44] The cell type storing histamine in rabbit fundic glands has not been clearly identified, although it has been hypothesized to be an endocrine cell. Although mast cells have not been identified in these gland preparations, the fixation and staining techniques may not have been optimized for staining mucosal mast cells; the component of histamine content in mast cells required further study. Using identical techniques, studies with gastric glands prepared from canine fundic mucosa found no indication of histamine release in response to gastrin or acetylcholine (Berglindh T, personal communication). No unifying concepts can be formulated based upon present data, other than an anticipation that histamine formation and release may vary as a function of the cell type storing histamine in the fundic mucosa in the species under consideration.

Overview

The canine parietal cell thus appears to have receptors for histamine, gastrin, and acetylcholine; potentiating interactions, reflecting convergence of cyclic AMP and calcium pathways, may be important modulators of parietal cell function. In addition, our present data obtained from studies with canine fundic cells indicate a complex model wherein both gastrin and acetylcholine have at least dual sets of receptors that are potentially involved in regulating acid-secretory function. (fig. 6) Gastrin interacts with receptors on the parietal cell and on the somatostatin cell, and, via these receptors, has opposing acid-stimulatory and acid-inhibitory actions. This wiring appears to be a short circuit, but several elements may modulate these opposing effects of gastrin on different cell types, thereby co-ordinating the regulatory process. Acetylcholine is probably a major modulating element, increasing the acid secretory response to gastrin by stimultaneously enhancing gastrin stimulating of parietal cell function and attenuating gastrin activation of the inhibitory mechanisms mediated by release of somatostatin. (fig. 7)

Therapeutic modalities for inhibiting acid secretion: Cellular mechanisms

Isolated parietal cells and gastric gland preparations provide a model for elucidating the mechanisms of action of antisecretory agents. Inhibitors presently exist that act directly on parietal cell function by three general mechanisms. (Table I)

SPECULATION

THE BALANCE OF GASTRIN CCK ACTIONS IN CANINE FUNDIC MUCOSA

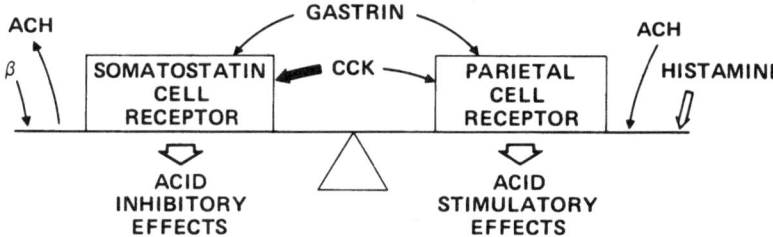

Figure 7. Modulation of inhibitory and stimulatory effects of gastric acid secretion. In the canine fundic mucosa, both CCK and gastrin interact with receptors on at least parietal and somatostatin cells, and thus these peptides may activate mechanisms either stimulating or inhibiting acid secretion. CCK8 more potently stimulates SLI release, thus possibly accounting for the impaired efficacy of this peptide as a stimulant of acid secretion *in vivo* in the dog. In addition, several factors may modulate the stimulatory or inhibitory effects of gastrin and CCK on parietal and somatostatin cells, thus shifting the balance of their actions. Acetylcholine inhibits SLI release in response to chemotransmitters but enhances parietal cell function; by both mechanisms acetylcholine will shift the balance to the acid-stimulatory side. β-adrenergic agents enhance CCK and gastrin action on SLI release, but appear to have no direct effect on canine parietal cell function; thus β-adrenergic agents shift the balance of CCK/gastrin action to the acid-inhibitory side. In contrast, histamine influences only the stimulatory limb, enhancing parietal cell response to gastrin and CCK8, but not influencing somatostatin release.[36]

Table I. Inhibitors of acid secretion acting on the parietal cell.

1. Receptor antagonists	Histamine H_2 receptor
	Muscarinic receptor
	Gastrin receptor
2. Inhibitors of cell activation	Prostaglandins E_2 and I_2
3. Inhibitors of H^+ pump	Substituted benziimidazoles

Receptor antagonists

Histamine H_2-receptor antagonists are clinically useful antisecretory agents that act directly and specifically on parietal cell receptors. These agents dispaly an apparent nonspecificity *in vivo* that may reflect several mechanisms, one of which is interference with the potentiating interactions that occur between secretagogues in their actions on parietal cell function. Histamine H_2-receptor antagonists are very effective inhibitors of gastrin- and meal-stimulated acid secretion. As noted above, this efficacy may result in part from inhibition of potentiating interactions at the parietal cell. Another element is that histamine does not alter release of somatostatin from fundic endocrine cells (unpublished observations), and therefore histamine H_2-receptor antagonists attentuate gastrin action on the parietal cell without impairing gastrin's acid-inhibitory effects mediated by release of somatostatin. Thus the presence of histamine H_2-receptor antagonists may shift the spectrum of gastrin action to the acid-inhibitory side. It is also possible that the profound effects of histamine H_2-receptor antagonists on gastrin action reflect a component of gastrin action due to histamine release, but this effect may be species variable and awaits direct confirmation.

Anti-muscarinic agents also act directly on parietal cell receptors, and serve to inhibit direct and potentiating effects of cholinergic agents on parietal cell function. Although there is no indication that the anti-secretory effects of histamine H_2-receptor antagonists are mediated by effects on cells other than parietal cells, muscarinic receptors are present on somatostatin cells and inhibition of release of this inhibitor may be an important component of cholinergic action. Therefore, administrating an anticholinergic agent will both block stimulation of parietal cell function and block cholinergic inhibition of somatostatin release. These dual actions will both serve to stimulate acid secretion and may account for a component of the interactions found between gastrin and vagal stimulation. Anticholinergic agents will shift gastrin action toward acid-inhibitory side by removing both endogenous muscarinic inhibition of somatostatin release (increasing release of this inhibitor) and blocking muscarinic stimulation at the parietal cell itself. The relative importance of these two effects to the antisecretory effects of muscarinic antagonists remains to be sorted out by *in vivo* studies.

The muscarinic antagonist pirenzepine potently inhibits acid secretion,[45] and is a clinically useful anti-ulcer agent. Although delivery to selective receptor sites may be an important determinant of the spectrum of action of this antagonist, there is indication that pirenzepine may preferentially interact with a subtype of muscarinic receptors regulating acid secretion. The interaction of pirenzepine with muscarinic receptors on both the somatostatin cells and on parietal cells has been studied. Pirenzepine inhibited both cholinergic stimulation of parietal cell function (unpublished observations) and cholinergic blockade of SLI release[35] with potency that was 80- to 100-fold less than atropine. This finding does not allow the identification of high affinity pirenzepine receptors, which may be present on other cell types. Alternatively, the apparent potency of the antisecretory actions of pirenzepine may reflect selective delivery to certain receptor sites.

Proglumide is a compound displaying selective antagonism of gastrin and cholecystokinin receptors. Although this agent inhibits acid secretion *in vivo*, the potency is low and it is unlikely that this compound will prove to be a clinically useful drug. However, more potent gastrin receptor antagonists may be of great interest both from a physiological and clinical perspective.

Inhibitors of cell activation

The antisecretory actions of prostaglandins probably reflect interference with histamine activation of adenylate cyclase activity. Several prostaglandins have been demonstrated to be clinically useful in healing duodenal and gastric ulcer. Although prostaglandins have been shown to prevent gastric mucosal injury by mechanisms independent of inhibition of acid secretion, clinical studies indicate that prostaglandin analogues heal duodenal ulcer as a function of their antisecretory potency.

Blocking calcium activation of parietal cell function by means of calcium channel blockers offers another theoretical therapeutic alternative. However, it is unlikely these Ca^{++} channel blockers will achieve sufficient selectivity and effectiveness to be clinically useful. Verapamil has only weak antisecretory properties *in vivo* against either pentagastrin or vagal stimulation by sham feeding.[46,47] The low effectiveness of these agents is in apparent contradiction with the hypothesis that cholinergic agents activate parietal cell function by enhancing calcium influx. The decreased efficacy of these calcium channel blockers may reflect heterogenity of calcium channels and low effectiveness against receptor-activated calcium channels in parietal cells. Alternatively calcium channel blockers may modulate secretory function at other sites with counterbalancing effects.

Direct inhibition of H^+/K^+-ATPase

A third mechanism of inhibition is the direct blockade of parietal cell H^+/K^+-ATPase by substituted benziimidazoles, such as omeprazole.[48] A specific H^+/K^+-ATPase is the pump that translocates H^+ for K^+ across the apical membrane of the parietal cells,[49,50] operating in concert with a K^+Cl^- cotransporter that is present in vesicles prepared from stimulated – but not resting – parietal cells.[49] This KCl-symport delivers K^+ to the apical surface for exchange with H^+ and Cl^- as the counter ion for H^+ secretion. H^+/K^+-ATPase inhibitors are potent inhibitors of acid secretion *in vivo* and they inhibit parietal cell function *in vitro*. These enzyme inhibitors are effective anti-ulcer agents, but their full spectrum of clinical usefulness will only become clear after more experience is gained with their use and the clinical implications of recently recognized effects on endocrine cell proliferation have been clarified.

Perspective

The apparent complexity of proposed regulatory mechanisms of acid secretion has increased dramatically with the acquisition of a relatively small amount of knowledge. As further knowledge is gained by reductionistic studies in *in vitro* systems and by studies in more integrated systems *in vivo*, the importance of the various regulatory receptors and elements may become clear and unifying hypotheses formulated. The regulation of histamine formation and release requires a great deal of additional study to clarify the interplay between the major pathways regulating acid secretion. There is no doubt that current models and knowledge will rapidly evolve, but the concept that the pathways mediating acid secretion both converge in parallel at the parietal cell and act in series, by modulating the release of paracrine transmitters, is attractive and likely to persist. Future therapeutic modalities may be developed that influence these nonparietal cell receptors and pathways increasing the versatility of the regimen used to treat ulcer disorders.

References

1. Grossman MI. Regulation of gastric acid secretion. In: Johnson LR (Ed). Physiology of the Gastrointestinal Tract. New York: Raven Press, 1980:659–671.
2. Feldman M. Gastric secretion. In: Sleisenger M, and Fordtran JS (Eds). Gastrointestinal Diseases. Saunders, Philadelphia. Third edition, 1983:541–558.
3. Code CF. Histamine and gastric secretion: A later look, 1955–1965. Fed Proc 1965;24:1311–21.
4. Johnson LR. Control of gastric secretion: No room for histamine. Gastroenterology 1971;61:106–118.
5. Black JW, Duncan WAM, Durant CJ, Ganellin CR, Parsons ME. Definition and antagonism of histamine H_2-receptors. Nature (Lond) 1972;236:385–90.
6. Grossman MI, Konturek SJ. Inhibition of acid secretion in dog by metiamide, a histamine antagonist acting on H_2 receptors. Gastroenterology 1974;66:517–21.
7. Gibson R, Hirschowitz BI, Hutchinson G. Actions of metiamide, an H_2-histamine receptor antagonist, on gastric H^+ and pepsin secretion in dogs. Gastroenterology 1974;67:93–99.
8. Berglindh T, Helander HF, Obrink KJ. Effects of secretagogues on oxygen consumption, aminopyrine accumulation, and morphology in isolated gastric glands. Acta Physiol Scand 1976;97:401–14.
9. Soll AH. The actions of secretagogues on oxygen uptake by isolated mammalian parietal cells. J Clin Invest 1978;61:370–380.
10. Lewin M, Cheret AM, Saumarmon A, Girodet J. Methode pour l'isolement et le tri des cellules de la muqueuse fundique du rat. Biol Gastroenterol 1974;7:139–44.
11. Ecknauer R, Dial E, Thompson WJ, Johnson LR, Rosenfeld GC. Isolated rat gastric parietal cells: Cholinergic response and pharmacology. Life Sci 1981;28:609–621.
12. Batzri S. Interaction of histamine with specific membrane receptors on gastric mucosal cells. Biochem Pharmacol 1981;30:3013–3016.
13. Sewing K-F, Harms P, Schulz G, Hannemann H. Effect of substituted benzimidazoles on acid secretion in isolated and enriched guinea pig parietal cells. Gut 1983;24:557–560.
14. Michelangeli F. Acid secretion and intracellular pH in isolated oxyntic cells. J Membrane Biol 1978;38:31–50.
15. Soll AH. Physiology of isolated canine parietal cells: Receptors and effectors regulating function. In: Johnson LR (Ed). Physiology of the Digestive Tract. New York: Raven Press, 1981:673–691.
16. Soll AH, Amirian DA, Thomas LP, Reedy TJ, Elashoff JD. Gastrin receptors on isolated canine parietal cells. J Clin Invest 1984;73:1434–1447.
17. Berglindh T, Dibona DR, Ito S, Sachs G. Probes of parietal cell function. Am J Physiol 1980;238(Gastrointest Liver Physiol 1):G165–G176.
18. Soll AH. Secretagogue stimulation of ^{14}C-aminopyrine accumulation by isolated canine parietal cells. Am J Physiol 1980;238:G366–375.
19. Chew CS, Hersey SJ, Sachs G, Berglindh T. Histamine responsiveness of isolated gastric glands. Am J Physiol 1980;238:G312–G320.
20. Dial E, Thompson WJ, Rosengeld GC. Isolated parietal cells: Histamine response and pharmacology. J Pharm Exp Ther 1981;219:585–90.

21. Berglindh T. Potentiation by carbachol and aminophylline of histamine- and dbcAMP-induced parietal cells activity in isolated gastric glands. Acta Physiol Scand 1977;99:75–84.

22. Chew CS, Hersey SJ. Gastrin stimulation of isolated gastric glands. Am J Physiol 1982;242(Gastrointest Liver Physiol):G504–512.

23. Berglindh T, Sachs G, Takeguchi N. Ca^+ dependent secretagogue stimulation in isolated rabbit gastric glands. Am J Physiol 1980;239:G90–G94.

24. Takeuchi K, Speir GR, Johnson LR. Mucosal gastrin receptor. I. Assay standardization and fulfillment of receptor criteria. Am J Physiol 1979;237:E284–E294.

25. Soll AH. The interaction of histamine with gastrin and carbamylcholine on oxygen uptake by isolated mammalian parietal cells. J Clin Invest 1978;61:381–389.

26. Soll AH. Potentiating interactions of gastric stimulants on ^{14}C-aminopyrine accumulation by isolated canine parietal cells. Gastroenterology 1982;83:216–223.

27. Berglindh T. Effects of common inhibitors of gastric acid secretion on secretagogue-induced respiration and aminopyrine accumulation in isolated gastric glands. Biochim Biophys Acta 1977;464:217–33.

28. Major JS, Scholes P. The localization of a histamine H_2-receptor adenylate cyclase system in canine parietal cells and its inhibition by prostaglandins. Agents and Actions 1978;8:324–31.

29. Wollin A, Soll AH, Samloff IM. Actions of histamine, secretin, and PGE_2 on cyclic AMP production by isolated canine fundic mucosal cells. Am J Physiol 1979;237:E437–E443.

30. Soll AH. Specific inhibition by prostaglandins EH_2 and IH_2 of histamine-stimulated $[^{14}C]$ aminopyrine accumulation and cyclic adenosine monophosphate generation by isolated canine parietal cells. J Clin Invest 1978;65:1222–1229.

31. Soll AH. Extracellular calcium and cholinergic stimulation of isolated canine parietal cells. J Clin Invest 1981;68:270–278.

32. Muallem S, Sachs G. Changes in cytostolic free Ca^{2+} in isolated parietal cells differential effects of secretagogues. Biochim Biophys Acta 1984;805:181–185.

33. Soll AH, Amirian DA, Thomas LP, Park J, Beaven MA, Yamada T. Gastrin receptors on nonparietal cells isolated from canine fundic mucosa. Am J Physiol 1984;247:G715–G723.

34. Soll AH, Yamada T, Park J, Thomas LP. Release of somatostatin-like immunoreactivity from canine fundic mucosal cells in primary culture. Am J Physiol 1984;247:G558–G566.

35. Yamada T, Soll AH, Park J, Elashoff J. Autonomic regulation of somatostatin release: Studies with primary cultures of canine fundic mucosal cells. Am J Physiol 1984;247:G567–G573.

36. Soll AH, Amirian DA, Thomas LP, Park J. CCK/gastrin receptors on somatostatin cells isolated from canine fundic mucosa. Am J Physiol 1985 (in press).

37. Soll AH, Lewin K, Beaven MA. Isolation of histamine containing cells from canine fundic mucosa. Gastroenterology 1979;77:1283–1290.

38. Thunberg R. Localization of cells containing and forming histamine in the gastric mucosa of the rat. Exp Cell Res 1967;47:108–15.

39. Soll AH, Lewin KJ, Beaven MA. Isolation of histamine-containing cells from rat gastric mucosa: Biochemical and morphologic differences from mast cells. Gastroenterology 1981;80:717–727.

40. Hakanson R, Lilja B, Owman Ch. Cellular localization of the histamine and monoamines in the gastric mucosa of man. Histochemie 1969;18:74–86.
41. Aures D, Hakanson R, Schauer A. Histidine decarboxylase and DOPA decarboxylase in the rat stomach. Properties and cellular localization. Eur J Pharmacol 1968;3:217–34.
42. Hakanson R, Liedberg G. The role of endogenous gastrin in the activation of gastric histidine decarboxylase in the rat. Effect of antrectomy and vagal denervation. Eur J Pharmacol 1970;12:94–103.
43. Berqvist E, Waller M, Hammar L, Obrink KJ. Histamine as the secretory mediator in isolated gastric glands. In: Schulz'I, Sachs G, Forte JG, Ullrich KJ (Eds). Hydrogen Ion Transport in Epithelia. Elsevier/North-Holland Biomedical Press, Amsterdam 1980:429–437.
44. Rangachari PK. Histamine release by gastric stimulants. Nature 1975;253: 53–55.
45. Hirschowitz BI, Fong J, Molina E. Effects of pirenzepine and atropine on vagal and cholinergic gastric secretion and gastric release and on heart rate in the dog. J Pharm Exp Ther 1983;225:263–268.
46. Kirkegaard P, Christiansen J, Petersen B. Sov Olsen P. Calcium and stimulus-secretion coupling in gastric fundic mucosa. Scand J Gastroenterol 1982;17:533–538.
47. Aadland E, Berstad A. Effect of verpamil on gastric secretion in man. Scand J Gastroenterol 1983;18:969–971.
48. Fellenius E, Elander B, Wallmark B, Hfelander HF, Berglindh T. Inhibition of acid secretion in isolated gastric glands by substituted benzimidazoles. Am J Physiol 1982;243(Gastrointest Liver Physiol 6):G505–G510.
49. Forte JG, Forte TM, Black JA, Okamoto C, Wolosin JM. Correlation of parietal cell structure and function. J Clin Gastroenterol 1983;5:17–27.
50. Sachs G, Berglindh T. Physiology of the parietal cell. In: Johnson LR (Ed). Physiology of the Gastrointestinal Tract, Chapter 19. New York: Raven Press 1981:567–602.

4. Aetiology of duodenal ulcer

K.G. WORMSLEY, M.D., D.Sc., F.R.C.P.

Department of Therapeutics, University of Dundee, Ninewells Hospital, Scotland

There are two conflicting views about the aetiology of ulcers: that ulcers of the stomach and duodenum (and sometimes of the oesophagus) are 'peptic' and somehow aetiologically unique or, much less popularly, that ulcers of the upper alimentary tract are nonspecific, like chronic ulcers elsewhere – for example, like varicose ulcers of the lower legs.

The basis for the proposal that gastric and duodenal ulcers are aetiologically unique depends on their anatomical localization and on the presence of what are assumed to be localized specific ulcerogenic factors. That is to say, localized ulcers are common in the duodenal bulb; are less common in the stomach and are very rare in the remainder of the small or large intestine. When the matter is considered further, it is clear that there are local factors in gastric juice, or in duodenal contents, which can be considered, a priori, to be sufficient to produce local mucosal ulcers. These latter factors have been viewed as 'aggressive' towards the local mucosa since the time when Claude Bernard demonstrated the powerful digestive capacity of gastric juice.

Two principal lines of study have strengthened the view that 'peptic ulceration' depends on the action of unique local 'aggressive' factors. In the first place, it has been frequently reported that ulcer disease – and especially duodenal ulcer disease – has a hereditary basis.[1] As with other hereditary abnormalities of metabolism, there has recently appeared a lot of information suggesting that there are definable increases in 'aggressive' potential, which are transmitted within families and which predispose to peptic ulceration.[2] When the prediction – that there is a familial incidence, which denotes an inherited functional defect which, in turn, can be defined – is translated into demonstrable fact, a powerful boost is given to this aetiological hypothesis of ulcer disease.

More important, perhaps, is the support provided for the hypothesis of 'local aggressive ulcerogens' by the demonstration that the positive and negative predictions of the hypothesis are apparently correct. An enormous number of studies have shown that there is an increase in the 'aggressive' factors in the stomach or duodenum of ulcer patients. These studies have been summarized[3] and include the demonstration that there is increased gastric juice in the duodenum of many patients with duodenal ulcer, or increased amount of duodenal contents in the stomach of many patients with gastric ulcer.

In addition, in the case of duodenal ulceration, a number of different mechanisms including increased production of gastric juice (because there are more secreting units, or the units work better, or are more sensitive than normal to stimulants) and abnormally rapid discharge of gastric juice from the stomach into the duodenum, have been demonstrated in affected patients.

Equally, or perhaps even more impressive has been the demonstration that ulcers apparently do not occur in the absence of these 'aggressive' factors, as duodenal ulceration does not occur in patients with severe impairment of gastric secretion. Indeed, much of the present succesful anti-ulcer therapy is based specifically on extrapolation from this type of 'negative' evidence. When we consider the frequent cure of ulcer disease by surgical techniques designed to decrease gastric secretion and the recent successes in healing ulcers by administration of drugs which inhibit gastric secretion, it seems permissible to conclude that the hypothesis, that ulcers are caused by 'aggressive factors', has been proven.

What about the alternative hypothesis, that duodenal and gastric ulcers are not unique or specific, but are just 'ordinary', albeit abnormally persistent, mucosal wounds or ulcers?

Much of the formidable collection of epidemiological information about ulcers[4] supports the view that exogenous ulcerogens are responsible for upper alimentary ulcers. For example, the dramatic changes in the incidence and prevalence of ulcers not only during the past century but even recently in countries like South Africa, indicate that apparently large sections of some populations have been, or are, exposed to environmental ulcerogens. Similar conclusions have been drawn from the very striking differences in the sex incidence of ulcers at different times and in different geographic areas, as well as some extraordinary changes in the age incidence of ulcers, from which it has been concluded that some population 'cohorts' have been especially exposed to environmental ulcerogenic factors.

Some hints are also becoming available concerning the nature of the environmental ulcerogens, which appear to be either infectious or chemical. Much recent evidence has pointed to the involvement of herpes simplex viruses in the acute exacerbations of duodenal ulcers. For example, not only are there marked clinical similarities between recurrent duodenal ulceration and infections with the herpes viruses[5] but increased blood levels of anti-herpes simplex type I antibodies have been found in patients with duodenal ulcer during acute exacerbations[6] and there are also increased levels of antiherpes simples IgA antibodies in the duodenal contents.[7] The main evidence for environmental chemical ulcerogens is derived from the production of experimental duodenal and gastric ulcers with chemicals. Many of the ulcers appear to be quite specific and restricted either to the duodenal or gastric mucosa.[8] Moreover, as has been pointed out,[9] some of these ulcerogenic chemicals are so ubiquitous that exposure must be common, although the noxious nature of the chemicals is not recognized. There are many chemicals which are known to damage the mucosa of the upper alimentary tract, but which are nevertheless consumed by large sections of the population because the chemicals have other pharmacological actions which are considered desirable, chemicals like the nonsterioidal anti-inflammatory drugs.

It might be asked: What of the evidence for endogenous ulcerogens? There have always been a number of problems with the plausibility of the hypothesis that 'aggressive' factors erode their way into and through the mucosa of the upper alimentary tract. There is, for example, the problem of the localized nature of the gastric and duodenal ulcers. While it is possible to envisage that local contact with a high concentration of an exogenous ulcerogen (a tablet of some ulcerogenic drug) can damage the mucosa at the point of contact, it has never been clear why contact with 'aggressive' gastric juice does not result in ulceration of the whole of the duodenal (and gastric) mucosa. Indeed, it is difficult to see how a focal lesion can arise from exposure to intraluminal ulcerogens. Not that most patients with duodenal ulcer are exposed to abnormal amounts of endogenous 'aggressive' factors, because all the 'pathophysiological disturbances' which have been identified in patients with duodenal ulcer have affected only small minorities of these patients. Most patients with duodenal ulcer do not appear to differ from individuals who have no ulcer, in their production of endogenous 'aggressive' factors.

It has therefore been suggested that patients with duodenal ulcer suffer, in some way, from defective 'defensive' barriers or processes. Despite much search, these 'deficiencies' have not been identified. To make matters worse, there is actually no evidence that there are any specific 'defensive' factors other than the usual ones against trauma or infection.

The success of therapy is really very difficult to explain in terms of the aetiology of ulcers. In this connection, though, it is necessary to emphasis that ulcer-curing operations and ulcer-healing drugs have effects which are not restricted to the inhibition of gastric secretion.[10]

As there are at present no indications which of the many effects of an operation, or drug, are involved in ulcer healing, it is not yet possible to interpret the results of successful therapy in terms of the aetiology of ulcers.

It seems to me that two recent endoscopic observations point to factors which may reflect aspects of the aetiology of ulcers. Almost every time an endoscopic examination is done, the stomach and duodenum are biopsied. Yet these traumatic post-biopsy ulcers do not become converted into 'clinical' ulcers, despite the presence of what are presumably sufficient 'aggressive' factors to produce the ulcers which are already presnt. It follows that intraluminal factors are not fundamentally involved in ulcerogenesis.

We have recently reported a study involving the follow up of asymptomatic ulcers.[11] One of the most extraordinary features of this type of ulcer is the tendency in about half of the affected patients for the ulcer to persist unhealed for many months. It is the failure to heal that is so remarkable and it seems to me that it is failure of the healing processes which is the fundamental aetiological problem in the pathogenesis of chronic gastric or duodenal ulcers. Unfortunately, we know too little about the processes involved in the repair of wounds and especially wounds of the mucosae: we know even less about abnormalities of these processes and about factors responsible for producing these abnormalities. It may be that when we obtain information about this latter aspect of the ulcer problem, we will be able to discuss more profitable the aetiology of ulcer disease.

References

1. McConnell RB. Peptic ulcer: Early genetic evidence – Families, twins and markers. In: Rotter JI, Samloff IM, Rimoin DL (Eds). Genetics and heterogeneity of common gastro-intestinal disorders. New York, Academic Press 1980:31–41.
2. Rotter JI. The genetics of peptic ulcer: More than one gene, more than one disease. In: Steinberg AG, Bearn AG, Motulsky AG, Childs B (Eds). Progress in Medical Genetics, Vol. 4. Philadelphia, WB Saunders 1980: 1–58.
3. Wormsley KG. Duodenal ulcer: Does pathophysiology equal aetiology? Gut 1983;24:775–780.
4. Boyd EJS, Wormsley KG. Etiology and pathogenesis of peptic ulcer. In: Haubrich WS, Kalser MH, Roth JLA, Schaffner F, Berk JE (Eds). Bockus Gastroenterology, 4th ed. Philadelphia, WB Saunders 1985;ch 66.
5. Borg I, Andren L. Herpes simplex virus as a cause of peptic ulcer. Scand J Gastroenterol 1980;15(supl 63):56–61.
6. Vestergaard BF, Rune SJ. Type-specific herpes simplex virus antibodies in patients with recurrent duodenal ulcer. Lancet 1980;I:1273–1275.
7. Rune SJ, Vestergaard BF. IgA antibodies to herpes simplex type I in duodenal juice and saliva from patients with duodenal ulcer and non-ulcer controls. Scand J Gastroenterol 1984;19:81–84.
8. Robert A. Experimental production of duodenal ulcers. Biol Gastroenterol (Paris) 1974;7:145–161.
9. Szabo S, Reynolds ES, Moslen MT. Chemical factors in aetiology of duodenal ulcer. Lancet 1975;2:73.
10. Wormsley KG. Duodenal ulcer: An update. Mt Sinai J Med 1981;48:391–396.
11. Boyd EJS, Wilson JA, Wormsley KG. The fate of asymptomatic recurrences of duodenal ulcer. Scand J Gastroenterol 1984;19.

5. Pyloric function and its role in the pathogenesis of gastric ulcer

A.G. JOHNSON, M.Chir., F.R.C.S.

University Surgical Unit, Royal Hallamshire Hospital, Sheffield, United Kingdom

Introduction

The pylorus (or 'gatekeeper') is the thickened muscle at the most distal end of the antrum. Its anatomy varies from species to species, but in man it consists of a thickened ring of circular muscle which is easily palpable at operation, or visible at endoscopy and which surrounds a pyloric canal of about 0.6 cm long. This most distal pyloric ring must be distinguished from the 2.5 cm length of increased thickness muscle which forms the terminal antrum. (fig. 1) This nomenclature is important as there has been much confusion: the term pyloric 'sphincter' is best avoided as it implies certain physiological characteristics which are not true of the pylorus. The pylorus is closely linked to the terminal antrum and duodenal cap, both anatomically and physiologically, and some writers refer to the antro-pyloro-duodenal segment as a whole. But we shall see the pyloric ring can sometimes function independently of both the antrum and the duodenum.

Function

The pylorus has three main functions.

1. Control of the size of food particles leaving the stomach.
Food particles that are too large to pass through the pylorus are powerfully retropelled into the body and fundus of the stomach for further digestion. The importance of this function of the pylorus can be seen when it is widened by a pyloroplasty or bypassed by a gastroenterostomy leading occasionally to bolus obstruction in the terminal ileum.

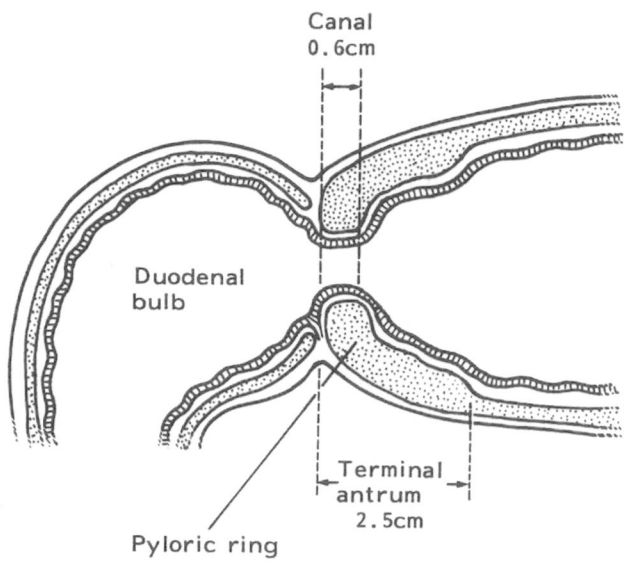

Figure 1. Diagram of the pylorus nomenclature.

2. *Limitation of the amount of chyme passing into the duodenum by contracting at the end of an antral contraction.*

During gastric emptying of solids, the closure of the pylorus with terminal antral contractions stops the passage of chyme into the duodenum and allows the rest to be returned to the body of the stomach. When this retropulsion is seen on a barium meal it can be confused with duodenogastric reflux. This function of the pylorus is seen, in one extreme form, in infantile hypertrophic pyloric stenosis with the strong, visible antral contractions and projectile vomiting.

3. *Prevention of duodenogastric reflux when the duodenal cap contracts*

The role of the pylorus in duodenogastric reflux will be discussed in detail in connection with the aetiology of gastric ulcer.

The characteristic myoelectrical activity in the fundic area is a slow depolarization of the membrane potential with slight amplitude and resulting in a tonic contraction. Depolarization never occurs spontaneously but is induced by extra-gastric factors only. In the antrum myoelectrical activity consists of slow wave pacesetter potentials (electrical control activity) on which spike potentials resulting in antral contractions can be superimposed (electrical response activity).

Gastric emptying rate is dependent on the pressure gradient divided by flow resistance. Because the flow resistance to liquids is very low, the result is that gastric emptying of liquids depends mainly on the static pressure of the fundus, the resting diameter of the pylorus and possibly the state of the duodenum, whereas emptying of solids depends on the strength and frequency of antral contractions and the coordinated opening and closing of the pylorus and contraction of the duodenal cap, as the flow resistance to solids is quite high.

Is there a high pressure zone at the pylorus in the resting individual? Early recordings from pull-through experiments using a catheter recording device with one hole demonstrated a high pressure zone (15 mm Hg above duodenal pressure) over a length of 2.5 cm. However, the problem with these devices is that if the side hole touches the wall it will register a closed pylorus. Any recording device has to have a system measuring pressure all the way round to show whether the pylorus is open, or closed. With these sort of devices the pylorus is found to be open for most of the time in the resting state.[2] (fig. 2)

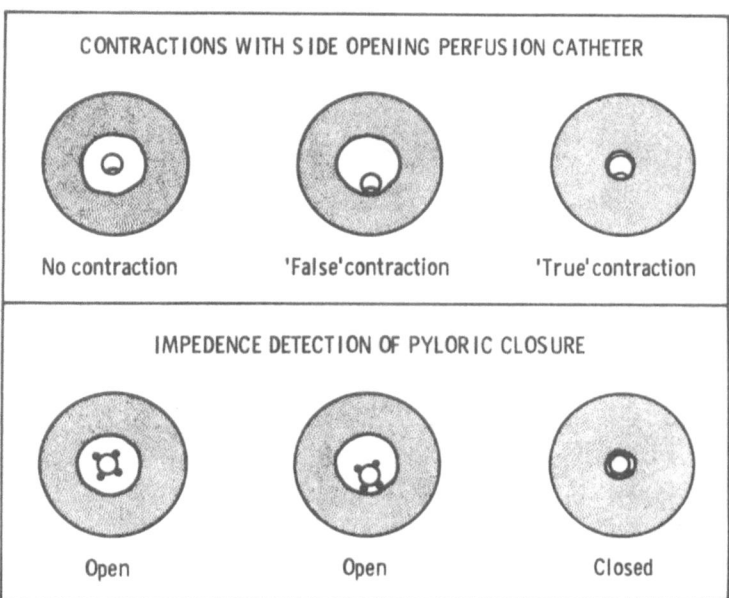

Figure 2. Measurement devices of pyloric closure. False-positive closure of the pylorus can be recorded with a 1-side hole catheter, but not with a 4-side impedance device.

62

Nervous and hormonal control

The nervous control of the pylorus is complicated and it does not have reciprocal innervation compared with the muscle either side as in the typical 'sphincter'. There are probably dopamine receptors in the pylorus. Intrinsic nerves enter the pyloric ring from the antral and also from the duodenal side. The submucosal plexus of nerves crosses the pylorus from the antrum to the duodenum whereas the muscle coats are nearly completely interrupted by a hypomuscular segment or 'septum'.

Hormones certainly influence antral contractions (e.g. cholecystokinin, CCK, inhibits them) and also affect the resting diameter of the pyloric ring. Our studies at endoscopy found that the 'resting' diameter of the pylorus (the maximum relaxation diameter between contractions) was widest in lesser curve gastric ulcer (GU) patients and smallest in duodenal ulcer (DU) patients with the normal subjects between. (Table I)

Table I. Endoscopic measurement of the maximal diameter of the pylorus; mean ± S.D.

	n	Diameter
Controls	10	11.4 ± 4 mm
Gastritis patients	10	10.1 ± 3 mm
Duodenal ulcer patients	10	7.3 ± 5 mm
Gastric ulcer patients	10	15.5 ± 3 mm

Moreover, the diameter correlated well with the serum level of cholecystokinin (measured by *in vitro* bioassay) (fig. 3) except in GU patients. After an intravenous bolus injection of CCK 1 U/kg the normal pylorus contracts sharply and stays in tonic concentration for about 3 minutes and then slowly relaxes again. (fig. 4)

It has been suggested that in GU patients the pylorus cannot contract completely. However, if CCK is administered in GU patients complete contraction of the pylorus is observed, as in normal controls. Probably another inhibitory hormone, for example gastrin, may produce the characteristically patulous pylorus of GU.[1]

In summary, it is probable, though not yet certain, that the resting diameter ('tone') of the pyloric ring is determined by the background level of various polypeptide hormones and contractions of the ring initiated by nervous or myogenic stimuli from antroduodenum, or more centrally.

63

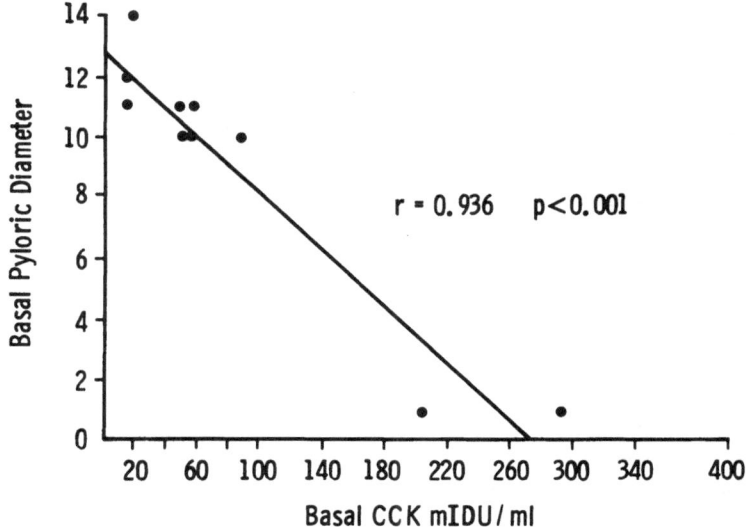

Figure 3. Correlation between resting pyloric diameter and serum concentration of CCK.

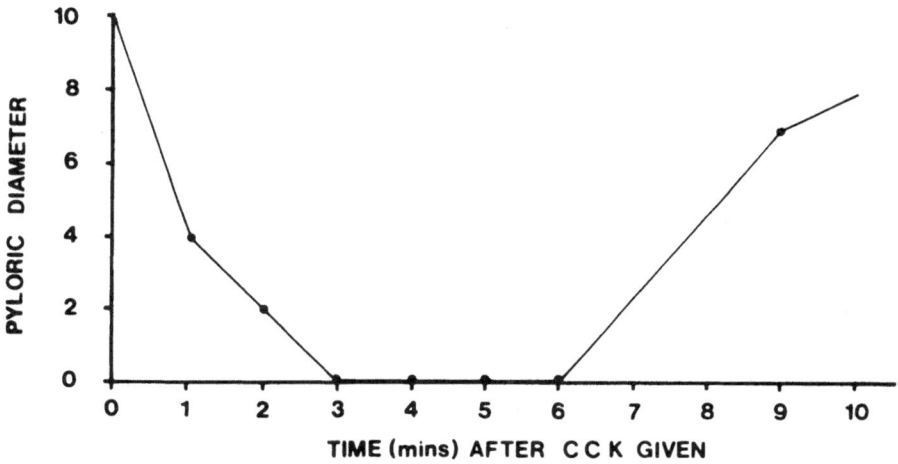

Figure 4. Pyloric diameter after intravenous bolus injection of exogenous CCK, 1 U/kg.

Movement of contents

Movement of gastric and duodenal contents across the pylorus does depend not only on whether the pylorus is open or closed, but also on the contractions and pressure on either side. If the whole antro-

Table II. Summary of studies of duodenogastric reflux in gastric ulcers.

Author	Method	Clinical state	Difference from controls
Capper (1966)	Radiological	Fasting	Highly significant
Flint (1970)	Radiological	Fasting	Highly significant
Cocking (1973)	Radiological	Fasting	Highly significant
DuPlessis (1965)	Bile acid concentrations (paper chromatography)	Fasting	Highly significant
Rhodes (1969)	^{14}C labelled bile salts	Fasting	$p < 0.05$
Black (1971)	Bile acids (steroid dehydrogenase)	Fasting	$p < 0.001$
Dewar (1983)	Bile acids (steroid dehydrogenase)	Fasting	Significant
Rhodes (1969)	^{14}C labelled bile salts	After Lundh meal	$p < 0.01$
Black (1971)	Bile acid	After Lundh meal	$p < 0.001$
Dewar (1983)	Bile acid	After Lundh meal	$p < 0.001$
Johnson (1974)	Lysolecithin (column and thin layer chromatography)	Nocturnal (fasting)	$p < 0.001$
Muller-Lissner (1983)	^{99}mTc HIDA	After intralipid meal	Not significant

Table III. Factors which are possibly important in duodenogastric reflux.

1. Frequency of duodenogastric reflux
2. Quantity of refluxed material
3. Length of time refluxed material stays in the stomach
4. Chemical composition of refluxed material (pH, bile salt composition, pancreatic juice)
5. State of the stomach at the moment of reflux (fasted, fed, at night)
6. Sex (gallstones predominantly in females, GU predominantly in males)

pyloro-duodenal segment is inhibited by a dose of atropine, no movement of contents will occur. If, however, the antrum is inhibited, the duodenum is very active and the pylorus open, the stage is set for duodenogastric reflux. For contents to pass from antrum to duodenum during gastric emptying the pylorus must be open (part of the time), the antrum contracting and the duodenal cap relaxed at the right time to accommodate the chyme.

Aetiology of GU

It is universally agreed that acid has to be present to produce a benign GU but as the acid secretion is often low, there must be some other factors reducing the natural resistance of the gastric mucosa, or prolonging the acid contact time. For many years there was conflict between two main theories: delayed gastric emptying on the one hand and duodenogastric reflux of bile on the other. More recently, we have come to realize that these are not opposing theories, but could be part of the same motility disorder and combine to produce more severe gastric mucosal damage: if duodenal juice does reflux, the time it stays in contact with the gastric mucosa may be critical.

Duodenogastric reflux

Table II summarizes the evidence from different studies of the importance of reflux measured by different methods under different conditions – fasting, during the night and after meals.

The early studies are radiological, which limits the time that observations can be made. The radiological studies by Capper (1966), Flint (1970) and Cocking (1973) demonstrated increased duodenogastric reflux of barium in fasting GU patients compared to controls.[3-5] Determination of bile salt concentrations in single fasting gastric juice samples, or in multiple samples before and after a standardized test meal all demonstrated increased concentrations in GU patients.[6-8]

It will be seen that many of these studies used a nasogastric tube, or even a tube through the pylorus. Although the same conditions were used for the controls, there is still an uneasy feeling that the tubes might contribute to the disturbed motility. Muller-Lissner et al[5] have failed to show significantly increased reflux in gastric ulcer

66

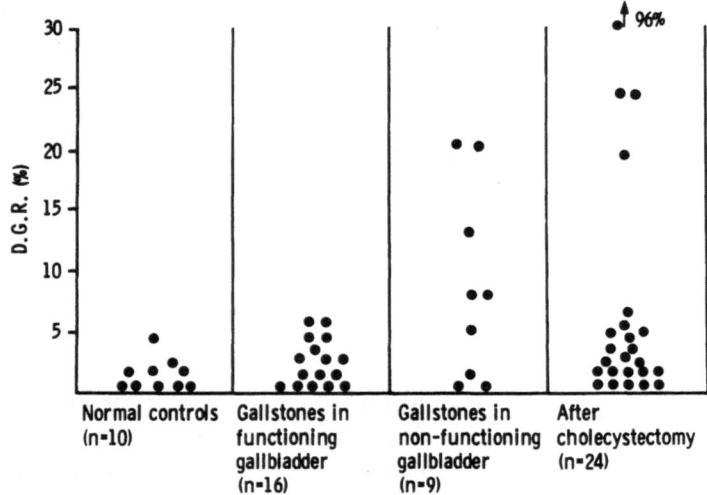

Figure 5. Percentage of duodenogastric reflux (DGR) in normal controls, gallstone patients and patients after cholecystectomy.

Table IV. Fasting and post-prandial intragastric bile acid concentration and pancreatic enzyme concentration in duodenogastric reflux.

	n	Bile acids (μmol/L)		Phospholipase (U/L)	
		fasting	post-prand	fasting	post-prand
Controls	6	24 ± 4	46 ± 8	5 ± 3	17 ± 7
Cholecystectomy	8	251 ± 168	448 ± 201	8 ± 5	41 ± 15
Gastric ulcer	11	277 ± 120	812 ± 383	169 ± 92	41 ± 15

patients after an intralipid meal but, they were using a continuous infusion of IDA and measuring reflux rates with gastric intubation: these are difficult to compare with other methods.

Surprisingly, there has been no good non-invasive study of reflux in GU. There is a continual problem of studying patients under physiological conditions particularly after 'normal' meals. Fat, for example, only releases some of the GI hormones and infusion of one hormone, such as CCK, may give spurious results.

Reflux in other conditions

Reflux has also been demonstrated in patients with gallstones before and after cholecystectomy by invasive and non-invasive methods.[11] (fig. 5)

An interesting question is that, if reflux is a cause of GU, why do patients after cholecystectomy not frequently develop a GU? Long-term follow-up studies after cholecystectomy and studies of patients with GUs have failed to show this connection.

Obviously duodenogastric reflux is not an all-or-non phenomenon and many factors may determine whether gastric mucosal lesions will develop as a consequence of increased reflux. (Table III) Recent studies from this department suggest that the relative concentration of the pancreatic components of the duodenal juice may be important.[12] (Table IV) In other words, the type of juice that refluxes may be as important as how much or how frequently it refluxes, for example taurine conjugated bile salts are more damaging to the gastric mucosa than glycine conjugated bile salts.

Delayed gastric emptying

In a well designed study, Millar et al[13] found that in gastric ulcer patients there is a delayed emptying of solids but normal emptying of liquids as well as increased reflux. This again shows the importance of checking what type of emptying is being studied.

The duodenal factor

Experiments in animals by Kelly,[14] and Monk[15] showed that duodenogastric reflux could be produced consistently during more than 80 – 90% of the evoked contractions by retrograde electrical pacing of the duodenum.

When the antrum was also contracting strongly, reflux was either blocked by the advancing terminal antral contraction, or the refluxed juice rapidly emptied. The pylorus itself appeared to play little part in the flow of contents. Studies with an impedance device to measure pyloric closure at endoscopy[2] have found that the pylorus can close with a terminal antral contraction, with a duodenal cap contraction, or independently.

In 11 normal controls with a total recording time of 127 minutes, 92 isolated duodenal contractions without linked antral contractions were observed. Of these 92 contractions, 2 occurred with an open pylorus, 7 induced pyloric opening, 30 induced pyloric closure and 49 occurred with a closed pylorus. So in 'normal' subjects, 90% of the isolated duodenal cap contractions were accompanied by pyloric closure. If this was not so, fasting reflux would be much more common in normal individuals than it is, because a large proportion of cap concentrations are unlinked. On the other hand, strong retroperistaltic contractions pushing the duodenal content ahead of the contraction would not close the pylorus until after the duodenal juice had refluxed.

The most recent studies have found that reflux is maximum at the end of duodenal phase III of the MMC, i.e. when the duodenum is contracting strongly and the antrum is quiet.[16] Figure 6 shows three types of antro-duodenal contractions recorded in one patient: retrograde duodenal contractions can either result in reflux, no reflux or very short-lived reflux.

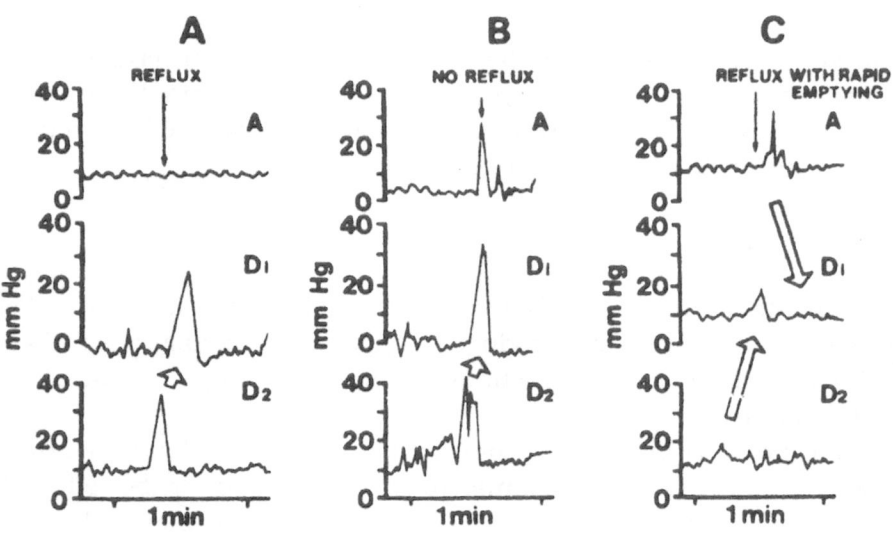

Figure 6. Three tracings of antral (A), proximal duodenal (D1) and distal duodenal (D2) contractions in one individual. Large arrows indicate movement of duodenal content.

The motility defect in GU causing reflux could be

a. an increase in the proportion of retroperistaltic duodenal contractions,

b. a failure of the pylorus to close in response to duodenal contractions, or

c. an incoordination between the bile and pancreatic secretion into the duodenum and the motility pattern so that refluxing patterns

occur when the duodenum is full of bile and/or pancreatic juice,
d. it has not been established as yet whether an 'inhibited' antrum plays a predominant role,
e. although a large resting pyloric diameter has been recorded in GU patients, this is probably not of importance as the pylorus can close in GU patients as effectively as in normal controls.

These hypotheses still wait to be tested but there is little doubt that we must look at the duodenum to find the remaining answers, as in the past we have concentrated exclusively on the stomach and pylorus.

Unfortunately duodenal motility studies are more difficult to perform.

Acknowledgements

Figure 1 has been reproduced from: Johnson AG. The pylorus. In: Thomas PA, Mann CV (Eds). Alimentary Sphincters and their Disorders. London, Macmillan Press 1984, with permission of the publishers.
Figure 6 has been reproduced from: Johnson AG. Peptic ulcer and the pylorus. Lancet 1979;1:710 – 2, with permission of the editor of the Lancet.

References

1. Johnson AG. The pylorus. In: Thomas PA, Mann CV (Eds). Alimentary Sphincters and their Disorders. London, Macmillan 1984.
2. Eyre-Brook IA, Smallwood RH, Linhardt GE, Johnson AG. Timing of pyloric closure in man. Studies with impedance electrodes. Dig Dis Sci 1983;28: 1106 – 15.
3. Capper WM, Airth GR, Kilby JO. A test for pyloric regurgitation. Lancet 1966;2:621 – 3.
4. Flint FJ, Grech P. Pyloric regurgitation and gastric ulcer. Gut 1970;11: 735 – 7.
5. Codking JB, Grech P. Pyloric reflux and the healing of gastric ulcer. Gut 1973;14:555 – 7.
6. DuPlesis DJ. Pathogenesis of gastric ulceration. Lancet 1965;1:974 – 8.
7. Black RB, Roberts G, Rhodes J. The effect of healing on bile reflux in gastric ulcer. Gut 1971;12:552 – 8.
8. Dewar P, King R, Johnston D (1983). Bile acid and lysolecithin concentrations in the stomach of patients with gastric ulcer: before and after treatment

by highly selective vagotomy, Billroth I partial gastrectomy and truncal vagotomy and pyloroplastry. Brit J Surg 1983;70:401 – 5.

9. Muller-Lissner SA, Fimmel CJ, Blum AL. Is there a relationship between duodenogastric reflux, gastric ulcer and gastritis? In: Akkermans LMA, Johnson AG, Read NW (Eds). Gastric and Gastroduodenal Motility. New York, Praeger 1984.

10. Johnson AG. Cholecystectomy and gallstone dyspepsia. Ann Roy Coll Surg Eng 1975;56:69 – 80.

11. Eyre-Brook IA, Holroyd AM, Johnson AG. A single isotope method of postprandial duodenogastric reflux assessment using ^{99m}Tc-labelled IDA in patients with gallstones. Clinical Physics and Physiological Measurement 1983;4:299 – 307.

12. Eyre-Brook IA, Smythe A, Bird NC, Mangnall YF, Johnson AG. Total bile acid and pancreatic phosphiliphase A_2 concentrations in the stomach in patients with gastric ulcer kand gallbladder disease. Brit J Surg (Abstract). In press.

13. Miller LJ, Malagelada L-R, Lengstreth GF, Go VLW. Dysfunction of the stomach with gastric ulceration. Dig Dis Sci 1980;25:857 – 64.

14. Kelly KA, Code CF. Duodenal-gastric reflux and slowed gastric emptying by electrical pacing of the canine duodenal pacesetter potential. Gastroenterology 1977;72:429 – 33.

15. Johnson AG. Peptic ulcer and the pylorus. Lancet 1979;1:710 – 2.

16. Eyre-Brook IA, Read NW, Brownson T, Johnson AG. The influence of chenodeoxycholic acid upon fasting antro-duodenal motility and reflux. Brit J Surg (Abstract). In press.

6. Pathogenesis of gastric mucosal damage: Contribution of the 'mucus-bicarbonate barrier'

W.D.W. REES, M.D., M.R.C.P. and LINDA GIBSONS,
Technical assistant

Hope Hospital, University of Manchester, Salford, United Kingdom

The unique ability of the gastroduodenal mucosa to resist the corrosive effects of gastric acid and pepsin has been the subject of considerable interest and speculation over the last century. Hypotheses have emerged and floundered with regular monotony and the precise mechanisms responsible for preserving epithelial integrity still remain a mystery.

The 'Davenport' hypothesis ascribed barrier function to the apical cell membrane and the tight intercellular junctions.[1] The demonstration of alkali secretion by epithelial cells of the stomach and proximal duodenum has reawakened interest in the protective functions of gastric mucus and non-parietal secretion and in this review the relative importance of the 'mucus-bicarbonate barrier' is discussed.

Components of the 'mucus-bicarbonate barrier' (fig. 1)

The 'mucus-bicarbonate barrier' consists of a thick, continuous layer of mucus gel overlying gastric and proximal duodenal mucosa, into which is secreted alkali from the underlying epithelium.[2] Within the unstirred zone produced by mucus gel this alkaline neutralizes acid diffusing from the lumen, resulting in a pH gradient across the gel layer and exposure of the epithelial cells to an alkaline environment. The viability of this hypothesis depends on the existence of both components as either alone would confer negligible protection. Mucus gel has little intrinsic buffering capacity and would not prevent acid from reaching the epithelium, while delivery of alkali directly into the

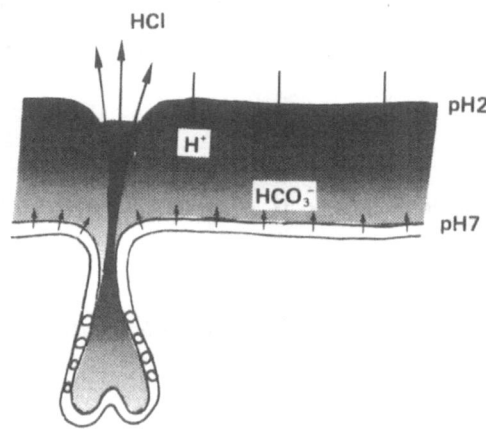

Figure 1. Diagram illustrating the components of the 'mucus-bicarbonate barrier'.

lumen would be overwhelmed by the larger concentration of hydro-chloric acid.

Mucus gel

Mucus is secreted by surface epithelial and foveolar pit cells of gastric mucosa and forms a continuous layer, some 5 to 10 times the height of epithelial cells, over the stomach and proximal duodenum.[3,4]

Using split lamp examinations of gastric resection specimens, mucus gel thickness (μm) was found to be 166 $\pm$ 10 in the rat, 500–652 in humans, 425 $\pm$ 17 in the dog and 234 $\pm$ 9 in the guinea pig.[2] This method measures probably the sum of mucus gel and an unstirred water layer and results in an overestimation of true gel thickness. Measurements with phase contrast microscopy may provide more information on the gel[3] and using this method mucus gel thickness (μm) was reported as 73 $\pm$ 5 in the rat, 192 $\pm$ 7 in humans and 75 $\pm$ 5 in the frog. In these studies mucus gel thickness (μm) was reduced by intra-gastric instillation of the mucolytic agent N-acetylcystein (from 167 $\pm$ 8 before instillation to 88 $\pm$ 2 after instillation). Dimethyl-prostaglandin E$_2$ (1 μg/ml) and carbenoxolone (2.5 mg/ml) increased gel thickness (301 $\pm$ 10 μm and 295 $\pm$ 11 μm respectively), but did not prevent its reduction by N-acetylcystein (81 $\pm$ 6 μm and 87 $\pm$ μm respectively).[3]

The principal organic component of mucus gel is glycoprotein which is present in tetrameric form with a molecular weight of 2×10^6. The glycoprotein concentration of secreted mucus exceeds 30 g/l and it has been shown that when this concentration exceeds 25 g/l, rotational[5,6] relaxation of the molecules is reduced resulting in gel formation. The gel layer appears to be in a dynamic state of equilibrium between synthesis and release from cells and erosion by luminal acid and pepsin.[7] The commonly measured luminal glycoprotein thus reflects breakdown products of the gel layer and does not necessarily correlate with synthesis rates, or indicate the integrity of the gel. Recent studies on mucus gel using a modified Ussing chamber suggest that it is capable of retarding small ion movement four times as much as a comparable layer of unstirred water.[8] However, despite these properties, it seems unlikely that mucus per se confers substantial protection to the underlying mucosa from the effects of luminal acid. The layer would of course provide an ideal zone for acid-alkali interaction, allowing the smaller amount of secreted alkali to be much more effective in neutralizing acid before contact with surface cells.

Gastric alkali secretion

The existence of an alkali component to gastric secretion was suggested almost a century ago by Schierbeck (1892) and Pavlov (1898). However, methodological difficulties related to the larger acid component, had prevented direct measurement of gastric alkali secretion until recently. The breakthrough was provided by the histamine H_2-receptor antagonists which allowed inhibition of acid output and the appearance of titratable alkalinity. Although the initial demonstration of gastric bicarbonate secretion was in amphibian gastric mucosa,[9,10] subsequent experiments have shown similar secretion in a variety of mammals and man *in vitro* and *in vivo*.[11-13]

Alkaline secretion is diminished by inhibitors of tissue metabolism such as dinitrophenol (10^{-4} M), potassium cyanide (10^{12} M) or tissue anoxia. This suggests that alkaline transport across mucosa is by a metabolically dependant process and not only by passive diffusion. (fig. 2) Application of acetazolamide to the serosal side of gastric mucosa reduced alkaline secretion significantly (to about 40% of baseline values) when applied in concentrations of 10^{-3}, but

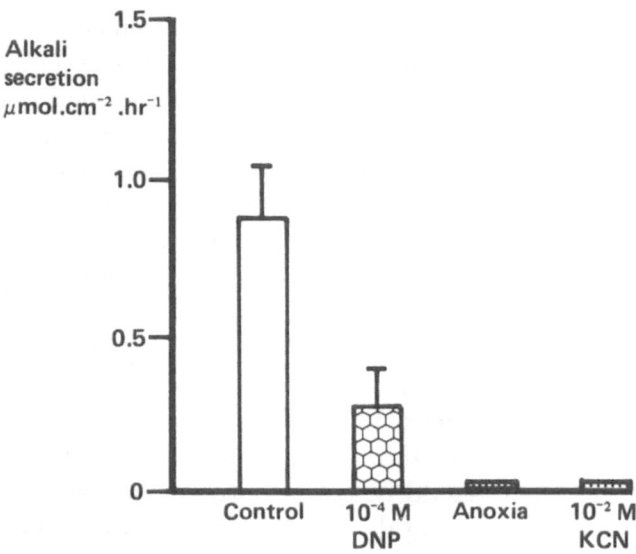

Figure 2. Effect of anoxia and metabolic inhibitors (DNP = dinitrophenol, KCN = potassium cyanide) on alkali secretion, by isolated rabbit fundic mucosa *in vitro*.

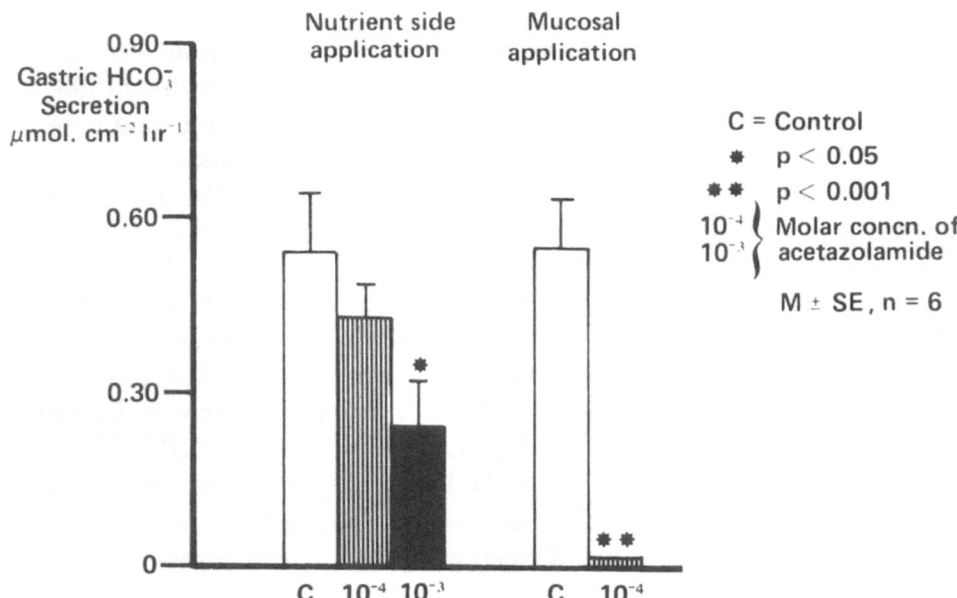

Figure 3. Effect of acetazolamide on alkali secretion by rabbit fundic mucosa *in vivo*.

not in concentrations of 10^{-4} M. However, when acetazolamide was applied to the mucosal side in a concentration of 10^{-4} M, alkaline secretion was completely abolished. (fig. 3)

Fundic mucosa is a very tight epithelium and is much less permeable to ions than antral mucosa. Thus fundic bicarbonate secretion is predominantly by a bicarbonate-chloride exchange mechanism. The bicarbonate is probably provided by the interaction between carbon dioxide and water, which is catalyzed by carbonic anhydrase. There is still some controversy about this transport mechanism. However, Silen's group supposes that the bicarbonate exchange mechanism is not at the apical membrane, but at the basolateral membrane, resulting in accumulation of bicarbonate in the cell and passive transport to the lumen along a concentration gradient. They suggest that endogenous production of bicarbonate within the cell is not important and that the bicarbonate supply is derived from serosal alkali.

The antral mucosa is more permeable and here the passive diffusion contributes substantially (up to 30%) to bicarbonate secretion. These and other *in vitro* experiments have established the likely cellular mechanism of bicarbonate transport (fig. 4) and a number of neurohumoral agents may regulate the magnitude of secretion. (Table I)

Table I. Stimulatory and inhibitory effects on gastric and duodenal bicarbonate secretion.

Bicarbonate secretion		Stimulatory	Inhibitory
Stomach		cholinergics glucagon, CCK prostaglandins	norepinephrine GIP parathyroid hormone
Duodenal	electrogenic	arichdonate prostaglandins	
	neutral	GIP, VIP glucagon neurotensin	glucagon (high doses)

The physiological significance of many of these observations has yet to be established. The existence of a local regulatory mechanism has been demonstrated recently. Using a canine Heidenhain pouch model, it was shown that perfusion of the gastric remnant with physiological concentrations of hydrochloric acid (10 mM) increased alkali secretion by the isolated pouch from 10 μmol/hr in the basal state to about 35 μmol/hr in the stimulated state.[15] This observation

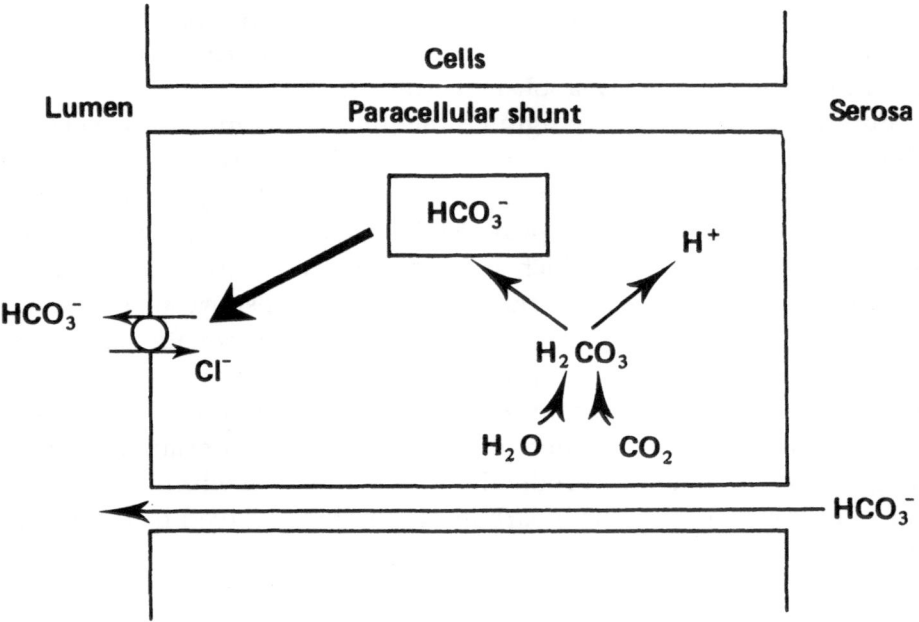

Figure 4. Cellular mechanisms of gastric bicarbonate transport.

was subsequently confirmed *in vitro* using pieces of gastric mucosa mounted in parallel in a specially constructed Ussing chamber, sharing a common serosal side solution.[16] In these experiments acidification of one of the luminal solutions stimulated bicarbonate secretion from the luminal surface of the parallel mucosa. Thus, exposure of gastric mucosa to a low pH increases alkali production. This may represent a 'protective' response, possibly mediated by local prostaglandin release in that the response was inhibited by indomethacin. Recently, bicarbonate secretion has been demonstrated from the intact human stomach[12] using an intubation technique in which the stomach was perfused with ^{3}H-polyethylene glycol as a non-absorbable marker and the duodenum with ^{14}C-polyethylene glycol as a second non-absorbable marker. The concentration of these markers was measured in gastroduodenal aspirates and the gastric volume and duodenogastric reflux calculated. By measuring the pH and pCO_2 of the aspirates total gastric bicarbonate concentration and output per unit time was calculated. During these experiments gastric acid secretion was inhibited by intravenous administration of cimetidine, which maintained gastric pH between 6 and 8. By determining amylase concentration in saliva, gastric and duodenal samples

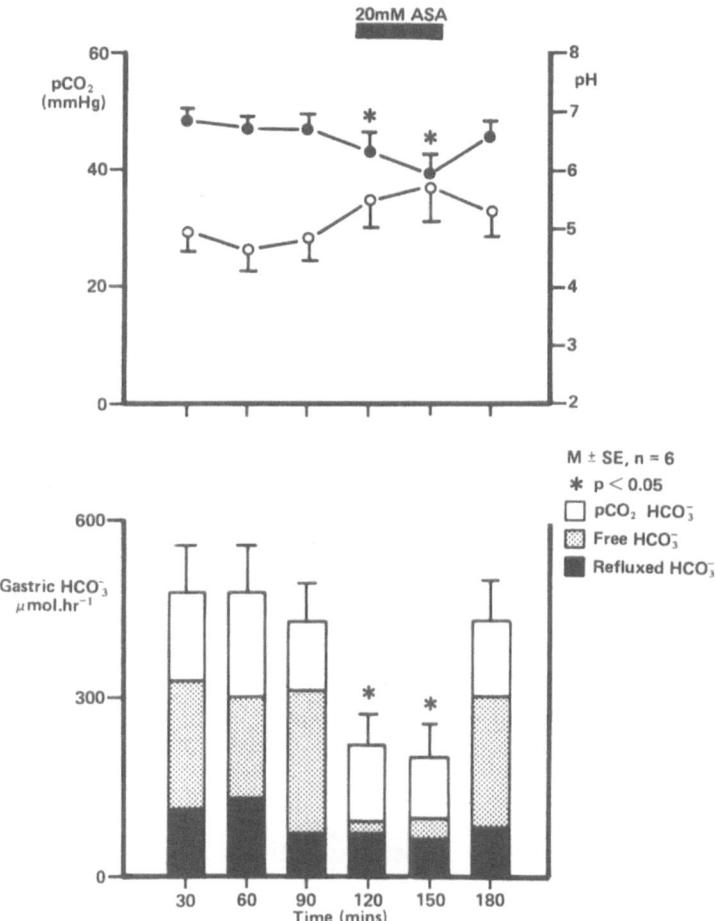

Figure 5. Effect of aspirin (ASA) on human gastric HCO$^-_3$ production. Closed circles represent pH and open circles pCO$_2$.

the contribution of swallowed saliva could be identified. The basal bicarbonate production calculated by this method was 400 μmol/hr of which only 5% was derived from saliva and 10% from the duodenum.

In these studies gastric alkali production was inhibited by aspirin (20 mM) and sodium taurocholate (10 mM). (figs 5 and 6) As in mammalian *in vitro* experiments, prostaglandin E$_2$ did not enhance

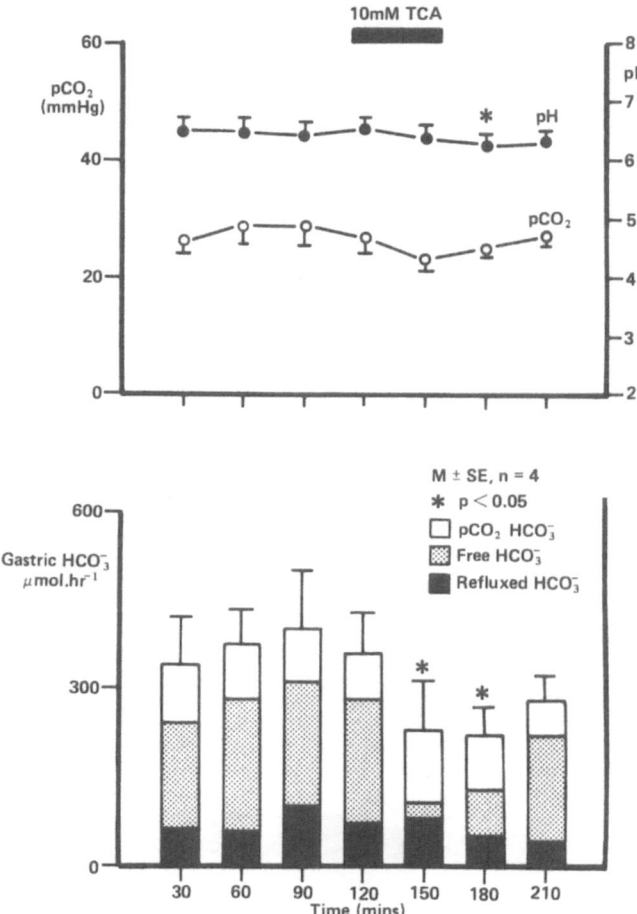

Figure 6. Effect of sodium taurocholate (TCA) on human gastric HCO^-_3 production.

basal secretion but did prevent its inhibition by aspirin (20 mM) and sodium taurocholate. (fig. 7) Since these concentrations of aspirin and taurocholate may be found in the human stomach after drug ingestion or bile reflux, these observations may be relevant to the pathogenesis of mucosal damage by these agents.

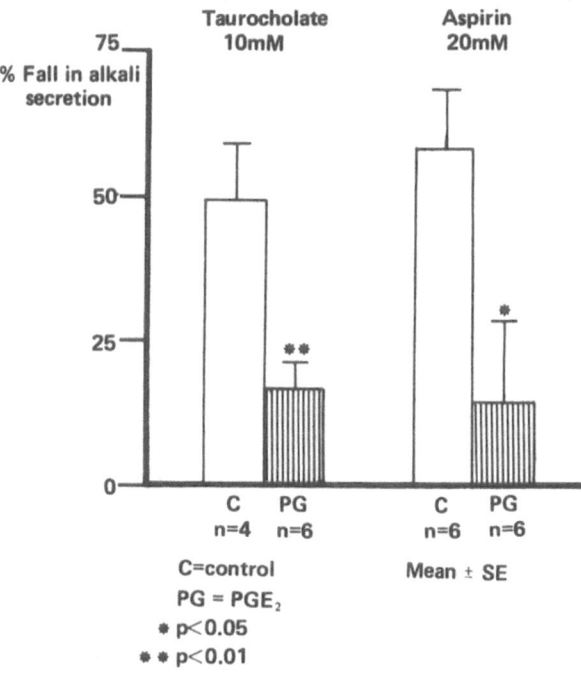

Figure 7. Effect of prostaglandin E_2 pre-treatment (5×10^{-7} M) on the fall in gastric HCO_3^- production by taurocholate and aspirin.

Mucus gel pH gradient

In 1959, Heatly proposed the existence of a pH gradient across gastric mucus gel which resulted from acid – alkali interaction within the unstirred layer.[18] According to his model, the epithelial cell surface could be maintained at pH 7.3 despite an intraluminal pH of 3. Almost 25 years later, Heatly's hypothesis was confirmed experimentally. Using antimony, pH sensitive microelectrodes, with a tip diameter of around 10 μm, a pH gradient was demonstrated *in vitro* and *in vivo*[19,20] across mammalian and human gastric mucus gel. (fig. 1) At luminal pH 2 to 3, the cell surface was maintained at pH 6 to 8. This gradient was reduced in rat as well as human gastric mucosa obtained from gastrectomy specimens by aspirin, bile salts and increasing luminal acidity from 1.6 to 1.2. (fig. 8 and Table II) Prostaglandins prevented the reduction of the pH gradient by aspirin.

More recently, a similar gradient has also been demonstrated across duodenal mucosa *in vitro* by Flemströms group.[21] The existence of a mucus gel pH gradient has provided definitive evidence for a 'mucus-bicarbonate barrier' preventing exposure of surface gastroduodenal epithelium to an acid environment. The contribution of the barrier to overall mucosal defence, however, remains to be established and it seems likely that other factors, such as apical cell membrane characteristics, cell migration and renewal, and mucosal blood flow providing oxygen and energy substrates, removal of hydrogen ions and delivery of bicarbonate to the cells, also play an important role.

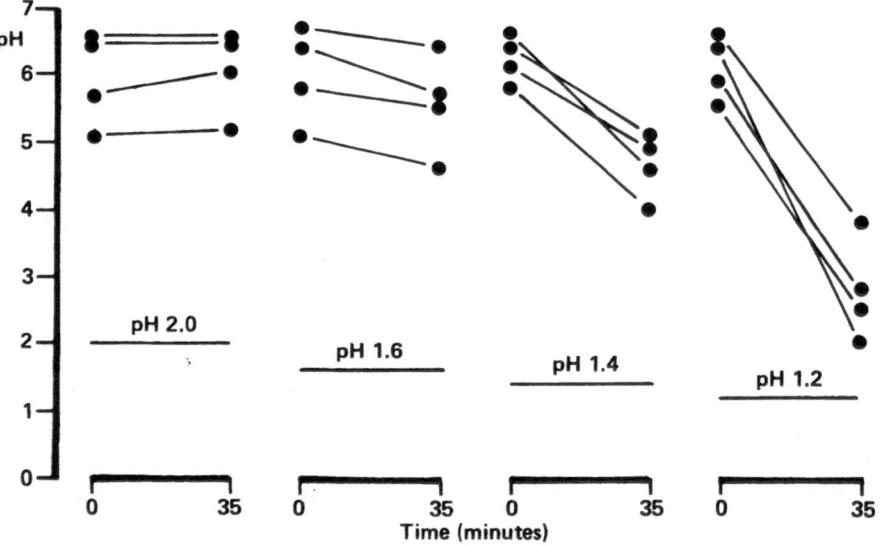

Figure 8. Influence of intragastric luminal pH on cell surface pH.

Table II. Maximal intramucus pH and the influence of barrier breakers, mean ± SD (or range).

	Rat	Man
Controls	6.68 (5.1–8.0)	6.96 (5.2–8.1)
Aspirin 10 mM	4.13 ± 0.84	4.90 (3.0–6.2)
Taurocholate 10 mM	4.51 ± 0.92	
N-acetylcystein 5%	4.18 ± 0.92	4.71 (3.3–6.0)

All experimental values are statistically significant different from control values (p < 0.001).

Clinical implications of the 'mucus-bicarbonate barrier'

There is circumstantial evidence that the barrier may be important in mucosal protection. Damaging agents, such as non-steroidal anti-inflammatory drugs, ethanol and bile salts reduces the effectiveness of the barrier, while it is enhanced by exogenous prostaglandins which protect gastric and duodenal mucosa and heal peptic ulcers.[1] Gastric mucus gel has been found to be defective in peptic ulcer patients, with an increased proportion of the monomeric glycoprotein in secreted mucus.[22] As yet there is no information available on the magnitude of alkali secretion or the integrity of the mucus gel pH gradient in these patients. Thus direct evidence for the involvement of defective mucus or bicarbonate production in the pathogenesis of peptic ulcer disease is not available at present. The influence of ulcer healing drugs on the barrier has also not been examined, although it is claimed that sucralfate may act by creating an artificial mucus layer over the ulcer crater, so establishing a pH gradient and allowing re-epithelialization to occur.

Conclusions

Recent experimental data has aroused considerable interest in the mechanisms of gastroduodenal mucosal protection and there is little doubt that a 'mucus-bicarbonate barrier' exists in the stomach and proximal duodenum. The role played by this barrier in protecting the normal stomach and in the development of peptic ulcers remains to be established. Attention is, however, firmly focussed on mucosal defence and it seems likely that future peptic ulcer therapy will be influenced by recent and anticipated developments in this area of intestinal physiology.

82

Acknowledgements

The authors are grateful to Mrs Julie Rostron for secretarial assistance and the Department of Medical Illustration, Hope Hospital for providing the figures.

References

1. Davenport HW. Salicylate damage to the gastric mucosal barrier. N Engl J Med 1967;267:1307–12.
2. Rees WDW, Turnberg LA. Mechanisms of gastric mucosal protection: a role for the mucus-bicarbonate barrier. Clin Sci 1982;62:343–348.
3. Bickel M, Kaufman G. Gastric gel mucus thickness: Effect of distension, 16,16dimethyl prostaglandin E_2 and carbenoxolone. Gastroenterology 1981; 80:770–775.
4. Kerss S, Allen A, Garner G. A simple method for measuring thickness of the mucus gel layer adherent to rat, frog and human gastric mucosa: Influence of feeding, prostaglandin, N-acetyl cysteine and other agents. Clin Sci 1982;63: 187–195.
5. Allen A. Structure of gastrointestinal mucus glycoproteins and the viscous and gel forming properties of mucus. Brit Med Bull 1978;34:28–33.
6. Allen A, Pain RH, Robson TR. Model for the structure of the gastric mucus gel. Nature 1976;264:88–89.
7. Pearson J, Allen A, Venables C. Gastric mucus: Isolation and polymeric structure of the undegraded glycoprotein: its breakdown by pepsin. Gastroentrology 1980;78:709–715.
8. Williams SE, Turnberg LA. Retardation of acid diffusion by pig gastric mucus: A potential role in mucosal protection. Gastroenterology 1980;79: 299–304.
9. Flemström G. Gastric secretion of bicarbonate. In: Johnson RL, Christensen H, Grossman MI, Jacobson ED, Schultz SG (Eds). Physiology of the Gastro intestinal Tract. New York, Raven Press 1981;vol 1:603–614.
10. Flemström G, Garner A. Gastroduodenal HCO^-_3 transport: Characteristics and proposed role in acidity regulation and mucosal protection. Am J Physiol 1982;242(Gastrointest Liver Physiol 5):G183–G193.
11. Rees WDW, Garner A, Turnberg LA, Gibbons LC. Studies of acid and alkali secretion by rabbit gastric fundus in vitro: Effect of low concentrations of sodium taurocholate. Gastroenterology 1982;83:435–440.
12. Rees WDW, Gibbons LC, Turnberg LA. Effects of non-steroidal anti-inflammatory drugs and prostaglandins on alkali secretion by rabbit gastric fundus in vitro. Gut 1983;24:784–789.
13. Rees WDW, Botham D, Turnberg LA. A demonstration of bicarbonate production by the normal human stomach in vivo. Dig Dis Sci 1982;27:961–966.
14. Flemström G, Heylings JR, Garner A. Gastric and duodenal HCO_3^- transport in vitro: Effects of hormones and local transmitters. Am J Physiol 1982; 242(Gastrointest Liver Physiol 5):G100–G110.
15. Garner A, Hurst BC. Alkaline secretion by the canine Heidenhain pouch in response to endogenous acid, some gastrointestinal hormones and prosta-

glandins. In: Gati T, Szollar LG, Ungvary CTY (Eds). Advances in Physiological Science, Vol 12. Nutrion, Digestion and Metabolism, 1981.

16. Heylings JR, Garner A, Flemström G. Regulation of gastroduodenal HCO_3^- transport by luminal acid in the frog *in vitro*. Am J Physiol 1984;246(Gastrointest Liver Physiol 9):G235–G242.

17. Rees WDW, Gibbons LC, Warhurst G, Turnberg LA. Studies of bicarbonate secretion in the normal human stomach *in vivo*: Effect of aspirin, sodium taurocholate and prostaglandin E_2. In: Allen A, Flemström G, Garner A, Silen W, Turnberg LA (Eds). Mechanisms of Mucosal Protection in the Upper Gastrointestinal Tract. New York, Raven Press, 1984.

18. Heatley NG. Mucosubstance as a barrier to diffusion. Gastroenterology 1959; 37:313–317.

19. Williams SE, Turnberg LA. Studies of the 'protective' properties of gastric mucus: Evidence for a 'mucus-bicarbonate' barrier. Gut 1981;22:94–96.

20. Ross IN, Bahari HMM, Turnberg LA. The pH gradient across mucus adherent to rat fundic mucus *in vivo* and effects of possible damaging agents. Gastroenterology 1981;81:713–718.

21. Flemström G, Kivilaakso E. Demonstration of a pH gradient at the luminal surface of rat duodenum *in vivo* and its dependence on mucosal alkali secretion. Gastroenterology 1983;84:787–794.

22. Younan F, Pearson J, Allen A, Venables C. Changes in the structure of the mucus gel on the mucosal surface of the stomach in association with peptic ulcer disease. Gastroenterology 1982;82:827–831.

7. Discussion I

Soll:

Drs Sanders, Ayalon and I have recently presented evidence suggesting that a barrier exists and should be included in the list of factors involved in allowing the mucosa to resist injury (Nature 1985; 313:52 – 4). In these studies, we placed chief cell-enriched elutriator fractions into short term cultures in the same conditions used for the somatostatin cells. In culture these cell formed a monoloayer consisting primarily of chief cells. This monolayer proved to be adequate for electrophysiologic studies (Proc Nat Acad Sci USA 1982;79:7009).

We mounted chief cell monolayers in Ussing chambers and determined the short-circuit current (I_{sc}), the potential difference (PD), and resistance (R) across the monolayer. Once stabilized the PD was 20 to 30 mV and the I_{sc} increased in response to prostaglandin E_2, an effect blocked by furosemide suggesting the I_{sc} may be dependent on chloride secretion from the basolateral to the apical cell surface. Apical application of amiloride reduces resting I_{sc}, suggesting Na^+ absorption via transcellular channels.

We studied the effects of acidifying the apical solution on the I_{sc} and the R across the barrier. When the apical pH was decreased to between 6.5 and 3.5, there was a rise in R and an increase of PD, while I_{sc} remained stable. As the pH dropped further to below 3, R increased further and now the I_{sc} decreased. There proved to be a two-phase rise in R upon acidification of the apical surface, probably reflecting sequential blockade of the paracellular 'shunt' pathway and transcellular Na^+ channels. This response of monolayers could be repeatedly obtained by recycling apical pH, and monolayers sustained themselves quite nicely with an apical pH < 2. With the apical surface acidified the addition of aspirin resulted in a marked decrease in resistance and the I_{sc}. These data indicated that the monolayer we studied was a model for the functional gastric barrier.

The barrier presented by the monolayers was polarized, because when the basolateral side of the monolayer was acidified, the PD and

I_{sc} rapidly decreased, and, after a short temporary rise, R fell to zero. Thus the basolateral surface cannot tolerate acidification at all, whereas the apical surface withstands high concentrations of H^+.

Ouabain has been used to study whether transcellular Na^+/K^+-ATPase-dependent transport is involved in this barrier function. Monolayers were treated with ouabain, producing the expected drop in PD and I_{sc}. The apical surface was then acidified and with acidification I_{sc} and PD further decreased essentially to zero and R rose to an even higher value. Despite a 100,000 fold pH gradient across the apical surface of the monolayer, essentially no H^+-ions permeated the monolayer; as indicated by the I_{sc} of near zero.

We conclude from these data that these canine chief cells are programmed to reform a monolayer with an apical surface which appears impermeable to H^+-ions. This barrier function of the apical surface must be an important component of mucosal defense, and one of the reasons why chief cells are able to withstand the high concentration of apical acid within the gastric pits. Chief cells do not have the benefit of bicarbonate or mucus secretion, but they do appear to have an apical barrier that allows them to survive without having to continually pump a large quantity of backdiffused H^+ out of the cell.

Rees:

What dr. Soll has shown us is very interesting. In fact this fits in beautifully with what we have demonstrated. You must bear in mind that dr. Soll was talking about the chief cells and not about the epithelial surface cells for which this kind of barrier function has not been shown as yet. The combination of the data presented by dr. Soll and my data provide an attractive hypothesis of the total gastric mucosal barrier. We have not shown as yet that the mucus-bicarbonate barrier is effective beyond the surface layer or that it dips down into the pits. So one of the major problems with the mucus-bicarbonate barrier hypothesis is how the cells within the pits, the chief cells, are protected against the large amount of acid present in the lumen of the pit. This shortcoming of the mucus-bicarbonate barrier hypothesis can be met with dr. Soll's hypothesis, that there is a specialized apical membrane covering the cells at this site. I think that there may also be a specialized apical membrane on the surface epithelial cells, but we have not any evidence at all for this as yet.

Soll:

It is certainly possible that mechanisms may be different in different cell types. We have had no success thus far in forming effective monolayers of surface cells. dr. W. Silen and coworkers have successfully studied surface cell monolayers from guinea pig; these monolayers do not appear to display the same degree of resistance to apical acidification as our chief cell monolayers. Whether this difference is due to different conditions or a true reflection of a different property of the cells remains to be established.

These mechanisms may differ among different cells. Surface cells are 'suicide' cells that are replaced by a rapidly replicating pool of cells, and because of mucus and bicarbonate secretion mucous cells may not have to face to the same kind of H^+ concentration as do parietal and chief cells.

Robert:

What could be the mechanism by which the apical sides of the chief cells in your monolayer can resist the effect of exposure to acid? Have you examined the ultra-structure of the apical and basolateral membranes to see whether there are any differences and do these cells resist acid even when they are exposed to indomethacin?

Soll:

We have not done comparative morphologic studies, or scanning electronmicroscopic studies, to see whether we can differentiate the apical surface of chief cells from other mucosal cells, such as the surface mucous cells, or other epithelial cells. We have compared chief cells to an epithelial cell line that has a high resistance and found that this latter cell line lacked a similar apical barrier to H^+. We do not know the nature of apical barrier to H^+, but I suspect that it represents specialization of the transcellular transport channels for sodium and of the paracellular shunt pathways, which allow H^+ to plug the door rather than get into the channels.

The second part of your question refers to the role of endogenous prostaglandins. We have incubated the monolayers with indomethacin at doses completely blocking prostaglandin production. And the barrier to acid does not change over two hours, in contrast with the acute change in barrier function after incubation with aspirin. Thus far, although we can see an electrical response to exogenous prosta glandins, there are no obvious effects of exogenous prostaglandins on the apical barrier of chief cells.

Meuwissen:

In the pits there are two populations which have been shown to contain pepsinogen, particularly pepsinogen I, but also pepsinogen II. They are the mucous neck cells and the chief cells. Most of the chief cells are at the bottom of the crypt and with an immunoperoxidase technique it has been demonstrated that they are largely clustered in the lower third of the pit. The question is: is the chief cell really in danger from H^+-ions? Have you ever measured by any micro-technique the pH-gradient in the deeper parts of the pit? Is the pH-gradient exactly the same at the bottom of the pit and at the top?

Rees:

We have no information on that. We have not measured the pH within the crypts and cells.

Guth:

Have you found a difference in mucus thickness over the corpus as opposed to the antrum? On ordinary PAS-stained histology sections there seems to be more mucus overlying the antrum than the corpus.

Rees:

These studies have been done by Bickel and Kaufman and also by Kerss and Adrian Allen's group. There are tremendous variations within the same specimen. If you look at the fundus alone and the antrum alone, there is tremendous variation; the values that they reported are somewhere in the region of 10 – 200 micrometers. The mean values for antrum and fundus and the degree of variation in antrum and fundus appeared roughly the same. You can not really extract this sort of information from Bickel and Kaufman's study, because they did not examine different parts of the specimen. All I can say is, that from the measurements that have been carried out comparing mucus thickness in different parts of the stomach, there is tremendous variation and there is no apparent difference in these *in vitro* studies. In studies on duodenal mucus from dr. Silen's group in the States and from Gunnar Flemström, it would appear that the thickness of mucus in the proximal duodenum is greater than in fundus and antrum.

Guth:

It would seem to me that the cell membrane that would have to be most resistant to acid back diffusion would be the parietal cell membrane; that membrane faces the highest H^+-ion concentration and I wonder if dr. Soll has done any monolayer studies with the parietal cells.

Soll:

Unfortunately we have been unable to develop techniques thus far for studying a parietal cell monolayer, so I cannot answer your question.

Zwaan (Rotterdam, the Netherlands):

What is the influence of smoking on acid production?

Johnson:

Can I extend on the question and ask about the effect of smoking on motility. There is some evidence that it does affect motility of the stomach and it certainly affects the lower oesophageal sphincter. Is there some evidence that smoking could be connected with ulcer disease aetiologically?

Wormsley:

This is totally controversial. There is nothing certain about smoking and ulcer disease, except a slower healing rate among smokers in therapeutic trials. This could be due to our finding, that smoking interferes with gastric acid inhibitory drugs. That has now been confirmed by André Blum. So that you don't need to stop your patients smoking, except after their nighttime pill, if you are treating them with a nighttime pill.

Soll:

Is not there also a reasonable suggestion that recurrence rates are increased in smokers compared with non-smokers?

Wormsley:

Yes, to a certain extent. But this is probably when they are being treated, because their drugs do not work. The position concerning recurrence in untreated individuals is by no means defined.

Soll:

But in untreated individuals healing is retarded by smoking.

Wormsley:

This has only been shown in trials where patients were treated with placebo.

Allgöwer:

I was very glad that Mr. Johnson raised the question of motility, because we talk mainly about secretion and we probably do not consider motility changes enough. I just wonder whether you have any observations which would separate the gastric ulcer patient in some way in motility patterns, particularly in the antrum, from controls.

Johnson:

I have not done this, but there is some work with large balloons in the antrum showing decreased antral motility in the gastric ulcer patient. The trouble with this is of course, that you put a device in the stomach which itself may be affecting motility. There is certainly evidence of delayed gastric emptying in gastric ulcer patients. We are mainly focussing on acid secretion, but the rate of delivery of gastric acid to the duodenum could well be more important than maximal acid secretory capacity. Dynamic studies of the pH in the duodenum are of great importance and we ought to obtain more data in that field.

We have not mentioned stress in aetiology. Studies of acute stress show that it can produce profound changes. It can produce inhibition of gastric emptying, increased reflux and, surprisingly, increased secretion. And that is a marvelous situation to produce a gastric ulcer: you have got three ulcer-promoting factors present. I was interested in the mechanism by which stress might increase gastric secretion, the effects of chronic stress and long-term changes. The most important point of getting a hypothesis for the aetiology of peptic ulcer is to be able to do something about it, either in prevention or treatment. It is not a problem of healing, it is a matter of preventing relapse. Could dr. Soll comment on how stress might produce acid secretion changes?

Soll:

I can only speculate as to where the end point of stress might be and I suspect there are probably multiple end points. One possibility would be adrenergic receptors. However, α- and β-adrenergic receptors will undoubtedly prove complex in their cellular distribution, with receptors on several cell types, probably producing counterbalancing effects. We have identified one of these receptors in our system; β-adrenergic receptors stimulate release of somatostatin from canine fundic cells and thereby potentially activate an inhibitory loop that would decrease acid secretion. The parietal cell may have a stimulatory β-adrenergic receptor, although we have not found evidence for this in canine parietal cells. No doubt, many other adrenergic receptors at other sites remain to be characterized. I suspect that the response to stress is mediated by a summation of factors, including the selective delivery of adrenergic stimuli, vagal cholinergic input and possibly the delivery of peptides, all of which will together determine the outcome. In the future, we may be able to answer your question with more than speculation.

Wormsley:

There are methodological problems regarding gastric bicarbonate secretion and the role of the mucus-bicarbonate barrier. Just one good swallow of saliva would provide as much bicarbonate as all those studies showed. You don't need gastric bicarbonate secretion, because you have got enough saliva. The gradient that we were shown was pH 2 to 7. Now, in gross gastric disease gastric juice that contains only 10 nmol/L of acid must be rare. Usually it is much higher. If we consider the mucus layer thickness, of 0.5 mm and the very rapid rate of diffusion of H^+-ions through it, these so-called barriers are really functionally negligible. The resistance of lipid membranes to H^+-ion passage is very great, unless there are a lot of water channels.

Rees:

We and other people have shown, that alkaline secretion does exist. I also showed that the contribution of saliva to total gastric bicarbonate is very small (10%) – this has been confirmed by others. The pH gradient can be overwhelmed if the intragastric pH falls below 1.5. At that point the barrier breaches, but we should keep in mind that the mucus-bicarbonate barrier is but one protecting factor. Below an intragastric pH of 1.5 the apical membrane barrier and mucosal blood flow remain as a second line of defense.

Moreover, I doubt that in the normal stomach the pH is below 1.5 for substantial periods during the day.

Wormsley:

Your figures showed a bicarbonate secretion of 400 μmol per hour. The bicarbonate concentration of saliva is about that of extracellular fluid, about 30 mmol/L, therefore 20 ml of saliva will contain 600 μmol. You see, it really does not need much saliva to give the same amount of bicarbonate which is secreted by the stomach apparently.

Let me just have a go at the reflux. You will have noticed the concentration of bile salts and of pancreatic contents in gastric juice from the graphs that were shown. We hear exactly the same about concentration of nitrosamines after histamine H_2-receptor antagonists. What is forgotten, is that in patients with gastric ulcer there is very little gastric juice, there is virtulaly no dilution of the material which is regurgitated. We all regurgitate duodenal contents at all times. If there is nothing to dilute them, then the concentration but not the amount of refluxed materials is going to be greater. Really there is no evidence (except for one very old paper from Mort Grossmann), that anything in duodenal contents damages the gastric mucosa. On the contrary, if bile salts are applied to the gastric mucosa repeatedly, the resistance of the gastric mucosa is influenced positively.

Johnson:

This could be the most important point: the high concentration of bile acids in the stomach could be much more damaging to the mucosa than larger total amounts in low concentration. Although continuous application of bile to the stomach might strengthen the mucosa, the alternative exposure to bile salts and acid might be highly damaging. In that sense motility might play a key role in the pathogenesis of gastric ulcer.

Rees:

It may well be right that chronic reflux could be protective. The work of Code and others has shown, that a single shot of bile salts to the gastric mucosa can result in disruption of the mucosal barrier, but re-application can result in an adaptive response: the mucosa does respond differently than to the first application. If aspirin is applied acutely to the gastric mucosa you will get damage. Yet we know that the incidence of aspirin-induced mucosal damage is very small. If you take patients with rheumatoid arthritis taking aspirin, the incidence of serious complication with gastric ulcer and bleeding is really very small: about 10 – 15/100,000 of heavy users per year. In the normal situation there may well be adaptation to damaging agents. If you take aspirin continuously you may get an adaptive response and the mucosa becomes more resistant to the effects. The development of gastric ulcer could be failure of this process of adaptation. Whether this adaptation takes the form of cell renewal, or changes in alkaline secretion or mucus production we do not know, but it could well be any of these factors which we have mentioned.

Johnson:

Just a comment on cell renewal. We have measured cell turnover in the duodenum in different conditions and it seems that the greater the degree of gastritis and the age of the ulcer, the greater the speed of amino-acid incorporation, which we could call a 'high output failure'. In fact it is going extremely rapidly at the edge of an ulcer and so purely in terms of cell renewal, that might be the problem. The problem of ulcer disease is not a problem of healing, it is a problem of staying healed.

8. Problems in the medical management of peptic ulcer

J.J. MISIEWICZ

Department of Gastroenterology and Nutrition, Central Middlesex Hospital, London NW10 7NS, United Kingdom

The aim of the opening paper of this session is to provide a background against which the subsequent presentations dealing in detail with various aspects of management of ulcer disease, can be discussed.

The development of the histamine H_2-receptor antagonists has provided effective treatment for the healing of duodenal ulcer (DU) during short-term treatment. At present there are a number of other drugs which have also been shown to be effective in the short-term treatment of DU. They include high-dose antacids, anticholinergic drugs such as pirenzepine, 'mucosal protective' drugs, such as bismuth, sulphated polysaccharide compounds and prostaglandins. None of these agents indisputably alter the subsequent natural history of duodenal ulcer diathesis. The illness is a chronic disease during which patients will relapse with varying frequency in the years following successful healing on acute therapy. Despite the availability of several drugs that are apparently effective in the acute healing of DU, at present only the histamine H_2-receptor antagonists ranitidine and cimetidine have been investigated sufficiently to show, that they are safe and effective in decreasing the incidence of duodenal ulcer relapse during prolonged periods of therapy, that is to say for periods longer than six months.

Duodenal ulcer can be classified as a chronic, relapsing condition. Some surveys show that approximately 90% of duodenal ulcers relapse within one year of healing. The population of duodenal ulcer patients will therefore need long-term maintenance therapy. Gastric ulcer is also chronic relapsing condition and, once the possibility of gastric carcinoma has been rigorously excluded by dilligent endoscopic multiple targeted biopsies and exfoliative brush cytology, medical maintenance therapy of GU may also be appropriate. Then problems of prolonged medical treatment of DU and GU encompass clinical care, monitoring of safety of long-term therapy, efficient arrangements for the diagnosis of relapses and the like. The initial requirement however, is the acquisition of reliable data on which to base decisions concerning the strategic options available that will govern long-term management of patients with peptic ulcer disease. Reliable data in this area have to be collected from the results of long term therapeutic maintenance trials and therefore the proper design of such trials is of great importance.Because the present experience of long-term medical treatment centres mainly on duodenal ulcer, results relating to the latter are discussed in this paper, but the principles should also be applicable to benign gastric ulcer.

Design of maintenance trials

The evaluation of maintenance treatment in controlled clinical trials consumes considerable time and resources. Substantial numbers of patients need to be studied for periods of at least six to twelve months, ensuring compliance with therapy and with the trial protocol. This is not easy to do. The results of treatment should be monitored by serial

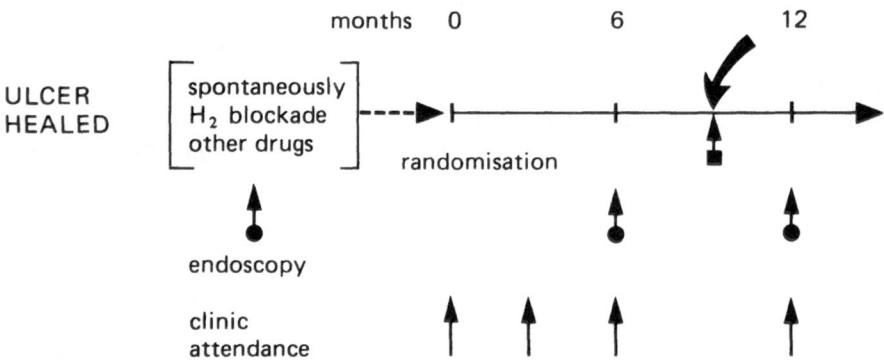

Figure 1. Design of trials of maintenance treatment for peptic ulcer.

endoscopy being triggered either by a predetermined time interval into the trial, and/or by the recurrence of ulcer symptoms at any time during the trial. The general design of a maintenance trial for DU is shown schematically in figure 1.

Comparisons of the many published maintenance trials are hampered by the lack of conformity in trial design. Hence when attempting to make comparisons between the widely differing ulcer recurrence rates reported, it is important to consider some of the main differences in trial protocols used. Some of these factors are now discussed.

Frequency of endoscopy

In initial maintenance trials endoscopy was done only when symptoms suggested ulcer recurrence. With increased endoscopic surveillance during long-term clinical trials it became apparent that ulcers could recur without accompanying symptoms: the so-called 'silent', or 'asymptomatic ulcer', or relapse. The frequency of endoscopy will therefore directly affect the ulcer recurrence rate reported. The trials in which only symptomatic patients are endoscoped will underestimate the ulcer recurrence rate, while frequent endoscopy will increase the chance of detection of the asymptomatic ulcers. Thus a conflict arises between the need for frequent endoscopy to reflect the true state of the disease, and acceptability of the procedure by the patients.

Frequency of clinical assessment

Regular and frequent clinic visits will help the detection of symptomatic relapse and encourage patient's compliance with the treatment.

Duration of study

The duration of the follow-up period may also influence the final quoted recurrence rate. It has been suggested that relapse rates decrease as the trial continues, so that recurrence rates during the second year are lower than during the first year. They may also be higher in the first few months of follow up. This presumably happens because the patients with severe disease who do not do well on conventional maintenance therapy, relapse early in the trial. The studies lasting six months may give misleading high recurrence rates, when compared with one and two year studies. Other studies suggest however, that recurrence rate on histamine H_2-receptor antagonists has a constant incidence with time. Placebo-treated patients probably relapse at a higher rate in the first few months after the initial healing of the DU.

Antacid consumption and timing of drug administration

It is usual to allow free antacids during maintenance studies. The type and amount of base consumed by the patients is rarely mentioned in the published reports. Moreover, patient's antacid consumption varies markedly in different countries. For example the daily consumption of antacids by patients in clinical trials of GU was 10 or 20 times higher in the United States than in England or France. Antacids have ulcer healing properties and if their use in trials is uncontrolled, this aspect should be considered when assessing the final recurrence rate reported. The dose of the active treatment given during maintenance trials in relation to the full dose used for acute healing, may also influence the results.

Extraenous factors

Extraenous factors relating to the patient's life style may seriously affect the outcome of prophylactic therapy in DU. The most important factor at present appears to be smoking of cigarettes. In one recent study, non-smoking appeared to be as good as cimetidine in the prevention of recurrence of DU. Smoking histories are generally sketchily reported in published maintenance trials and differences in ways in which cigarette consumption is recorded and reported makes comparisons between trials difficult (Sontag et al, 1984).

Definition of ulcer relapse/remission

Some investigators specify clearly the definition of ulcer healing and ulcer relapse, but this may vary from centre to centre. In other studies clear definition of these entities is lacking. It is difficult to agree on precise definitions of endoscopic criteria of ulcer healing, and the difference between an ulcer crater and an erosion is very subtle. Observer error must therefore be appreciable in many studies. No studies have adopted the technique of several observers inspecting the ulcer site at endoscopy and recording their conclusions independently. Definitions of symptomatic recurrence of DU are also low-precision data, based on the patient's subjective experience. The number of days with recurrent ulcer pain necessary for this symptom to trigger an extra endoscopy varies in different trials; nor is it always specified. The problem of measuring the symptoms of DU may be eased by having the patients record them on diary cards. If this method is adopted, careful instructions have to be given to each patient and it is to be expected that a proportion of the subjects studied will be unable to comply adequately. If diary cards are to be used for recording of symptoms, they should be as simple as possible. The average patient finds it difficult to differentiate between subtle gradations of epigastric pain, or heartburn. In general, data based on patient's records of symptoms or antacid consumption are bound to be inaccurate. This begs the question of how reliable is the information relating to symptomatic relapse of DU collected in the course of maintenance trials. The inescapable conclusion is that the data are of low precision, but it is difficult to see how they could be improved.

Diagnosis of ulcer

Difficulties of adopting uniform criteria attending the diagnosis of DU healed, or unhealed have already been mentioned. Studies of GU should ideally be stratified according to the anatomical location of the ulcer within the stomach. Pre-pyloric ulcers probably need to be considered separately from DU and GU.

Calculation of recurrence rates

The methods used for calculating ulcer recurrence rates in maintenance trials vary. Most commonly the recurrence is expressed as
the total number of patients relapsing (symptomatic and asymptomatic with endoscopically verified recurrent DU craters) as a percentage of the evaluable patients completing the trial: this is sometimes called the cumulative recurrence rate. Alternatively, life table
analysis may be used as a more rigorous statistical evaluation of the
results, and this is a preferable technique to employ.

Withdrawals

In general, the number of patients reported as withdrawn for various
clinical reasons (which may include untoward effects of medication,
or non-compliance with the protocol, or intercurrent illness, or complications of the ulcer), or 'dropped out' (term usually reserved for
those who fail to attend for follow-up visits), are similar in each group
in comparative trials. However, failure to attend for repeated serial
endoscopies is a common problem in maintenance trials. This problem
increases with the duration of the trial and the number of endoscopies. Unless sufficiently large numbers of patients are recruited at
the start, the final numbers are too small. Unfortunately, this problem
is reflected in the many small, inconclusive trials reported in the literature. Life-table analysis will allow patients who have not completed
the whole period of the trial, but in whom some follow-up endoscopic
data have been recorded, to be included in calculation of results, increasing the number available for analysis.

Compliance

Comparisons of treatments in maintenance trials are dependent on
the patient's compliance with therapy. In most trials this is assumed
rather than assessed. Counts of returned tablets are a simple, but not
very reliable way of assessing compliance. Analysis of urine for drug
metabolites is better, but expensive in large studies. Compliance is a
very neglected aspect of maintenance trial methodology. Patients
with severe ulcer disease may be more assidous in taking the medica-

tion, than those with few symptoms. On the other hand, those with severe DU may have a life style which militates against the taking of medication regurlarly.

Geographical variations

Healing rates of duodenal ulcer during short-term treatment with cimetidine vary considerably from country to country and even from centre to centre in the same country (Fig. 2, Blum et al 1978) Several factors probably conspire to produce these differences, including variations in age, race and cultural habits of the recruited population, availability of endoscopic facilities, waiting lists for endoscopy, local referral patterns to specialist centres, constraints of trial protocols and the like. Whatever the explanation, the data suggest that the geographical location of the study may have a bearing on the results of trials. It also emphasises the value of large multicentre trials with a common protocol and the need to view the results obtained as pertaining to that particular study, rather than as applying across the board. The more patients in the trial, the more confident the interpretation of results.

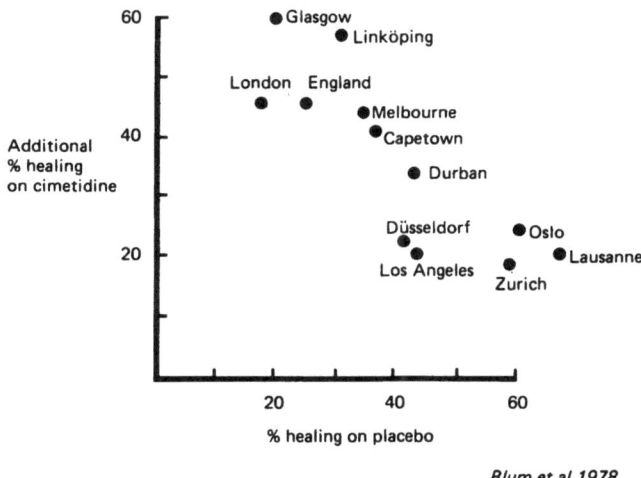

Figure 2. Variation in duodenal ulcer healing rates in short-term trials. (Modified from Blum et al, 1978)

Recruitment of patients

By definition, patients recruited into a maintenance trial will have a recently healed duodenal ulcer. In most trials patients enter a maintenance trial immediately following successful healing on short-term full dose therapy. The nature of the treatment in the acute ulcer healing phase may vary widely and often includes a placebo. A long delay between the end of successful acute therapy and entry into the maintenance trial may influence results, but there is no evidence to decide if the nature of the acute treatment can affect the subsequent cause of the DU within maintenance trials.

Exclusion of patients

Various criteria for exclusion of patients from entry into the trial have been used. For example, patients receiving concurrent medication with potentially ulcerogenic drugs are usually excluded. It is often difficult to control concurrent medication in prolonged clinical trials, particularly if there is a change in medication during the course of the trial. Such information is often poorly documented.

Duodenitis

In some trials patients with duodenitis are included, in others they are not. It is not known whether duodenitis affects the outcome of maintenance therapy, but its incidence should be recorded.

General considerations

In designing the 'ideal' maintenance study, all these points should be considered. On the other hand rigid criteria of trial protocol and strict exclusion rules select the trial population to an artificial degree, not representative of everyday clinical practice.

Table I. 1 Year maintenance cimetidine 400 mg at night vs placebo

Reference	Frequency of endoscopy	Relapse data		
		Drug	No. of patients	Total recurrence
Bianchi Porro et al 1979 (i)	6 & 12 months	Cim 400 mg nocte	25	39%
		placebo	25	83%
Massarat et al 1982	6 & 12 months	CIM 400 mg nocte	29	51%
		placebo	14	71%
Sontag et al 1981	6 & 12 months	Cim 400 mg nocte	46	13%
		placebo	49	53%
Sonnenberg et al 1981 (i)	1 year	Cim 400 mg nocte	29	24%
		placebo	27	62%
Sonnenberg et al 1979 (ii)	1 year	Cim 400 mg nocte	20	15%
		placebo	18	61%
Weber et al 1978	1 year	Cim 400 mg nocte	20	15%
		placebo	18	61%
Walters* et al 1981	5 & 11 months	Cim 400 mg nocte	34	38%
		placebo	37	70%

* 11 months

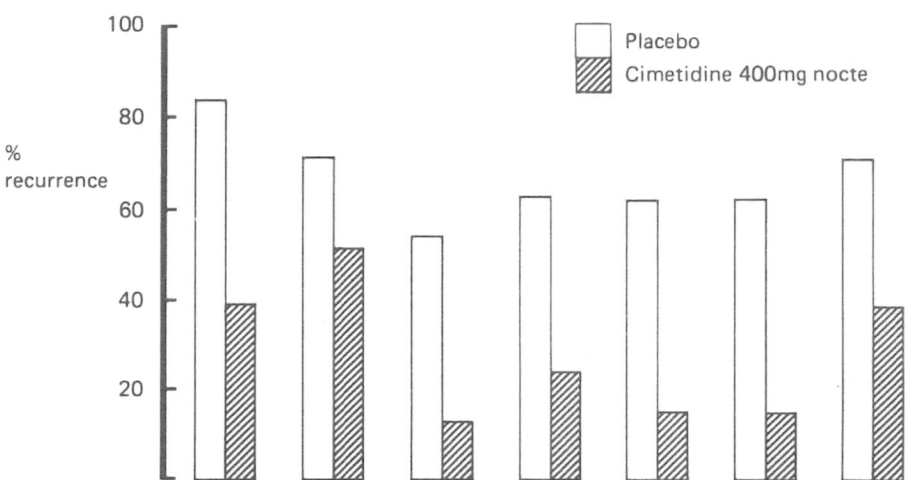

Figure 3. Recurrence rates of duodenal ulcer in 1 year trials comparing cimetidine 400 mg nocte with placebo. (Cimetidine results in obliquely hatched bows)

Results of maintenance trials in duodenal ulcers

Table I lists the results of one year maintenance treatment of duodenal ulcer with cimetidine 400 mg at night – the recommended dose of this drug for maintenance therapy. The results contained in Table I are graphically summarized in figure 3. It will be seen that although the relapse rate of duodenal ulcer is lower on the active, than on the control therapy in all instances, the results are somewhat variable, the

Table II. Ranitidine 150 mg night vs placebo or antacid 1 year maintenance studies.

| Reference | Frequency of endoscopy | Relapse data | | |
		Drug	No. of patients	Total recurrence
Alstead et al 1983	1 year	Ran 150 mg nocte	20	35%
		placebo	17	87%
Boyd et al (v)	Not stated	Ran 150 mg nocte	21	18%
		placebo	26	87%
		(NB 2nd year following successful 1st year maintenance therapy)		
Di Mario et al 1982	6 & 12 months	Ran 150 mg nocte	31	26%
		low dose antacid	30	60%

Table III. 1 Year maintenance ranitidine 150 mg at night vs cimetidine 400 mg nocte.

| Reference | Frequency of endoscopy | Relapse data | | |
		Drug	No. of patients	Total recurrence
Bolin et al 1983	4 monthly	Ran 150 mg nocte	26	12%
		Cim 400 mg nocte	12	17%
Hunt et al 1981	6& 12 months	Ran 150 mg nocte	28	25%
		Cim 400 mg nocte	33	24%
Van Dommelen et al 1982	1 year	Ran 150 mg nocte	24	17%
		Cim 400 mg nocte	22	27%

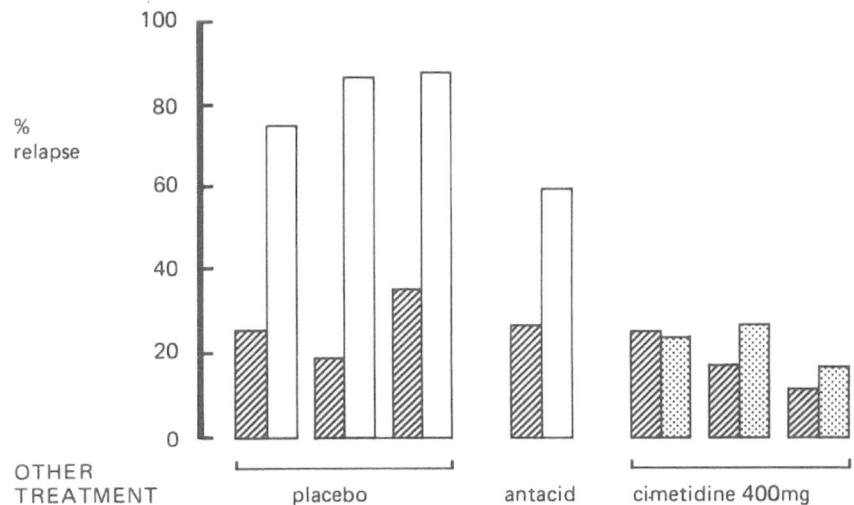

DU MAINTENANCE : RANITIDINE 150mg FOR 1 YR

Figure 4. Recurrence rates of duodenal ulcer in 1 year trials comparing ranitidine 150 mg nocte with placebo, low-dose antacid, or cimetidine

reported percentage relapse rate for cimetidine ranging from 15 to 51%.

Results of maintenance treatment with ranitidine 150 mg at night are shown in tables II and III. Table II presents comparisons of ranitidine treatment with placebo, or low-dose antacid. Table III shows results of studies comparing ranitidine 150 mg at night with cimetidine 400 mg at night, in the maintenance treatment of duodenal ulcer for one year. The results in tables II and III are summarized in figure 4. The data obtained in these 1 year studies of maintenance treatment of duodenal ulcer with ranitidine show a cumulative relapse rate on ranitidine therapy ranging from 12 to 35%

Other comparisons

Figure 5 shows the relapse rate on ranitidine 150 mg at night, or placebo, in patients with duodenal ulcer treated for one year. This illustrates the difference between the relapse on treatment with ranitidine compared with the control group. The data also make the point that although therapy with an histamine H_2-receptor antagonist does significantly decrease the relapse rate, there is nevertheless an appre-

106

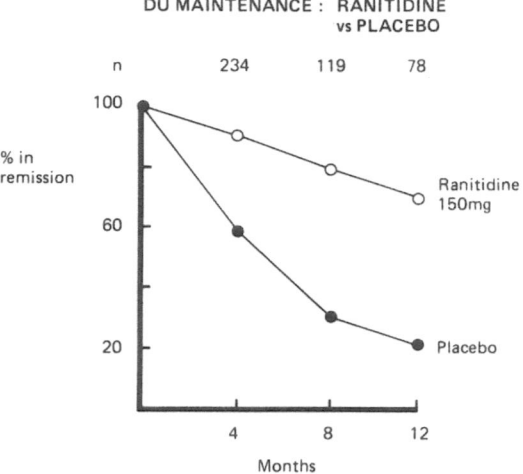

Figure 5. Recurrence rates of duodenal ulcer during 12 months maintenance treatment with ranitidine or placebo.

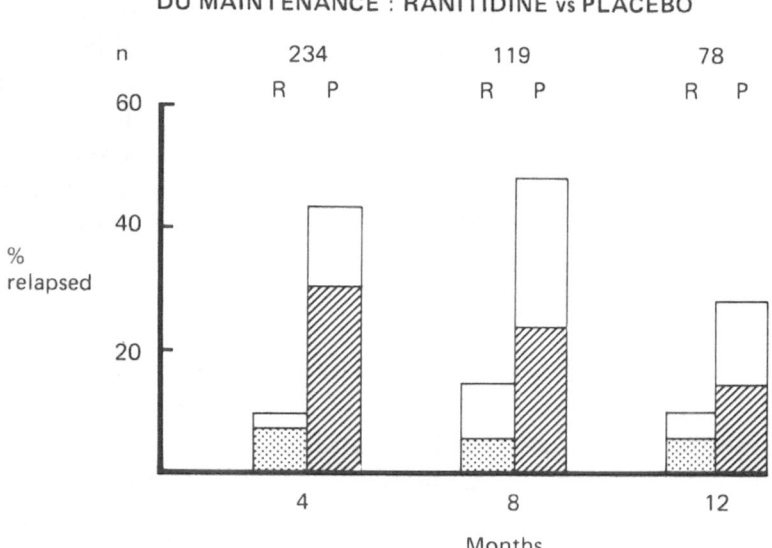

Figure 6. Recurrence rates of duodenal ulcer during 12 months maintenance treatment with ranitidine (R) or placebo (P). Hatched blocks show symptomatic recurrences.

MEAN 24 HOUR H+ ACTIVITY (mmol. l^{-1})

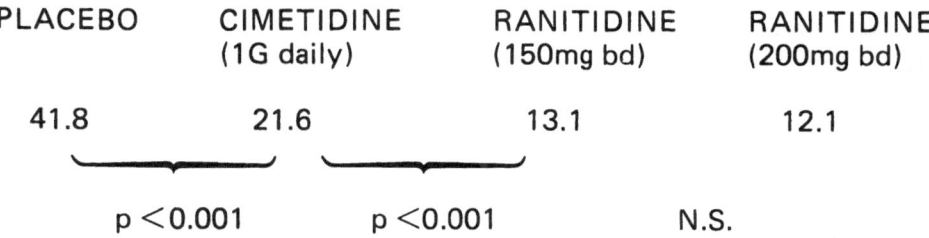

PLACEBO	CIMETIDINE (1G daily)	RANITIDINE (150mg bd)	RANITIDINE (200mg bd)
41.8	21.6	13.1	12.1

p $<$ 0.001   p $<$ 0.001   N.S.

% INHIBITION OF 24 HOUR H+ ACTIVITY

48%   69%   71%

Figure 7. Mean 24 hr intragastric H$^+$ activity in duodenal ulcer patients on various doses of ranitidine, or cimetidine (from Walt et al 1981).

MEAN OVERNIGHT ACID SECRETION (0100—0700) mmol. h^{-1}

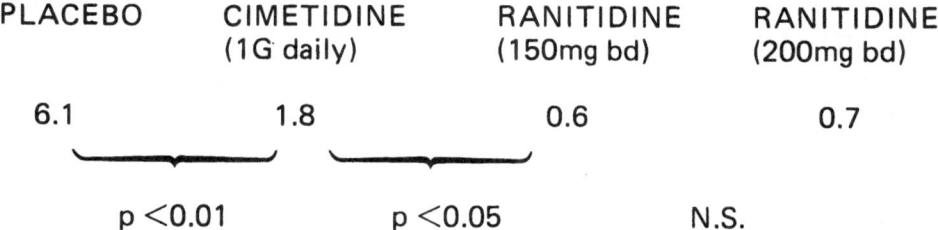

PLACEBO	CIMETIDINE (1G daily)	RANITIDINE (150mg bd)	RANITIDINE (200mg bd)
6.1	1.8	0.6	0.7

p $<$ 0.01   p $<$ 0.05   N.S.

% INHIBITION OF OVERNIGHT ACID OUTPUT

70%   90%   89%

Figure 8. Mean overnight acid output in duodenal ulcer patients on various doses of ranitidine, or cimetidine (from Walt et al 1981).

ciable rate of occurrence of duodenal ulcer during the treatment period. The reasons for this slow rate of recurrence are not clear, although it is reasonable to assume that failure to comply with the treatment regimen must play a part. It is notoriously difficult to persuade well people to take tablets regularly.

Figure 6 presents the results in a form that shows the relative proportions of symptomatic and asymptomatic relapses of duodenal ulcer to be seen. Treatment with ranitidine, or with placebo, is associated with an appreciable incidence of asymptomatic relapses of duodenal ulcer.

Comparative potency of ranitidine and cimetidine

In doses recommended for short-term therapy, (ranitidine 150 mg twice daily; cimetidine 200 mg three times a day and 400 mg at night), studies of 24 hour intragastric acidity (fig. 7) and overnight acid (fig. 8) in patients with duodenal ulcer, show ranitidine to be a significant more potent inhibitor of acid than cimetidine (Walt et al 1981). Nocturnal acid secretion, which tends to be high in patients with duodenal ulcer disease, is probably an important factor in maintaining chronicity, or producing a relapse of duodenal ulcer. The greater potency of recommended maintenance dose of ranitidine (150 mg at night) over that of cimetidine (400 mg at night) in long-term therapy is likely to be important. This contention is borne out by the results of long-term multicentre maintenance trials comparing the efficacy of ranitidine with cimetidine at these dose levels, which show ranitidine to be more effective. In a trial involving 484 patients with DU, the relapse rate was significantly lower in those given ranitidine 150 mg at night, than in those treated with cimetidine 400 mg (8% versus 21% at 4 months; 14 versus 34% at 8 months and 23% versus 37% at 12 months; Gough et al 1984). Similar results have been obtained in another trial employing an identical protocol and method of analysis. These considerations may also be relevant to long-term management of gastric ulcer.

Rebound re-ulceration after prolonged treatment

Rebound re-ulceration after prolonged inhibition of gastric acid secretion with histamine H_2-receptor antagonists do not appear to be

a problem. Neither ranitidine nor cimetidine at recommended therapeutic or maintenance doses produce complete suppression of gastric
acid output, the intragastric pH remaining low for an appreciable
fraction of each 24 hour period of therapy. Gross hyper-secretion of
gastrin from the antral G-cells therefore does not occur and thus
hyperplasia of the parietal cell mass does not take place. Relapse rates
recorded after 1 year treatment with cimetidine 400 mg twice daily,
were very similar to those recorded when placebo was given immediately after initial ulcer healing. (fig. 9)

Surgical or medical therapy

As figure 10 shows, the number of patients undergoing surgery for
duodenal ulcer has markedly diminished in the United Kingdom
following the introduction of cimetidine; this trend is likely to be
reinforced with the availability of ranitidine, and reflects the
widespread adoption of, and demand by the patients for, long-term
maintenance therapy. It is as yet too early to say whether the decrease
in the incidence of surgery for peptic ulcer is a temporary, or
permanent.

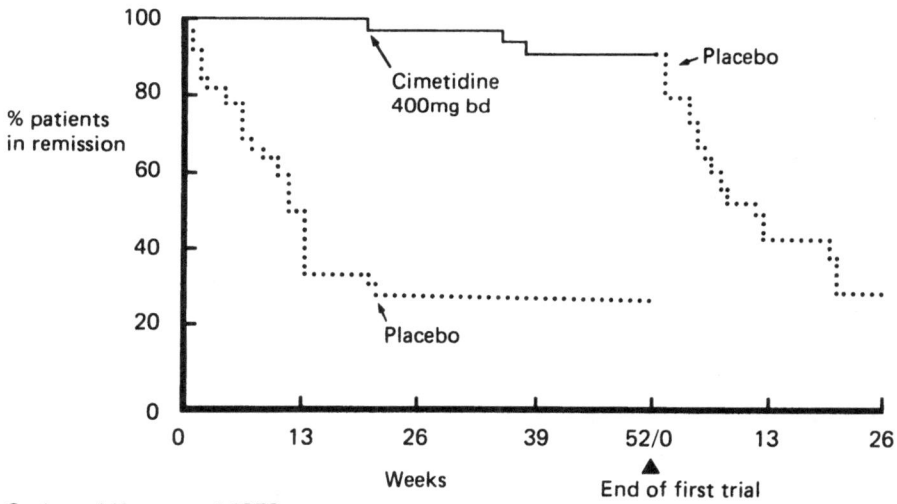

Gudmand-Hoyer et al 1978

Figure 9. Recurrence rates in duodenal ulcer before and after 1 year's maintenance therapy
(from Gudmand-Hoyer et al 1978).

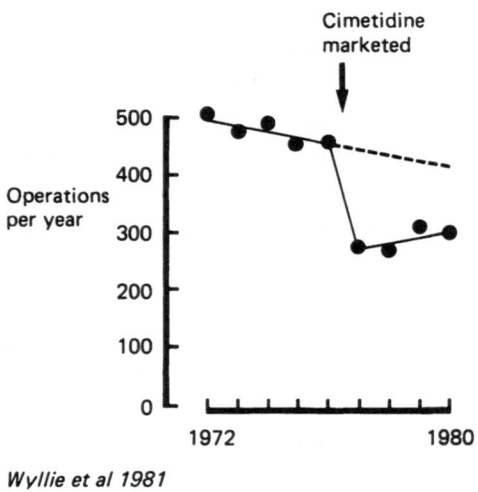

Wyllie et al 1981

Figure 10. Number of ulcer operations per year in relation to marketing of cimetidine (from Wyllie et al 1981).

Patients with complications of chronic ulcer, such as pyloric outlet obstruction, recurrent or relentless haemorrhage, or perforation, will need surgical treatment. It will also be necessary in those who do not respond well to ranitidine and whose symptoms are severe, or in those who live and work in areas where adequate medical facilities are not readily available. On the other hand patients in whom surgery carries an excessive risk of mortality or morbidity because of age, concurrent disease, or who are psychologically unsuitable for it, and also those with mild symptoms, would seem suitable for prolonged medical management.

Medical treatment carries with it a risk of recurrence, but so do operations for peptic ulcer. Recurrent ulcer can be operated on, but repeated operations are risky. Even elective surgery for peptic ulcer carries a definite, if low, mortality.

Modes of maintenance therapy that have been investigated mainly in Europe and in North America comprise continuous prophylactic administration of ranitidine, or cimetidine. Available evidence suggests that the benefit of maintenance treatment lasts only as long as the treatment itself. An alternative to this mode of drug administration consists of intermittent short courses of histamine H_2-receptor antagonists, especially for patients with well defined symptomatic relapses, which would be expected to respond rapidly to each period of administration of an H_2-blocker. These ideas are supported by studies which showed that more than two thirds of patients were satisfactorily managed by intermittent H_2-receptor blockade (Bardhan 1980; Rune, Mollman and Rahbek 1980).

Histamine H_2-receptor antagonists now provide effective therapy for the long-term management of peptic ulcer diathesis, appreciably decreasing the relapse rate. The design of maintenance trials and the interpretation of results have had a profound influence of the way peptic ulcers are managed by physicians and surgeons. The better the design and the more rigorous the analysis of results, the better will be the treatment available to our patients.

References

Alstead EM, Ryan FP, Holdsworth CD, Ashton MG, Moore M. Ranitidine in the prevention of gastric and duodenal ulcer relapse. Gut 1983;24:418 – 420.

Bardhan KD. Intermittent treatment of duodenal ulcer with cimetidine. Brit Med J 1980;2:20 – 22.

Bianchi Porro G, Petrillo M. Long-term prophylactic treatment with cimetidine in duodenal ulceration. Ital J Gastroenterol 1979;11:181 – 183.

Blum AL, Siewert JR, Holter F. Ulkustherapie mit Cimetidin. Dtsch Med Wochenschr 1978;103:135 – 138.

Bolin TD, Billington BP, Davis AE. Comparison of ranitidine and cimetidine as maintenance therapy in the prevention of duodenal ulcer recurrence. 25th Annual Scientific Meeting. Gastroenterological Society of Australia. Perth 2 – 4th May 1983;25:12.

Boyd EJS, Wilson JA, Wormsley KG. A double blind comparison of continuous ranitidine with placebo after one years successful maintenance of duodenal ulcer healing with ranitidine 150 mg nocte. Gastroenterology 1983;84(Part 2):113.

DiMario F, Albano O, Angelini G, Cavallini G. Dorenzo F, Farini R, Francavilla A, Naccarato R, Scuro LA, Vianello F. Ranitidine in long-term duodenal ulcer treatment: a multicentre trial. Digestion 1982;24:260 – 263.

Gough KR, Bardhan KD, Crowe JP, Korman MG, Lee FI, Reed PL, Smith RN. Ranitidine and cimetidine in prevention of duodenal ulcer relapse. A double blind randomised multi-centre comparative trial. Lancet 1984;ii:659 – 662.

Gudmand-Hayer E, Jensen KB, Krage E, Rask-Madsen J, Rahbek I, Rune SJ, Wuif HR. Prophylactic effect of cimetidine in duodenal ulcer disease. Brit Med J 1978;1:1095 – 1097.

Hunt RH, Walt RP, Trotman IF, Colley S, Bewar EP, Frost RA, Shepherd TH, Golding PL, Colin-Jones DG, Misiewicz JJ, Milton-Thompson GJ. Comparison of ranitidine 150 mg nocte with cimetidine 400 mg nocte in the maintenance treatment of duodenal ulcer in the clinical use of ranitidine. In: Misiewicz JJ, Wormsley KG (Eds). Proceedings of the 2nd International Symposium on Ranitidine. Oxford, Medicine Publishing Foundation, 1981:192 – 195.

Massarrat S, Heuser E, Hausmann L, Schubotz R. Long-term prevention of duodenal ulcer with cimetidine. Effect of the rhythm of ingestion and drug compliance in the incidence of recurrences. Dtsch Med Wochenschr 1982;107:1085–1088.

Rune SJ, Mollman KM, Rahbek J. Frequency of relapses in duodenal ulcer patients treated with cimetidine during symptomatic periods. Scand J Gastroenterol 1980;14(Suppl 58):85–92.

Sonnenberg A et al. Prevention of duodenal ulcer recurrence with cimetidine. Dtsch Med Wochenschr 1979;104:725–730.

Sonnenberg A, Muller-Lissner SA, Vogel E, Schmid P, Gonvers JJ, Peter P, Strohmeyer G, Blum AL. Predictors of duodenal ulcer healing and relapse. Gastroenterology 1981;81:1061–1067.

Sontag S, Graham D, Belsito A, Weiss J, Kinnear D, Farley A, Grunt R, Cohen N, Archambault A, Davis W, Thayer J, Archard J, Dyck W, Gillies P, Mann J, Sidorov J, Fleshier B, Cleator I, Wenger J. Three cimetidine dose schedules versus placebo in preventing duodenal ulcer recurrence. A multicentre doubleblind study. Gastroenterology 1981;80(abstract):1290.

Sontag S, Graham D, Belsito A et al. Cimetidine, cigarette smoking and recurrence of duodenal ulcer. New Engl J of Med 1984;311:689–693.

Van Dommelen CKV, Stalder FH, Boekhorst JC. Comparison of ranitidine with cimetidine in the treatment of duodenal ulcer. In: Misiewicz JJ, Wormsley KG (Eds). Proceedings of the 2nd International Symposium on Ranitidine. Oxford, Medicine Publishing Foundation 1982:154–156.

Walt RP, Male PJ, Rawlings J, Hunt RH, Milton-Thompson GJ, Misiewicz JJ. Comparison of the effects of ranitidine, cimetidine and placebo on the 24-hour intragastric acidity and nocturnal acid secretion in patients with duodenal ulcer. Gut 1981;22:49–54.

Walters JM, Crean P, Kelly D, Cahill B, Cole TS, Whelton M, Wier D, McCarthy CF. Cimetidine and duodenal ulcer, a study of initial and low dose maintenance treatment in Ireland. Irish J Med Sci 1980;149(7):270–274.

Weber KB, Giger M, Sonnenberg A et al. Therapy and long-term prophylaxis of duodenal ulcer with cimetidine. Z Gastroenterol 1978;16/11:697–698.

Wyllie JH, Clark CG, Alexander-Williams J, Bell RF, Kennedy TL, Kirk RM, MacKay C. Effect of cimetidine on surgery for duodenal ulcer. Letter. Lancet 1981;1:1307–1308.

9. 1976 – 1984: How should we use histamine H$_2$-receptor antagonists?

R. POUNDER, M.A., M.D., F.R.C.P.

Academic Department of Medicine, Royal Free Hospital, London, United Kingdom

Black and his colleagues described the discovery of an histamine H$_2$-receptor antagonist in 1972.[1] The first duodenal ulcer patient received cimetidine in June 1975, and the drug was marketed for general use in the United Kingdom in November 1976.

The histamine H$_2$-receptor antagonists have been not only a therapeutic, but also a commercial success: they provided the first decisive and safe medical treatment for peptic ulceration and millions of patients have benefited from their use. Cimetidine and ranitidine are now the biggest selling drugs in the world.

Changing dose regimens of histamine H$_2$-receptor antagonists

During the last eight years there has been a gradual change in the way that histamine H$_2$-receptor antagonists are used, evolving from a four times a day regimen to a once daily tablet.

When cimetidine was introduced as a treatment for duodenal ulceration in 1976, it was recommended that the patient should receive a 200 mg tablet three times a day with meals, taking 400 mg at bedtime.[2] The aim of this complicated regimen was to provide optimal control of intragastric acidity throughout the 24 hours. Early studies of 24 hour intragastric acidity had demonstrated that the best daytime control of intragastric acidity was achieved by the three doses of cimetidine 200 mg with meals, but a larger dose was required to control nocturnal acidity.[3] Even with this regimen unexpectedly low intragastric pH was still recorded in the stomach during the day and during the night. Cimetidine 1 g per day in four divided doses speeded

114

ulcer healing, improving average four week ulcer healing rates from 43% on placebo to 77% on cimetidine.[4]

When ranitidine was discovered, the drug was soon shown to be a powerful antisecretory agent. Twenty-four intragastric acidity experiments showed that ranitidine 150 mg taken at breakfast and at bedtime could provide control of intragastric acidity, superior to convetional cimetidine 1 g per day in four divided doses.[5] Ranitidine was marketed in 1981 with a recommended dose of 150 mg twice a day. Encouraged by this simple regimen, studies with cimetidine soon demonstrated that a similar twice a day regimen, using cimetidine 400 mg morning and evening could also speed ulcer healing.[6]

Perhaps encouraged by the prospect of omeprazole, which could be a once-a-day ulcer healing drug,[7], 24 hour intragastric acidity experiments showed that either cimetidine 800 mg, or ranitidine 300 mg at bedtime could effect a profound decrease of nocturnal acidity, with a lesser control of acidity during the day.[8] (fig. 1) Clinical trials soon demonstrated that such a once-a-day regimen with either histamine H_2-receptor antagonists could produce ulcer healing rates equivalent to the same dose of drug taken in two divided doses.[9-12] (Table I)

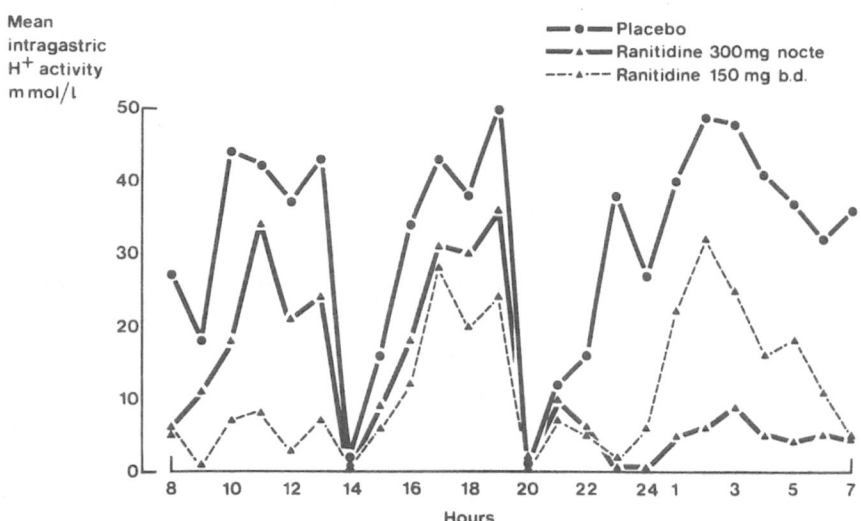

Figure 1. Mean hourly intragastric hydrogen ion activity during treatment with ranitidine 150 mg bd and ranitidine 300 mg nocte.[8]

Table I. Endoscopic healing rates of duodenal ulcer after 4 and 8 weeks of treatment with histamine H_2-receptor antagonists, either as a bd dosage or a single night time schedule.[11,12]

Treatment	n	Healing rates (percentage)	
		4 weeks	8 weeks
Cimetidine 400 mg bd	273	74	94
Ranitidine 150 mg bd	301	82	95
Cimetidine 800 mg nocte	274	79	96
Ranitidine 300 mg nocte	304	76	94

Hence, control of nocturnal acidity by a large bedtime dose of an histamine H_2-receptor antagonists speeds duodenal ulcer healing, despite continuing acidity during the day. Perhaps the advantages of improved compliance are balanced by the poor control of daytime acidity.

Why do 20% of duodenal ulcers fail to heal at one month?

Whatever the regimen, a full dose of either cimetidine or ranitidine will heal approximately 80% of ulcers at the end of one month. Why is it that 20% of ulcers remain unhealed?

The first problem may be compliance – as soon as some patients obtain relief of symptomes they stop taking the tablets, before there is healing of the ulceration. This is probably more of a problem in clincial practice than in clinical trials, where compliance is encouraged by careful supervision of the patients.

The second possibility is that every duodenal ulcer does not have the same cause – some ulcers may only heal during control of acid secretion, whereas other ulcers will heal only when assisted by one of the 'mucosal protective' agents such as tripotassium dicitrato bismuthate, or sucralfate.

The third possibility is that the conventional histamine H_2-receptor antagonists are not sufficiently strong – could stronger antisecretory agents provide more rapid and complete ulcer healing?

Do we want more potent antisecretory drugs?

Walt and his colleagues demonstrated that cimetidine 1 g per day in four divided doses was not as potent as ranitidine 300 mg a day

116

MEAN HOURLY INTRAGASTRIC ACIDITY

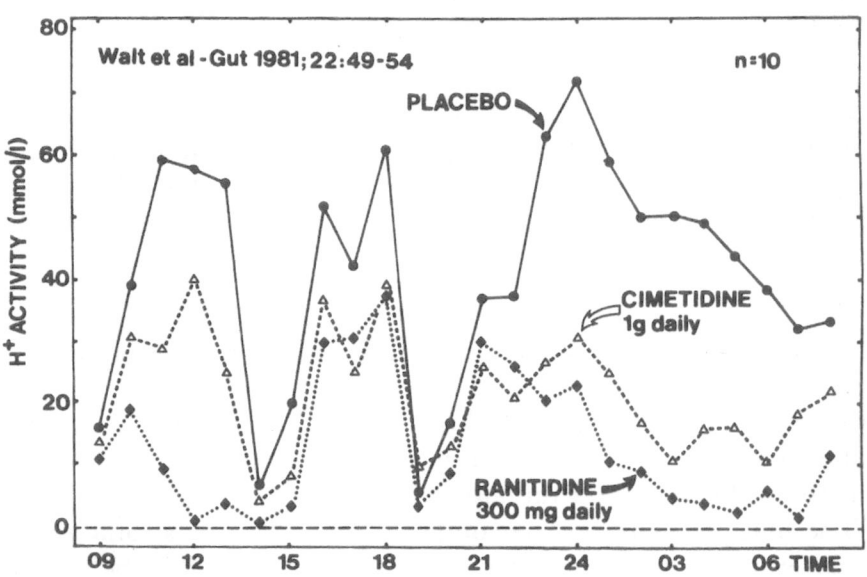

Figure 2. Mean hourly intragastric hydrogen ion activity during treatment with placebo, cimetidine 1 g daily and ranitidine 300 mg daily (N = 10).[5]

divided in two doses.[5] (figs 2 and 3) In terms of 24 hour median intragastric pH, treatment with cimetidine moved median pH from 1.4 to 1.7(a two-fold decrease of acidity), whereas ranitidine moved median pH from 1.4 to 2.4 (a ten-fold decrease).[13] Hence in conventional doses ranitidine is five times as potent as cimetidine, yet no difference in acute ulcer healing rates has been observed.

Omeprazole provides not only a profound decrease of acidity, but also a decrease that is sustained for several days. For example, omeprazole 30 mg daily causes a 97% decrease of mean intragastric acidity (shifting 24 hour median intragastric pH from 1.4 to 5.3 — an 8,000-fold decrease of acidity) and omeprazole 20 mg per day

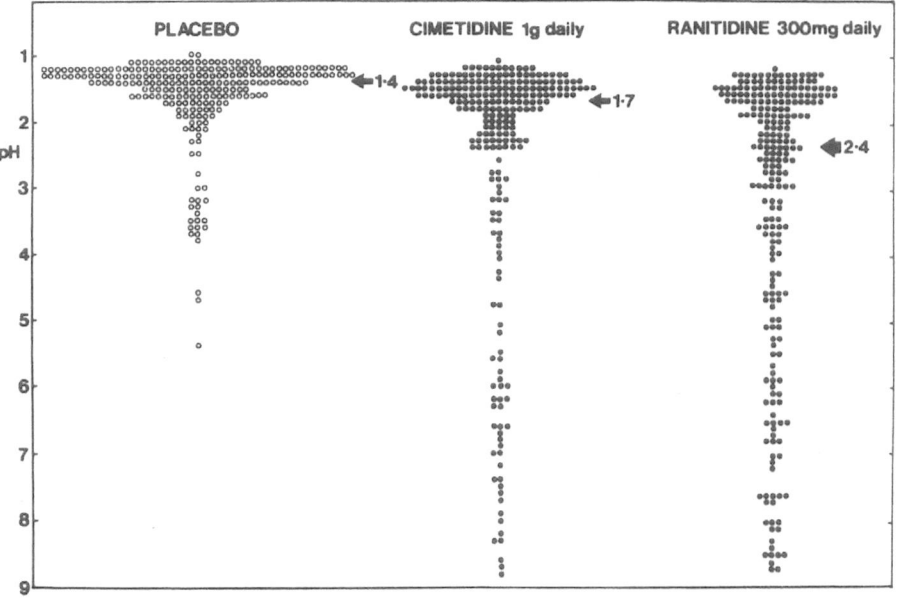

Figure 3. pH values of gastric aspirate obtained hourly from ten patients with duodenal ulcers receiving placebo, cimetidine 1 g, ranitidine 300 mg daily. Arrows indicate median pH.[5]

causes a 90% decrease.[7] (figs 4 and 5 There is only one published controlled trial comparing ranitidine 150 mg bd with omeprazole 20 mg om when, after two weeks of treatment, the percentage of ulcers healed were 59 and 72% respectively, and after four weeks of treatment 92 and 96% respectively.[14] Hence, even a major increase of antisecretory potency has not been rewarded by an improved ulcer healing rate – albeit that in this study ranitidine achieved its best-ever result.

A profound decrease of 24 hour acidity is not without theoretical disadvantages.[15,16] Rebound acid secretion after discontinuation of

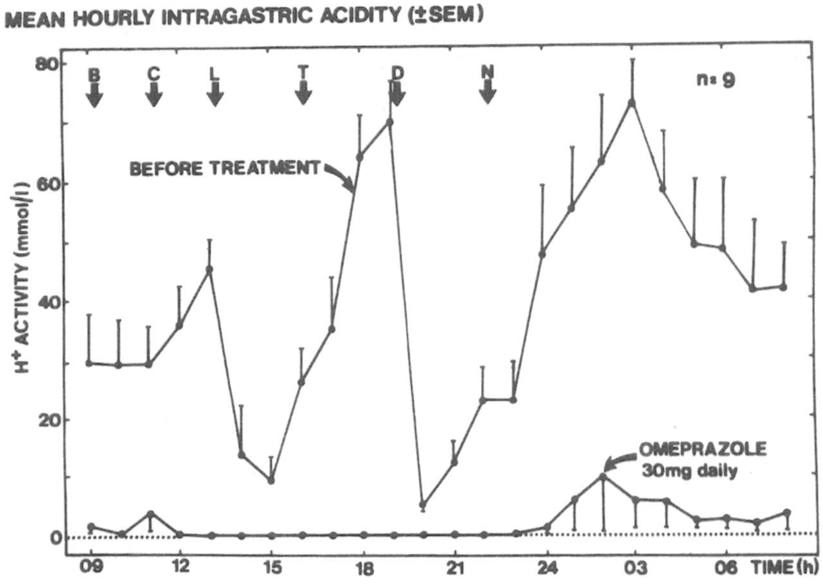

MEAN HOURLY INTRAGASTRIC ACIDITY (±SEM)

Figure 4. Mean hourly intragastric hydrogen ion activity before and during treatment with omeprazole 30 mg daily (n = 9). Omeprazole 30 mg was taken at 09.00 h.[13]

drug therapy has been suggested, but has never been demonstrated. Virtual anacidity may leave the intestine vulnerable to enteric infections: – it certainly allows bacterial overgrowth with the transient production of nitrosamines. Drug-induced hypergastrinaemia may cause hyperplasia of enterochromaffin cells in the body of the stomach.

What is the ideal decrease of intragastric acidity for duodenal ulcer healing? Should a new antisecretory drug be more or less potent than the conventional histamine H_2-receptor antagonists?

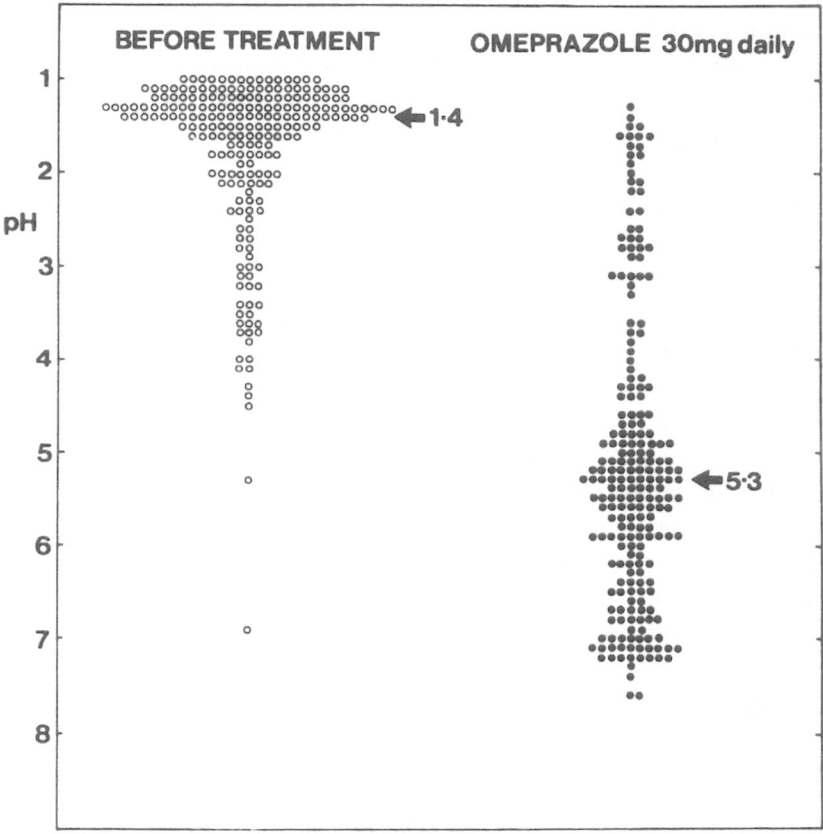

Figure 5. pH values of gastric aspirate obtained hourly from nine patients with duodenal ulcer before and during treatment with omeprazole 30 mg daily. Arrows indicate median pH.[13]

Ulcer symptoms after eight weeks of treatment

After eight weeks of treatment with a full dose of either cimetidine or ranitidine, 5 to 10% of patients will have continuing symptoms. How should they be managed?

The first step is to check on the patient's compliance, as a considerable proportion of treatment failures might be due to inadequate intake of the prescribed drugs. The second step is to determine whether the continuing symptoms are due to active duodenal ulceration –

and this can only be determined accurately by endoscopy. A barium meal might demonstrate continuing dudodenal deformity, yet the mucosa may be intact. Endoscopy will demonstrate whether pain is due to continuing ulceration – if no ulcer is found then histamine H_2-receptor antagonist can be stopped, and other diagnoses considered. An accurate history should be taken of the use of anti-inflammatory drugs and the abuse of either nicotine or alcohol.

If continuing duodenal ulceration is present, the patient should be identified as a problem, deserving further investigation. The duodenal mucosa should probably be biopsied, to exclude rare conditions, such as tuberculosis, carcinoma, lymphoma, or Crohn's disease of the duodenum. A blood sample should be taken for measurement of the fasting plasma gastrin concentration, to eliminate the Zollinger-Ellison syndrome.

What treatment should be offered to the patient with continuing duodenal ulceration? Surgery should be considered. However, the patients that are not responding well to standard treatment with histamine H_2-receptor antagonists are probably less suitable for surgery. Bardhan explored the possibility of increasing the dose of cimetidine for many months – he demonstrated that 66 of 495 episodes of duodenal ulceration were not healed after three months of treatment with cimetidine 1 g per day.[17] Thirty-seven of these patients were finally healed after a mean of 7.4 months of treatment, but 29 never healed despite mean 9.4 months of treatment – usually using increased doses of cimetidine.

If continuing with cimetidine treatment is unsuccessful, is changing to ranitidine useful? A recent Italian study of 40 patients who had not healed their duodenal ulcers after six weeks of treatment with cimetidine 1 g per day, showed that 63% had healed after a further six weeks of treatment with the same dose of cimetidine, and 62% healed after six weeks of treatment with ranitidine 150 mg bd.[18] There seems to be no benefit from changing to the more potent histamine H_2-receptor antagonist.

A study from Hong Kong investigating 25 patients whose duodenal ulcer had not improved after one month of treatment with cimetidine 1 g per day, showed that changing from an histamine H_2-receptor antagonist to tripotassium dicitrato bismuthate would usually result in ulcer healing – 85% of ulcers healed during bismuth treatment, whereas only 40% healed during further treatment with an increased dose of cimetidine (400 mg four times a day).[19]

If a duodenal ulcer has not healed after eight weeks of treatment with full-dose histamine H_2-receptor blockade, it seems sensible to switch to treatment with tripotassium dicitrato bismuthate, or perhaps sucralfate.[20]

Duodenal ulceration is a chronic illness

During the early development of cimetidine it soon became clear that although ulcers would heal with an histamine H_2-receptor antagonist, they soon returned. During one year maintenance studies, two-thirds of patients receiving placebo treatment relapsed within one year of ulcer healing.[21] Treatment with cimetidine 400 mg at bedtime decreased the rate of ulcer relapse. 8.5% of duodenal ulcers receiving placebo maintenance treatment relapse each months, whereas only 2.5% relapse each month when receiving cimetidine 400 mg at bedtime. Even a full year of treatment with cimetidine 400 mg bd does not eliminate the tendency for ulcers to return – duodenal ulceration is controlled during histamine H_2-receptor blockade, but when treatment is stopped the ulcers tend to return.[22] There is no modern evidence that patients 'grow out' of duodenal ulceration – it appears to be a chronic illness.

Long-term treatment of duodenal ulceration

As duodenal ulceration is a chronic illness, each patient requires a long-term strategy. A model of duodenal ulceration, using accepted healing and relapsing rates, demonstrates the dramatic benefit of maintenance histamine H_2-receptor blockade.[4] (fig. 6)

Due to spontaneous healing and recurrence of duodenal ulcer, 17% of an untreated ulcer population will have an active ulcer at any one time. If patients only receive treatment at times of ulcer relapse, 10% will have an ulcer at any one time – because intermittent treatment does not deal with the tendency of ulceration to relapse, and 8.5% of untreated ulcer patients relapse every month. Alternatively, if patients receive maintenance histamine H_2-receptor antagonists using a low dose at bedtime, with full-dose treatment at times of rare ulcer relapse, only 3 in 100 patients will be expected to have an ulcer at any one time. A recent study of maintenance treatment in 484 pa-

122

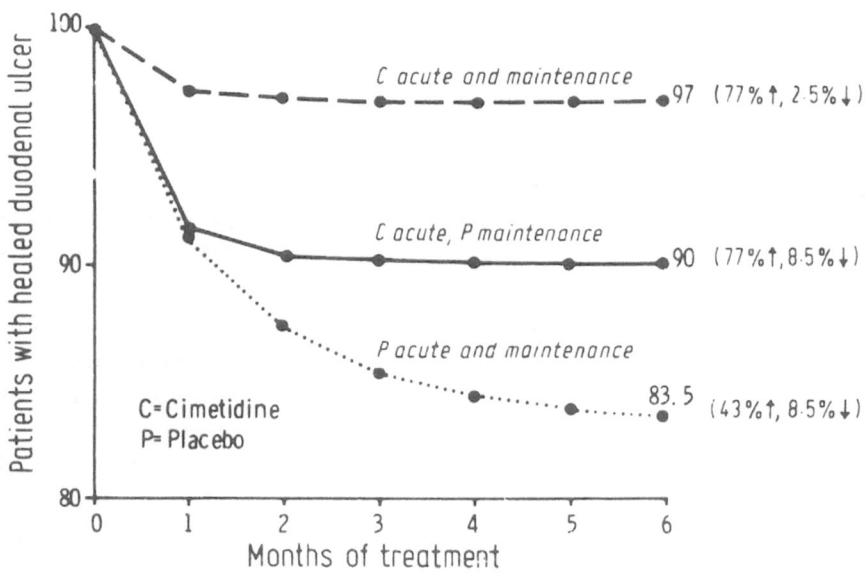

Figure 6. Models for the treatment of duodenal ulcer.[4]

tients showed a superior effect of ranitidine 150 mg nocte over cimetidine 400 mg nocte.[23] At the end of one year, the percentage of patients with healed ulcers were 77% and 63%, respectively.

Obviously not every duodenal ulcer patient requires continuous histamine H_2-receptor blockade. It should be reserved for those with aggressive ulceration, who rapidly redevelop symptoms when treatment is withdrawn, or who have a history of repeated haemorrhage or over-sewn perforation. It should also be used by those patients who could not risk a complication of duodenal ulceration because of other medical illness – the patient with severe liver, renal, heart or lung disease, or the elderly patient may be put at great risk by gastrointestinal haemorrhage or perforation. Such patients deserve maintenance treatment with histamine H_2-receptor antagonists.

Although patients on maintenance histamine H_2-receptor blockade receive daily treatment, in fact this provides only a short-lived control of intragastric acidity. Patients receiving ranitidine 150 mg at night have decrease in acidity during the night and early morning (from midnight to 9 am), but for most of the day the intragastric acidity is normal.[24] The presence of normal acid during most of the day should greatly decrease the risk of long-term complications.

In an endoscopically controlled trial of maintenance treatment, asymptomatic ulcers were shown to be present in 39 of 134 patients on placebo (29%), in 102 of 1328 patients on ranitidine (8%), and in 8 of 100 patients on cimetidine (8%).[25] It is not known how much of a hazard these asymptomatic ulcers present.

An alternative possibility would be on-demand treatment. Properly selected patients could be allowed to take a full-dose of an histamine H_2-receptor antagonist during clinical relapse until 2 weeks after complete symptomatic relief. As soon as symptoms recur a further course of full-dose treatment would be taken.

The advantages of this regimen are:
– prompt relief of symptoms,
– early initiation of treatment and hence presumably less risk of complications,
– less exposure to drug.

However, the disadvantages of this schedule are that the 29% of asymptomatic ulcers remain at risk, and repeated relapses might discourage the patients from taking further courses of treatment.

Conclusions

There is no non-infectious chronic medical illness that is cured by a single course of treatment with tablets. During the last eight years we have learned that histamine H_2-receptor antagonists are a treatment for duodenal ulceration and not a cure.

It is now clear that control of nocturnal acidity will not only speed ulcer healing, but will protect from ulcer relapse. Most patients will respond to full dose treatment with an histamine H_2-receptor antagonist at times of ulcer relapse.
Maintenance treatment should be reserved for those with aggressive ulceration, the ill and the elderly.

References

1. Black JW, Duncan WAM, Durant CJ, Ganellin CR, Parsons ME. Definition and antagonism of histamine H_2-receptors. Nature 1972;236:385 – 390.
2. Gray GR, McKenzie I, Smith IŠ, Crean GP, Gillespie G. Oral cimetidine in severe duodenal ulceration. Lancet 1977;i:4 – 6.
3. Pounder RE, Williams JG, Milton-Thompson GJ, Misiewicz JJ. 24 hour control of intragastric acidity by cimetidine in duodenal ulcer patients. Lancet 1975;22:1069 – 72.
4. Pounder RE. Model of medical treatment for duodenal ulcer. Lancet 1981;i:29 – 30.
5. Walt RP, Male PJ, Rawlings J, Hunt R, Milton-Thompson GJ, Misiewicz JJ. Comparison of the effects of ranitidine, cimetidine and placebo on the 24 hour intragastric acidity and nocturnal acid secretion in patients with duodenal ulcer. Gut 1981;22:49 – 54.
6. Kerr GD. Cimetidine: twice daily administration in duodenal ulcer – results of a UK and Ireland multicentre study. In: Baron JH (Ed). Cimetidine in the 80s. Edinburgh, Churchill Livingstone, pp 9 – 13.
7. Sharma BK, Walt RP, Pounder RE, Gomes MdeFA, Wood EC, Logan LH. Optimal dose of oral omeprazole for maximal 24 hour decrease of intragastric acidity. Gut 1984;25:957 – 964.
8. Gledhill T, Howard DM, Buck M, Hunt RH. Single nocturnal dose of an H_2-receptor antagonist for the treatment of duodenal ulcer. Gut 1973;24: 904 – 8.
9. Capurso L, Dale Monte PR, Mazzeo F et al. Comparison of cimetidine 800 mg once daily and 400 mg twice daily in acute duodenal ulceration. Brit Med J 289:1418 – 20.
10. Ireland A, Gear P, Colin-Jones DG et al. Ranitidine 150 mg twice daily versus 300 mg nightly in treamtnet of duodenal ulcers. Lancet 1984;ii:274 – 5.
11. Lambert R. In: Tagamet: New dimensions. Proceedings of a symposium. Windemere Communications Inc. 1984:15 – 23.
12. Walt RP, Gomes MdeFA, Wood EC, Logan LH, Pounder RE. Effect of daily oral omeprazole on 24 hour intragastric acidity. Brit Med J 1983;287:12 – 14.
13. Danman H-G, Classen M, Domschke W et al. Ulcera Duodeni heilen unter Omeprazole nach zwei Wochen schneller ab als unter Ranitidin. Z Gastroenterol 1984;22:500.
14. Sharma BK, Santana IA, Wood EC, Walt RP, Pereira M, Noone P, Smith PLR, Walters CL, Pounder RE. Intragastric bacterial acitvity and nitrosation before, during and after treatment with omeprazole. Brit Med J 1984;289:717 – 719.
15. Pouder RE. Duodenal ulcers that will not heal. Gut 1984;25:697 – 702.
16. Bardhan KD. Intermittent treatment of duodenal ulcer with cimetidine. Brit Med J 1980;2:20 – 2.
17. Quatrini M, Basilisco G, Bianchi PA. Treatment of 'cimetidine-resistant' chronic duodenal ulcers with ranitidine or cimetidine: a randomised multicentre study. Gut 1984;25:1113 – 7.
19. Lam SK, Lee NW, Koo J, Hui WM, Fok KH, Ng M. A randomised crossover trial of tripotassium dicitrato bismuthate vs high dose cimetidine for duodenal ulcers resistant to standard dose of cimetidine. Gut 1984;25:703 – 6.
20. Guslandi M, Ballarin E. Tittobello A. Sucralfate bei Cimetidin- und Ranitidin-Resistenten Duodenalgeschwuren. Therapie Woche 1984;34:653 – 4.

21. Burland WL, Hawkins BW, Beresford J. Cimetidine treatment for the prevention of recurrence of duodenal lulcer: an International Collaborative study. Postgrad Med J 1980;56:173 – 6.
22. Gudmand-Hoyer E, Birger-Jensen K, Krag E, Rask-Madsen K, Rahbed I, Rune SK, Wulff HR. Prophylactic effect of cimetidine in duodenal ulcer disease. Brit Med J 1978;1:1095 – 7.
23. Santana IA, Sharma BK, Pounder RE, Wood EC, Masters S, Talbot M. 24 hour intragastric acidity during maintenance treatment with ranitidine. Brit Med J 1984;289:1420.
24. Record CO. Maintenance treatment with ranitidine in peptic ulceration. In: Tijtgat GN (Ed). Ranitidine, a selective new H_2 antagonist. Guildford, Theracom, p 20.

10. Omeprazole: A review of its pharmacological and clinical properties

H.P.M. Festen, H.A.R.E. Tuynman and S.G.M. Meuwissen

Department of Gastroenterology, Free University Hospital, 1117, De Boelelaan, 1081 HV Amsterdam, The Netherlands

Introduction

Before the discovery of the histamine H_2-receptor antagonists the classical anticholinergics were the only inhibitors of gastric acid secretion available. Their clinical use, however, was limited by unwanted effects and the results of treatment disappointing. This picture changed completely in the seventies with the advent of the histamine H_2-receptor antagonist, cimetidine. An overwhelming number of studies showed that suppression of gastric acid secretion is indeed the mainstay in the treatment of acid peptic diseases. However safe these compounds proved to be, H_2-receptors are not limited to the parietal cell and neither are the effects of the antagonists. Anticholinergics and histamine H_2-receptor antagonists act systemically by blocking their specific receptors throughout the body.

In those days it was already known that the secretion of acid into the gastric lumen is finally effected by one enzyme: the H^+-K^+ ATP-ase. In man this enzyme is found in the parietal cell membrane and nowhere else in the body. The ability to block this so called proton pump would therefore provide a very specific inhibitor of gastric acid secretion. A Swedish group of investigators succeeded in synthesizing a new class of compounds with this property: the substituted benzimidazoles.

In vitro and animal studies

Fellenius and coworkers showed in isolated rabbit gastric glands that the substituted benzimidazole picoprazole inhibits acid secretion stimulated by histamine, dibutyryl cyclic AMP and high doses of K^+, whereas cimetidine inhibited the effect of histamine only.[1] They also demonstrated a specific antagonizing effect of this compound on the activity of isolated H^+-K^+ ATP-ase in an *in vitro* model. Their study shows therefore that substituted benzimidazoles act somewhere in the parietal cell, beyond the receptors on the cell surface and most probably by blocking the enzyme H^+-K^+ ATP-ase in the apical membrane.

Omeprazole, the successor of picoprazole, is 5-10 times more potent on a molar base. It is the compound chosen for further clinical evaluation. Omeprazole has the same properties as picoprazole and both act in a non-competitive way.[2] In isolated gastric glands omeprazole inhibits acid secretion mediated through gastrinergic, histaminergic and cholinergic stimulation as well as stimulated by cyclic AMP.[3] The specificity of omeprazole was suggested by the lack of effect on basal, cholinergic and cyclic AMP-stimulated pepsinogen release in enriched chief cell fractions.[4]

The effect of omeprazole on gastric acid secretion is much longer than its presence in the blood. This is due to the fact that omeprazole, being a weak base, accumulates in the acid environment of the secretory canaliculi of the parietal cells. In non-ionized form it is trapped there and unable to leave the cell. This also contributes to the specificity of action of omeprazole as it is quickly eliminated from all other compartments in the body. In a very elegant study using whole body auto-radiography in the mouse, Helander and Ramsay showed that 16 hours after oral administration of ^{14}C labelled omeprazole activity was present only in the gastric mucosa. Using electron microscopy, this activity was localized to the secretory membrane and tubulovesicles of the parietal cells.[5]

Pharmacokinetics

Omeprazole is acid labile. To protect the drug from degradation by gastric acid it was administered orally in earlier studies together with a sodium bicarbonate suspension. Peak blood levels are reached 30-40 minutes after oral administration and decline thereafter with a half-life ($T\frac{1}{2}$) of about 50 minutes. The area under the plasma concentration curve (AUC) increased with increasing dose.[6,7] For clinical practice an enteric coated preparation of omeprazole was developed. Peak blood levels appeared from 1 to 6 hours after oral dosing in a fasted subject and the AUC varied widely after a given dose.[8,9,10] Omeprazole facilitates its own absorption during repeated dosing, probably as a result of the increased intragastric pH: peak blood levels and the AUC increase significantly, reaching a steady-state after about 5 days of treatment.[8,9] (Table I) Omeprazole is almost completely metabolized before elimination, mainly through the kidneys. Unchanged drug has not been recovered in the urine.[8] Three metabolites, hydroxy-omeprazole, the sulfone and sulfide of omeprazole, have been identified in human blood.

Table I. Oral pharmacokinetics of omeprazole EC 40 mg/day in 8 healthy subjects (values are mean ± SEM).[8]

	Morning dose	
Pharmacokinetic parameter	day 1	day 5
C_{max} (ng/ml)	644 ± 110	936 ± 177
AUC (ng.h/ml)	1187 ± 246	2223 ± 1425
T_{max} (h)	3.0 ± 0.4	2.9 ± 0.3
$T_{1/2}$ (h)	0.7 ± 0.1	1.1 ± 0.1

Pharmacodynamics

Effects on gastric acid secretion

The inhibition of acid secretion by omeprazole does not correlate with the peak plasma level, or plasma concentration, but correlates with the AUC.[6,7,10] In dogs it was shown that the inhibitory effect of omeprazole and the AUC are related to the concentration of omeprazole in the gastric mucosa.[11] In one study in man the calculated mean AUC for 50% inhibition of gastric acid secretion was 1.5 ± 0.02 μmol.h/l and this was achieved after administration of one dose of omeprazole 30-40 mg as a buffered solution.[6] The mean inhibition of acid secretion stimulated by a peptone meal and pentagastrin ranged from 36 to 99% after single oral administration of buffered suspensions of omeprazole, 20 to 90 mg.[6,7] The effect of omeprazole on acid secretion is not only strong but also prolonged, much longer than its presence in the blood: one 40 mg oral dose still produced a significant effect 3 days after administration while omeprazole was no longer detectable in plasma after 24 hours. After 14 days no effect was measurable any more.[7]

130

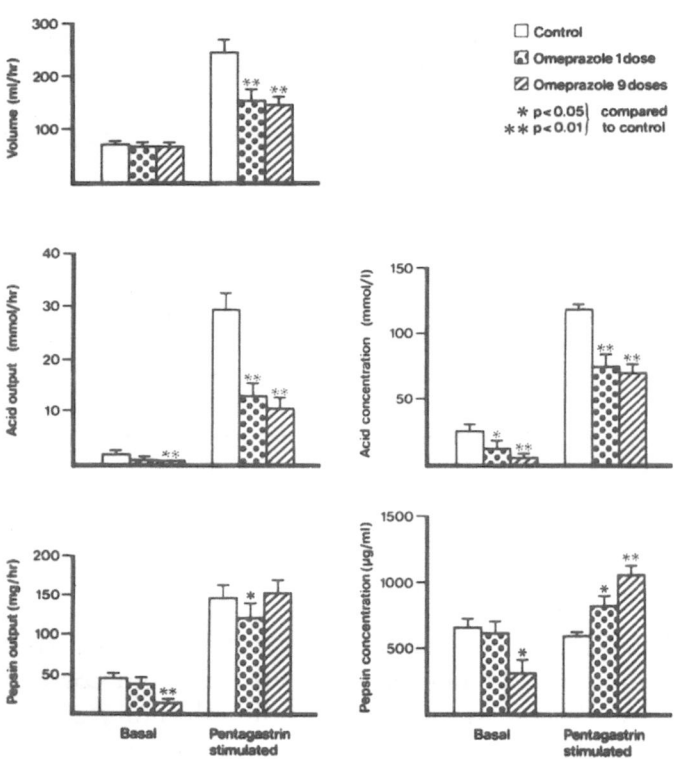

Figure 1. The effect of one and nine days administration of omeprazole 40 mg daily on volume, acid and pepsin secretion (mean ± SEM) basal during 1 hour (represented as 'basal') and subsequently during 90 minutes of continuous pentagastrin stimulation (1.5 μg/kg.h), (the last hour of stimulation is represented as 'pentagastrin stimulated') in 12 healthy volunteers.

Administered as enteric coated (EC) granules omeprazole produces a very variable effect on gastric acid secretion, as expected from the variation in bioavailability. This effect increases after repeated dosing with the increase in bioavailability, reaching a plateau after 3 to 5 days.[12] Repeated doses of omeprazole EC up to 10 mg have hardly any effect on acid secretion.[10,13,14,15] After 20 mg of omeprazole EC a variable effect is recorded.[10,15,16] A 30 mg dose produces a 45 to 94% inhibition of pentagastrin stimulated acid secretion when measured 24 hours after repeated dosing.[12,13,15,16] We studied the effect of omeprazole EC 40 mg and found that basal acid secretion was decreased by 72% after one dose and by 89% after 9 doses. Pentagastrin stimulated acid secretion decreased by 55% and 62% respectively.[17] (fig. 1) In other studies a 67-91% inhibition of pentagastrin stimulated acid output was recorded after omeprazole 40 mg EC.[15,16,18,19] Omeprazole also inhibits vagally stimulated acid secretion after sham feeding.[20] The volume of secretion is also reduced by omeprazole, although to a lesser extent than gastric acid. In our study no effect on volume of basal secretion was documented, but pentagastrin-stimulated volume decreased by 40%.[17] (fig. 1)

In duodenal ulcer patients 24 hour intragastric acidity was measured during administration of omeprazole EC. Here again 10 and 20 mg doses showed considerable interindividual fluctuations.[10] A once daily 30 mg dose for one week caused a 95% decrease of intragastric acidity and a rise of the median pH from 1.4 to 5.3.[21] With 40 mg the inhibition was more than 99%.[22] One week after stopping treatment some decrease of nightly intragastric acidity was observed. However, after eight weeks there was complete return to pre-treatment levels.[10] Rebound hyperacidity was not observed in any subject.

An intravenous preparation of omeprazole became available recently. Two studies showed a rapid rise of the gastric pH > 4 within one hour after infusion, but unexpectedly large doses of intravenous omeprazole compared with oral omeprazole were needed to achieve an effect.[23,24]

In summary, omeprazole is the most potent known inhibitor of gastric acid secretion with a long duration of action. With doses of 30 and 40 mg, 24 hour intragastric acidity is virtually abolished. After stopping the drug there is no rebound acid hypersecretion and a gradual return to pre-treatment levels. The wide interindividual variation of the effect after lower doses of the drug is at least partly due to variable bioavailability, but also to the steep slope of the dose-response curve. This makes it difficult to achieve a partial decrease of intragastric acidity with omeprazole.

132

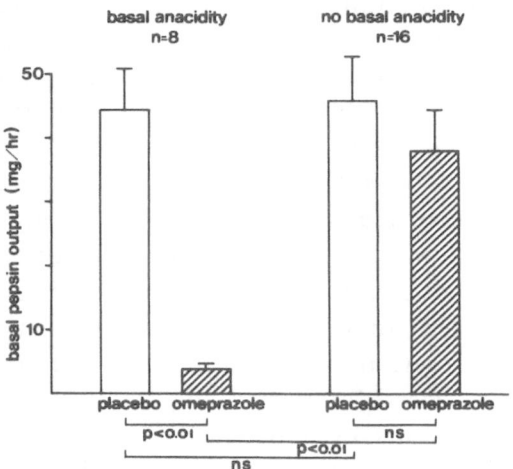

Figure 2. Basal pepsin output (mg/h; mean ± SEM) during placebo and omeprazole in sub-jects with concomitant basal anacidity during omeprazole administration (left) and no basal anacidity during omeprazole (right).

Effects on pepsin secretion

In several studies a decrease of pepsin secretion during treatment with omeprazole has been reported.[20,25,26] In our study basal pepsin output was unchanged after a single dose of omeprazole but was significantly reduced after repeated doses. Pentagastrin stimulated pepsin output was slightly decreased after a single dose of omeprazole and unaffected by repeated doses.[17] (fig. 1) The decrease in basal pepsin output after repeated doses was entirely due to findings in subjects with total basal anacidity during omeprazole: in those subjects basal pepsin output was significantly reduced by more than 90%, whereas in all other subjects, with no basal anacidity, basal pepsin output did not change significantly.[17] (fig. 2) It seems therefore that in the absence of gastric acid, no pepsin is secreted. In one of the studies mentioned earlier[15] pentagastrin stimulated pepsin secretion was measured after different doses of omeprazole and no change was observed (C. Cederberg, personal communication). Omeprazole in itself has therefore probably no effect on pepsin secretion. This is corroborated by the finding already cited that omeprazole had no effect on pepsinogen secretion in isolated chief cell preparations.[4]

Effects on intrinsic factor secretion

So far one study has been published reporting the effect of omeprazole on intrinsic factor secretion. No change in either basal or pentagastrin stimulated intrinsic factor secretion was measured.[25] This observation underlines the specificity of action of omeprazole: gastric acid and intrinsic factor are produced by the parietal cell and both are stimulated by pentagastrin, but only acid secretion is inhibited by omeprazole.

Effects on serum gastrin

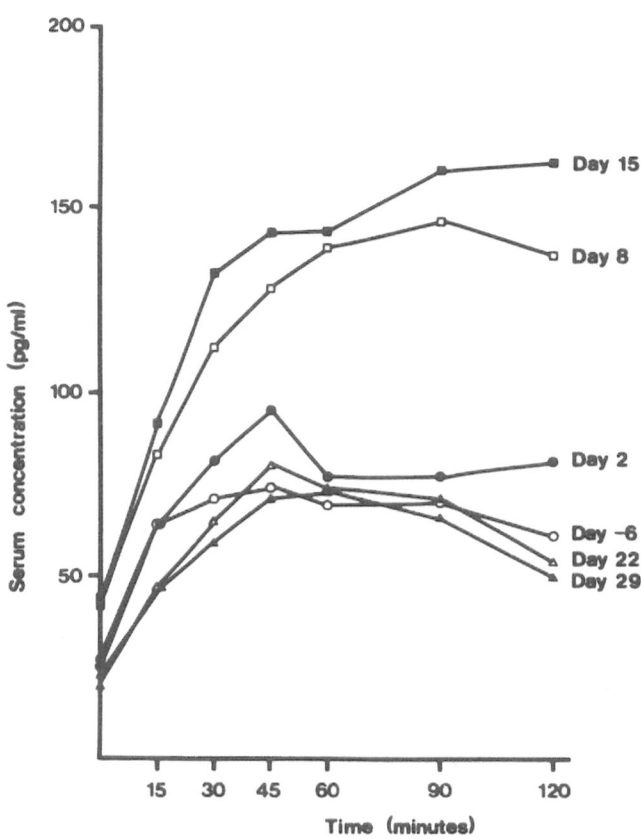

SERUM GASTRIN LEVELS AFTER A TEST MEAL

Figure 3. Mean serum gastrin levels (pg/ml) fasting and in response to a test meal in 8 healthy volunteers. Omeprazole, 30 mg daily, was administered for 14 days starting on day one.

As a result of the striking inhibition of intragastric acidity caused by omeprazole it was likely that serum gastrin levels would increase during treatment. This was indeed reported by several investigators.[10,17,27,28] More important is the question whether such a rise persists after stopping treatment, because if it does, it may cause rebound acid hypersecretion. During treatment with omeprazole 30 mg we found a rise of 63% of fasting concentration and of 138% of meal stimulated serum gastrin. After stopping treatment, serum gastrin levels normalized within one week, which parallels the duration of the inhibitory effect of omeprazole on acid secretion.[28] (fig. 3) Another study showed no rebound acid hypersecretion after treatment with omeprazole.[29]

No effect was seen on a variety of other gastrointestinal hormones after a single dose of omeprazole.[27]

Other effects

A rise in fasting serum pepsinogen I levels was seen during omeprazole treatment which normalized after stopping.[28] The clinical significance of this phenomenon is not clear, as it is not known how and why pepsinogens are released to the blood.

In rats omeprazole proved to have cytoprotective properties, but only after oral and not after intravenous, or intraperitoneal administration. This action of omeprazole seems not to be mediated by endogenous prostaglandin stimulation, as the effect was not blocked by indomethacin.[30,31]

Clinical studies

Expectations for the treatment of acid-peptic disease with omeprazole were pitched high. Indeed healing rates in duodenal ulcer reported up to now are high. After 4 weeks treatment with single daily doses of 20 mg or more ulcer healing was well above 90%. (Table II) Interestingly, healing rates after 2 weeks treatment were also very high and over 90% with a 40 and 60 mg dose.[32,33] Most studies published up to now are open studies,[18,19,33,36] some are double-blind dose findings trials[16,32,34] and all but one have rather low numbers of patients. One large double-blind study compared omeprazole 20 mg with ranitidine 300 mg in 334 patients.[35] In this study healing rates after

Table II. Results of treatment of duodenal ulcer with omeprazole.

Author (ref.)	n	Dose	% healed	
			2 wk	4 wk
Uusitalo[18]	15	40 mg	–	100
Damman[35]	146	20 mg	72	96
Vezzadini[36]	16	30 mg	94	100
Gustavsson[32]	16	20 mg	63	93
	16	60 mg	100	–
Br Coop Study[16]	10	20 mg	–	90
	12	30 mg	–	100
	10	40 mg	–	90
	11	60 mg	–	100
Prichard[34]	30	10 mg	53	83
	36	30 mg	78	90
Walan[33]	44	40 mg	93	100
Scand Multic St[19]	26	40 mg	–	96

two weeks treatment with omeprazole were 72% and with ranitidine 59% (p <0.02) and after 4 weeks treatment 96% and 92% respectively (NS). More large trials are needed to define the optimal dose and optimal length of treatment of duodenal ulcer with omeprazole. In all clinical trials the enteric coated formulation of omeprazole was used. From the pharmacological data of this preparation it seems logical to choose a dose for the treatment of acute duodenal ulcer of at least 20 mg daily or more as the effect on acid secretion of lower doses is too unpredictable.[10,13,14,15,16]

To date only two studies on the treatment of gastric ulcer with omeprazole have been published.

In one study the effect of omeprazole 20 mg was compared with ranitidine 300 mg in 183 patients.[37] Healing rates were comparable after 2, 4 and 8 weeks therapy (omeprazole: 43, 81, 95%; ranitidine 45, 80 and 90%). In another study 32 patients were treated openly with a 30 mg daily dose and healing rates were 22% after two, 72% after four and 100% after 8 weeks.[38]

Omeprazole is the drug of choice in the treatment of the Zollinger-Ellison syndrome.[39,40] It is not only very effective in reducing acid hypersecretion and relieving symptoms, but it also allows the patient to take drugs only once, or twice a day. The high potency of omeprazole and its non-competitive action are responsible for this remarkable result. Because of the latter, the high levels of endogenous

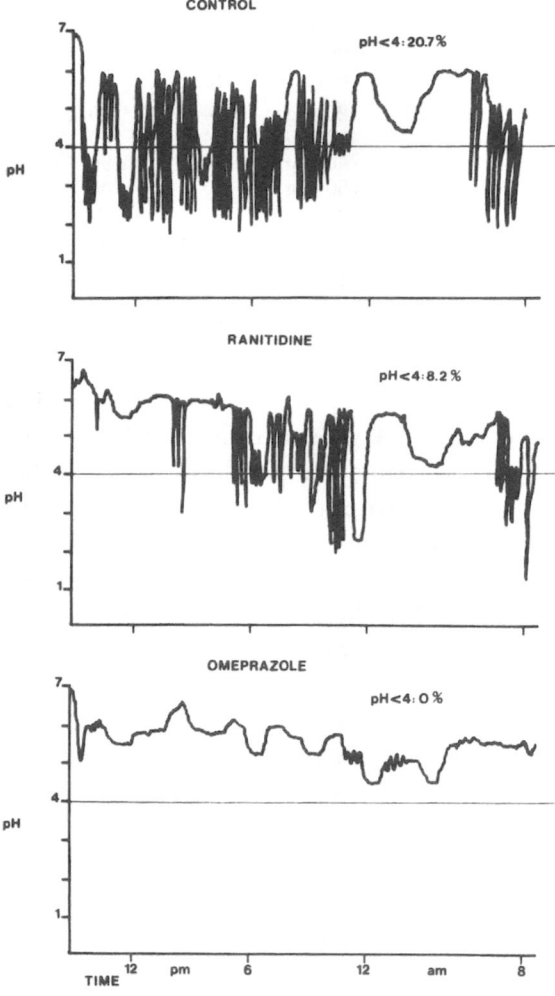

Figure 4. 24 Hour pH measurement in the oesophagus in one patient, studied before treatment (upper panel), during treatment with ranitidine 2 x 150 mg daily (middle panel) and during treatment with omeprazole 60 mg daily (lower panel).

gastrin, present in these patients, cannot overcome the blockade of acid secretion by omeprazole, whereas histamine H_2-receptor antagonists, acting competitively, are displaced from the receptors.

At present there is only one preliminary report on the treatment of reflux oesophagitis with omeprazole, showing a beneficial effect.[41] In our department 24 hour pH measurements in the oesophagus have been performed in a double-blind cross-over study in patients with severe reflux oesophagitis before and after 2 weeks treatment with ranitidine 2 x 150 mg and omeprazole 60 mg daily. Preliminary results are impressive for omeprazole. (Dr. E.C. Klinkenberg-Knol, personal communication). Figure 4 shows the results in one such a patient. These promising results warrant further study with omeprazole in reflux oesophagistis.

Safety

Because of its specific mode of action there were good hopes that omeprazole would be devoid of side-effects. Indeed in most trials no adverse effects have been reported. One study reported changes in liver function tests.[32] However, this finding was not confirmed by others[42] and could not be reproduced by the authors in follow-up studies.[43]

The sequelae of profound inhibition of gastric acid secretion, such as a rise in serum gastrin levels[28] and an increase in the gastric bacterial flora with endogenous production of N-nitroso compounds do take place.[44] However, after stopping the drug serum gastrin levels rapidly return to normal[28] and there is no indication of rebound acid hypersecretion.[10,29] Similarly the intragastric bacterial flora returns to pre-treatment values soon after omeprazole is discontinued.[44] It is not likely that these changes will be clinically important during short-term treatment with omeprazole, but caution is warranted during long-term use and further studies are needed. Intermittent treatment with omeprazole for benign conditions may be a solution for these problems.

Omeprazole interferes with the excretion of drugs through the cytochrome P450 system in the liver. There is, however, no consensus about the degree of this interference. In man, the elimination of diazepam is substantially inhibited.[45] Other studies show a much lesser degree of inhibition of aminopyrine and antipyrine elimination in man[46] and antipyrine and pentobarbitone elimination in the rat.[47,48] A possible explanation for this discrepancy is that cytochrome P450 consists of a multiplicity of enzymes and that omeprazole selectively binds to only some of them. Further studies will have to clarify the clinical significance of this interference of omeprazole.

Castric emptying is not influenced by omeprazole.[49]

Omeprazole does not interfere with renal electrolyte turnover and urinary acidification.[50] This provides further evidence for its specificity of action.

An important observation, however, led to a temporary suspension of clinical studies with omeprazole. In 2 year toxicity studies in rats an increase in enterochromaffin-like cells (ECL cells) and gastric carcinoids has been observed, predominantly in female rats and only in animals treated with very high doses of omeprazole (A.B. Hässle, personal communication). Similar abnormalities were not seen in dogs, or mice. It seems that the enormously increased serum gastrin levels in these rats are responsible for this phenomenon: it is known that antrum exclusion in rats leads to hypergastrinemia and subsequently to hyperplasia of oxyntic ECL cells.[51] In antrectomized rats treated with omeprazole no such increases in ECL cells were seen (A.B. Hässle, personal communication). ECL cells are much more frequent in rats than in man and serum gastrin levels during omeprazole treatment are 10 times lower in man than in rats. Furthermore gastric carcinoids are very rare in man even in coditions associated with hypergastrineamia such as the Zollinger-Ellison syndrome and pernicious aneamia.[52] Therefore there are no indications that treatment of patients with omeprazole will imply a risk for the development of carcinoids. Recently omeprazole was re-released for use in clinical trials.

Summary and future outlook

Omeprazole is a potent and very selective inhibitor of gastric acid secretion. No side-effects have been reported in man. It is effective in healing duodenal ulcer and the best drug currently available for the treatment of the Zollinger-Ellison syndrome. Results of treatment of gastric ulcer and reflux oesophagitis are promising, but need further study. Without doubt it is the drug of choice in conditions requiring a strong inhibition of gastric acid secretion, therefore its role in the prevention of stress ulceration needs to be evaluated. Short-term treatment with omeprazole seems safe, but potential deleterious effects of long-term pronounced inhibition of acid secretion have to be taken into account during maintenance treatment. Intermittent treatment may prove preferable in certain conditions. Possible interference with the excretion of other drugs has to be studied.

References

1. Fellenius E, Berglindh T, Sachs G, et al. Substituted benzimidazoles inhibit gastric acid secretion by blocking H^+-K^+ ATP-ase. Nature 1981;290: 159–161.
2. Sjöstrand SE, Ryberg B, Olbe L. Stimulation and inhibition of acid secretion in the isolated guinea pig gastric mucosa. Acta Physiol Scand 1978;spec. suppl.:181 – 5.
3. Wallmark B, Jaresten BM, Larsson H, Ryberg B, Brändström A, Fellenius E. Differentiation among inhibitory actions of omeprazole, cimetidine, and SCN^- on gastric acid secretion. Am J Physiol 1983;245:G64–71.
4. Fryklund J, Wallmark B, Larsson H, Helander HF. Effect of omeprazole on gastric secretion in H^+-K^+ ATP-ase and in pepsinogen-rich cell fractions from rabbit gastric mucosa. Biochem Pharmacol 1984;33:273–80.
5. Helander HF, Ramsay CH. Localization of omeprazole in the mouse. Gastroenterology 1984;86(2):1109.
6. Londong W, Londong V, Cederberg C, Steffen H. Dose-response study of omeprazole on meal-stimulated gastric acid secretion and gastrin release. Gastroenterology 1983;85:1373–8.
7. Lind T, Cederberg C, Ekenved G, Haglund U, Olbe L. Effect of omeprazole – a gastric proton pump inhibitor – on pentagastrin stimulated acid secretion in man. Gut 1983;24:270–6.
8. Prichard PJ, Yeomans ND, Mihaly GW, et al. Omeprazole: A study of its inhibition of gastric pH and oral pharmacokinetics after morning or evening dosage. Gastroenterology 1985;88:64–9.
9. Howden CW, Meredith PA, Forrest JAH, Reid JL. Oral pharmacokinetics of omeprazole. Eur J Clin Pharmacol 1984;26:641–3.
10. Sharma BK, Walt RP, Pounder RE, Gomes M de FA, Wood EC, Logan LH. Optimal dose of oral omeprazole for maximal 24 hour decrease of intragastric acidity. Gut 1984;25:957–64.
11. Carlsson E, Karlsson A, Larsson H, Löfberg I, Sundell G, Skånberg I. Concentration of omeprazole in blood and gastric mucosa and the relation to inhibition of gastric acid secretion. Gastroenterology 1984;86(2):1041.
12. Müller P, Dammann HG, Seitz H, Simon B. Effect of repeated, once daily, oral omeprazole on gastric secretion. Lancet 1983;1:66.
13. Stenderup J, Mertz A, Wandall JH, Bonnevie O. The inhibition of gastric-acid secretion by omeprazole in daily doses of 10 and 20 mg. Scand J Gastroenterol 1984;19(suppl 98):48.
14. Prichard PJ, Yeomans ND, Jones DB, McNeil JJ, Louis WJ, Smallwood RA. Effect of morning or evening dosage with 10 mg omeprazole on 24 H gastric pH in duodenal ulcer patients in remission. Gastroenterology 1984;86(2):1213.

15. Cederberg C, Lind T, Axelson M, Olbe L. Long term acid inhibitory effect of different daily doses of omeprazole 24 hours after dosing. Gastroenterology 1984;86(2):1043.
16. Cooperative study. Omeprazole in duodenal ulceration: Acid inhibition, symptom relief, endoscopic healing, and recurrence. Br Med J 1984;289: 525 – 8.
17. Festen HPM, Tuynman HARE, Défize J, Frants RR, Straub JP, Meuwissen SGM. The effect of single and repeated doses of oral omeprazole on gastric acid and pepsin secretion and fasting serum gastrin and serum pepsinogen I levels. Gastroenterology.
18. Uusitalo A, Keyriläinen O, Salaspuro M, Tarpila S. Effect of omeprazole on duodenal ulcer healing and acid secretion. XII International Congress of Gastroenterology Lisbon, Portugal 1984; abstract 31.
19. Scandinavian multicenter study. Gastric acid secretion and duodenal ulcer healing during treatment with omeprazole. Scand J Gastroenterol 1984;19: 882 – 4.
20. Konturek SJ, Kweicien N, Obtulowicz W, Kopp B, Olesky J. Action of omeprazole (a benzimidazole derivate) on secretory responses to sham feeding and pentagastrin and upon serum gastrin and pancreatic polypeptide in duodenal ulcer patients. Gut 1984;25:14 – 8.
21. Walt RP, Gomes M de FA, Wood EC, Logan LH, Pounder RE. Effect of daily oral omeprazole on 24 hour intragastric acidity. Br Med J 1983;287: 12 – 4.
22. Naesdal J, Bodeman G, Walan A. Effect of omeprazole, a substituted benzimidazole, on 24-H intragastric acidity in patients with peptic ulcer disease. Scand J Gastroenterol 1984;19:916 – 22.
23. Walt RP, Reynolds JR, Langman MJS, et al. Intravenous omeprazole rapidly raises intragastric pH. Gut 1984;25:1139 – 40.
24. Lind T, Moore M, Olbe L. Intravenous omeprazole: Effect on 24-hour intragastric pH. XII International Congress of Gastroenterology Lisbon, Portugal 1984, abstract 651.
25. Kittang E, Aadland E, Schjønsby H. Effect of omeprazole on acid, pepsin and intrinsic factor (IF) secretion in healthy subjects. Scand J Gastroenterol 1984;19(suppl 98):2.
26. Wilson Ja, Boyd EJS, Wormsley KG. Effect of intraduodenal omeprazole on gastric acid and pepsin secretion. Gut 1983;24:A497 – 8.
27. Allen JM, Adrian TE, Webster J, Howe A, Bloom SR. Effect of single dose of omeprazole on the gastrointestinal peptide response to food. Hepato-Gastroenterol 1984;31:44 – 6.
28. Festen HPM, Thijs JC, Lamers CBHW, et al. Effect of oral omeprazole on serum gastrin and serum pepsinogen I levels. Gastroenterology 1984;87: 1030 – 4.
29. Sharma BK, Lundborg P, Pounder RE, et al. Acid secretory capacity after treatment with omeprazole. Gastroenterology 1984;86(2):1246.
30. Mattsson H, Anderson K, Larsson H. Omeprazole provides protection against experimentally induced gastrin mucosal lesions. Eur J Pharmacol 1983;91:111 – 4.
31. Kollberg B, Isenberg JI, Johansson C. Cytoprotective effect of omeprazole on the rat gastric mucosa. In: Allen A, et al (Eds). Mechanisms of mucosal protection in the upper gastrointestinal tract. Raven Press, New York 1984:351 – 5.
32. Gustavsson S, Adami HO, Lööf L, Nyberg A, Nyrén O. Rapid healing of

duodenal ulcers with omeprazole: double-blind dose-comparative trial. Lancet 1983;2:124 – 5.

33. Walan A, Bergsaker-Aspöy J, Farup P, et al. Four week study of the rate of duodenal ulcer healing with omeprazole. Gut 1983;24:A972.

34. Prichard PJ, Rubinstein D, Jones DB, et al. Omeprazole: Double-blind comparison of 10 mg versus 30 mg for healing duodenal ulcers. Gastroenterology 1984;86(2):1213.

35. Dammann HG, Classen M, Domschke W, et al. Omeprazole is superior to ranitidine within two weeks' treatment of duodenal ulcer. XII International Congress of Gastroenterology Lisbon, Portugal 1984, abstract 1274.

36. Vezzadini P, Rinetti M, Tomassetti P, et al. Healing of duodenal ulcer with omeprazole. XII International Congress of Gastroenterology Lisbon, Portugal 1984, abstract 431.

37. Londong W, Classen M, Dammann HG, et al. Omeprazole versus ranitidine for gastric ulcer – results of a german multicenter trial. XII International Congress of Gastroenterology Lisbon, Portugal 1984, abstract 1299.

38. Hütteman W. Kurzzeitbehandlung des Ulcus ventriculi mit Omeprazol in einmal täglicher dosierung. Dtsch med Wschr 1985;110:38 – 9.

39. Lamers CBHW, Lind T, Moberg S, Jansen JBMJ, Olbe L. Omeprazole in Zollinger-Ellison syndrome. Effects of a single dose and of long-term treatment in patients resistant to histamine H_2-receptor antagonists. New Engl J Med 1984;310:758 – 61.

40. McArthur KE, Collen MJ, Cherner JA, et al. Omeprazole as a single daily dose is effective therapy in Zollinger-Ellison syndrome. Gastroenterology 1984;86(2):1178.

41. Dent J, Heddle R, Downton J, Mackinnon M, Toouli J, Lewis I. Omeprazole heals ulcerative peptic oesophagitis. Gastroenterology 1984;86(2):1062.

42. Sharma BK, Santana IA, Walt RP, Pounder RE. Omeprazole and liver function tests. Lancet 1983;2:346.

43. Lööf L, Adami HO, Gustavsson S, Nyberg A, Nyren O, Lundborg P. Omeprazole: no evidence for frequent hepatic reactions. Lancet 1984;1:1347 – 8.

44. Sharma BK, Santana IA, Wood EC, et al. Intragastric bacterial activity and nitrosation before, during, and after treatment with omeprazole. Br Med J 1984;289:717 – 9.

45. Gugler R, Jensen JC. Omeprazole inhibits elimination of diazepam. Lancet 1984;1:969.

46. Henry DA, Somerville KW, Kitchingman G, Langman JS. Omeprazole: Effects on oxidative drug metabolism. Br J Clin Pharmacol 1984;18:195 – 200.

47. Webster LK, Jones DB, Mihaly GW, Smallwood RA. Effect of omeprazole in polyethylene glycol-400 on antipyrine elimination by the isolated perfused rat liver. J Pharm Pharmacol 1984;36:470 – 2.

48. Henry DA, Gerkens JF, Brent P, Somerville K. Inhibition of drug metabolism by omeprazole. Lancet 1984;2:46.

49. Horowitz M, Hetzel DJ, Buckle PJ, Chatterton BE, Shearman DJC. The effect of omeprazole on gastric emptying in patients with duodenal ulcer disease. Br J Clin Pharmacol 1984;18:791 – 4.

50. Howden CW, Reid JL. Omeprazole, a gastric 'proton pump inhibitor': Lack of effect on renal handling of electrolytes and urinary acidification. Eur J Clin Pharmacol 1984;26:639 – 40.

51. Alumets J, El Munshid HA, Håkanson R, et al. Effect of antrum exclusion on endocrine cells of rat stomach. J Physiol 1979;286:145 – 55.

52. Wilander E. Achylia and the development of gastric carcinoids. Virchows Arch (pathol Anat) 1981;394:151 – 60.

11. Medical treatment of peptic ulcer with prostaglandins

G.N.J. TIJTGAT, M.D.

Division of Gastroenterology-Hepatology, University of Amsterdam, Academic Medical Center, Amsterdam, The Netherlands

Several prostaglandins have been shown to inhibit the secretion of acid and pepsin by the stomach of various species. They possess anti-ulcer acitivity in the upper gastrointestinal tract in animal models and have beneficial 'cytoprotective' effects on the integrity of the gastric mucosa when it is exposed to noxious stimuli in animals and man. The 'cytoprotective' effect of prostaglandins is independent of the anti-secretory action.[1]

Patients with peptic ulcer disease have therefore been investigated because of the anti-secretory, anti-ulcer and 'cytoprotective' properties of prostaglandins.

Effects of prostaglandins upon the human stomach mucosa

After administration of 15(R)-15-methyl-PG E_2 (arbaprostil) to healthy volunteers in anti-secretory doses for two months, the mucosal lining of the antrum and fundus becomes thicker.[2] Similar observations have been made in animal studies.[3,4] We investigated the morphological changes in the gastric mucosa with oral administration of arbaprostil to 25 healthy male volunteers. The volunteers were randomized into two groups: a prostaglandin and a placebo group. The prostaglandin group was given arbaprostil 100 μg q.i.d. for two months and placebo for another two months. The placebo group was given placebo only throughout the four months period. Arbaprostil and placebo capsules were taken one hour before each meal and at bed time.

Endoscopic forceps biopsies using a large calibre endoscope (Olympus Gif-1T and FB-13U) were obtained immediately before treatment and at the end of each two months period. Biopsies were

144

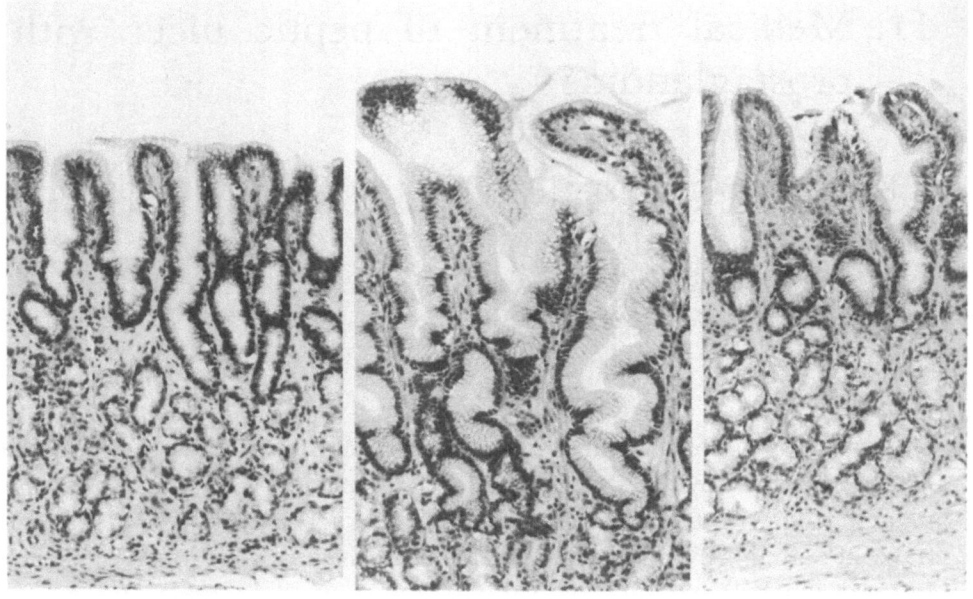

Figure 1. Low toner photograph of antral mucosa baseline after two months of prostaglandin therapy and after two further months of placebo. Note the thickening of the mucosal layer after prostaglandin therapy.

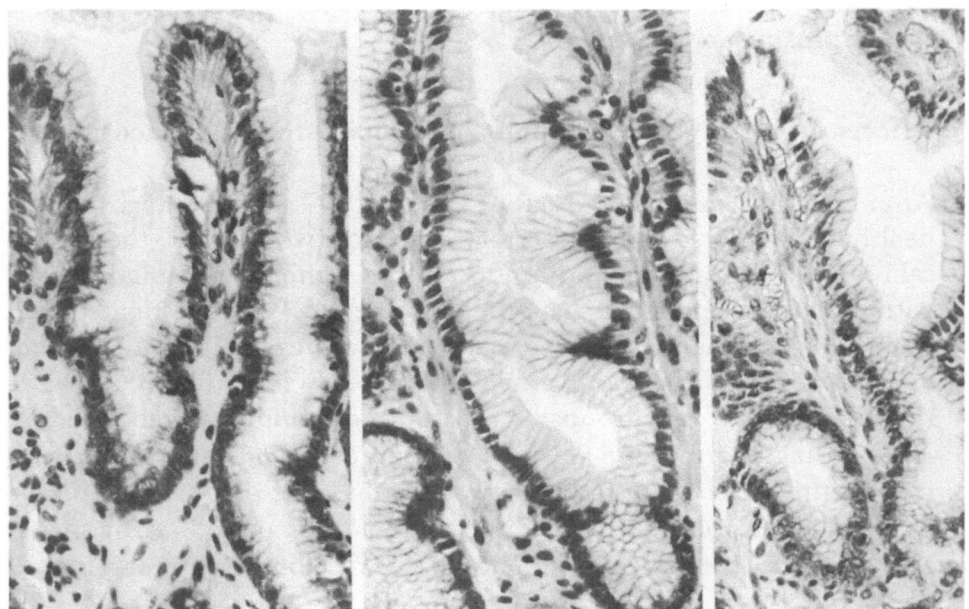

Figure 2. High toner photograph of antral mucosa, before, after two months of prostaglandin therapy, followed by two months of placebo. Note the enlargement of the mucus secreting layer.

taken from the antrum and the fundus and immediately processed for histology, electron microscopy and cell kinetic studies.

In the histology sections the total mucosal and total foveolar height, number foveolar cells and foveolar cell height at the mid-position of the foveolae were measured with a calibrated eye piece micrometer. The biopsies were incubated for cell kinetic studies with 25 μCi tritiated thymidine and studied by autoradiography. The approximate boundaries of the proliferative zone (PZ) were defined by the localization of the uppermost and lowermost labelled cell in the cell column. The labelling index (LI) was defined as the ratio between the number of labelled cells and the total number of cells in the proliferative zone $\times$ 100%.[5] The localization of the labelled cells in the gastric pits was determined in relation to a reference position (R = 0), which was the limit between the last foveolar, or neck cell and the first specialized glandular cell.[6]

After prostaglandin administration for two months the total antral mucosal thickness and the antral and fundic foveolar thickness increased by 36%, 44%, and 51% respectively. Not only the number of the cells increased, but also their height and width. After stopping treatment there was a complete return to pre-treatment values within two months. (figs. 1 and 2) In the placebo group no changes were detected.

In the electron microscopy study no changes in the ultrastructure of the parietal cell were observed after prostaglandin treatment. The labelling index, representing cell proliferation, of the placebo and prostaglandin group are summarized in Table I.

The labelling index after two months prostaglandin treatment is not statistically significantly different from the pre-treatment and placebo values. Neither did the localization of the proliferative zone differ in the autoradiographic studies.

Because the morphologic changes demonstrated above cannot be attributed to alterations of proliferative activity (Table I), it seems

Table I. Determination of labelling index (LI) after prostaglandin (PGE$_2$) or placebo (p) therapy (mean $\pm$ SD).[7,8]

		0	2 months	4 months
LI antrum	PGE$_2$	7.75 $\pm$ 2.75	6.68 $\pm$ 2.37	7.82 $\pm$ 2.40
	p	7.38 $\pm$ 2.16	7.48 $\pm$ 1.81	8.06 $\pm$ 2.87
LI fundus	PGE$_2$	6.20 $\pm$ 2.58	6.13 $\pm$ 2.36	8.90 $\pm$ 3.05
	p	7.91 $\pm$ 1.41	8.42 $\pm$ 2.94	8.28 $\pm$ 1.88

logical to explain the foveolar expansion by retarded senescence and retarded exfoliation of the surface epithelium, presumably as a consequence of the protective action of the prostaglandin against luminal noxious factors.[7,8]

A similar retarded cell shedding due to prostaglandin therapy has been demonstrated in animals[9] and in humans after ethanol damage.[10]

The absence of enhanced proliferative activity observed in humans is at variance with the slight increase in labelling index at the end of three weeks PGE_2 administration in the rat.[11,12]

Prostaglandins and the pathogenesis of peptic ulcer

The local generation of some prostaglandins from arachidonic acid, via the cyclooxygenase pathway[13,14] has been shown to enhance bicarbonate and mucus secretion, mucosal blood flow and other factors that strengthen mucosal resistance.[15-18] Several *in vivo* studies have shown that the pathogenesis of peptic ulcer disease may involve a lack of, or a decrease in endogenous prostanoids.[19] Normally, prostaglandin synthesis by duodenal mucosa increases proportionally to the duodenal acid load.[20] In patients with duodenal ulcer disease this activation of prostaglandin synthesis seems to fail. Decreased gastric prostanoid content in patients with gastric ulcer has also been reported.[21] Whether these changes are of primary pathogenic importance, or secondary to mucosal damage and inflammation, is uncertain at present.

Prostaglandins used in peptic ulcer disease

Not only native prostaglandins such as PGE_2, but also prostaglandin analogues have been used in the therapy of peptic ulcer disease. These analogues have been found not only to be more potent than natural prostaglandins as inhibitors of gastric acid secretion, but also to be effective when administered orally.

Drugs most commonly used in the therapy of peptic ulcer disease at present are PGE_2, 15(R)-15-methyl PGE_2 (arbaprostil, Arbacet®), 15-deoxy, 16-hydroxy, 16-methyl PGE_1 methyl esther (misoprostol, Cytotec®), and trimethyl PGE_2 (trimopostil). Arbaprostil and misoprostol have been evaluated most extensively.

Initially it was thought that the action of PGE_2, given orally, was mainly cytoprotective. However, recent studies have shown that oral PGE_2 in man is anti-secretory with an ED_{50} of 1.1 mg.[22] Overall PGE_2 is not as potent an inhibitor of gastric acid production as a number of chemically modified analogues.

In addition the anti-secretory activity starts to wane at the end of one hour. This difference in anti-secretory activity may be related to a difference in metabolism. PGE_2 is first metabolized by oxidation of the 15-hydroxyl to a ketone, followed by reduction of the 13 – 14 double bond.[23] With the addition of one or two methyl groups at the 15 or 16 position, this series of metabolic steps is inhibited.[24]

Arbaprostil is not only a potent inhibitor of gastric acid and pepsin secretion,[25-28] but is also a powerful stimulant of gastric mucus production when given orally.[29] In the presence of acid, arbaprostil is rapidly converted to a mixture of 15(R) and 15(S)-15-methyl PGE_2 which has both anti-secretory and cytoprotective properties. Arbaprostil inhibits about 50% of meal-stimulated gastric acid secretion in normal volunteers at a dose of 10 μg.[30]

Misoprostol also has been shown to inhibit the gastric secretion of acid and pepsin[31-33] and has cytoprotective effects upon the gastric mucosa of animals and man.[34-37] Anti-ulcer activity has been demonstrated in animal models.[38]

Therapeutic efficacy of prostaglandins in peptic ulcer disease

Several clinical studies have evaluated the therapeutic efficacy of prostaglandins in peptic ulcer disease. The studies were based on the observation that prostaglandins have marked inhibitory effects on gastric acid and pepsin secretion and a stimulatory effect on gastric secretion of mucus together with cytoprotective properties. Some of the early studies, summarized in Table II and more extensively discussed elsewhere[39] suggest that gastric and duodenal ulcer healing may be obtained with various prostaglandins.

The more recent results with natural PGE_2 are summarized in Table III. PGE_2 was given in a dose of 2.5 mg per day (0.5 mg t.i.d. and 1 mg nocte). Both Kollberg et al[30] and Johansson et al[3] obtained duodenal ulcer healing in a large percentage of patients. The results obtained by Chen et al[44] were somewhat less convincing.

Table II. Endoscopic healing rates (%) of duodenal ulcer (DU) and gastric ulcer (GU) on prostaglandins (PG) and placebo (p).

Author	No		Dose	Dur (w)	% healing PG	p	Statistically sign.
Karim et al[25]	19	GU	600 mcg 15(R)-15-methyl PGE$_2$	2	70	22	+
Fung et al[40]	20	GU	600 mcg 15(R)-15-methyl PGE$_2$	2	63	17	+
Fung et al[41]	20	GU	4 mg PGE$_2$	2	42	14	+
Gibinski et al[42]	77	DU + GU	~5 mcg 15(R)-15-methyl PGE$_2$	2	65	46	+
			~6 mcg 15(R)-15-methyl PGE$_2$	2	65	46	–
Rybicka et al[43]	117	DU + GU	PGE$_2$ methylanlologues	2	65	46	+

Table III. Endoscopic healing rates (%) of duodenal ulcer after 4 weeks treatment with prostaglandin E$_2$ (PG) and placebo (p).

Author	No	Dose	Dur (w)	% healing PG	p	Statistically sing.
Kollberg et al[30]	28	2.5 mg	4	86	43	+
Johansson et al[3]	25	2.5 mg	4	91	46	+
Chen et all[44]	35	1.5	4	73	50	

Table IV. Endoscopic healing rates (%) of duodenal ulcer after 4 weeks treatment with 15(R)-15-methyl prostaglandin E$_2$ (PG) and placebo (p).

Author	No	Dose	Dur (w)	% healing PG	p	Statistically sing.	Increased bowel frequency (%)
Tijtgat et al[45]	40	4 × 100 mcg	4	69	33	+	
Vantrappen et al[46]	173	4 × 100 mcg	4	67	39	+	33

Table IV summarizes the results obtained with arbaprostil 100 µg q.i.d. which significantly accelerated healing rates when compared with placebo.

With the dose of 100 μg four times daily for a 4-week period, a substantial proportion of patients noticed increased bowel frequency and even occasional diarrhea. Since then, arbaprostil has been administered to over 1000 patients with acute upper GI-bleeding (50 μg q.i.d. for 7 days), gastric ulcer (10 and 25 μg q.i.d. for 42 days), duodenal ulcer (10 and 25 μg q.i.d. for 28 days) and NSAID-induced gastric mucosal damage (10 and 25 μg q.i.d. for 28 days) with no statistically significant unwanted effects.

Table V. Endoscopic healing rates (%) of duodenal ulcer and gastric ulcer comparing 16-methyl esther PGE_1 (PGE_1) therapy with placebo (p) and cimetidine (CIM).

Author	No	Dose	Dur (w)	% healing PGE_1	p	CIM (1.2 g)	Statistically sign.	Increased bowel frequency (%)
Duodenal ulcer								
Brand et al[47]	207	4 × 200 mcg	4	77	51	–	+	13
Arvanitakis et al[48]	36	4 × 200 mcg	4	75	–	91	–	
Multicenter[49,50]	467	4 × 200 mcg	4	60	–	67	–	13
Gastric ulcer								
Multicenter[51]	266	4 × 200 mcg	4	58	–	60	–	

The results obtained with misoprostol are summarized in Table V. Only the data obtained with a dose of 200 μg q.i.d. are shown, because a dose of 50 μg q.i.d. was ineffective in all trials. In two of three trials where misoprostol was compared with cimetidine, the healing rates were similar with the histamine H_2-receptor antagonist and the prostaglandin. In one multicenter gastric ulcer study, healing was recorded in 58% of misoprostol treated patients, compared with 60% with cimetidine. In two of the studies, increased bowel frequency was noted in 13% of the patients.

Table VI. Endoscopic healing rates (%) of duodenal ulcer on trimethyl prostaglandin E_2 (PG) compared with cimetidine (CIM).

Author	No	Dose	Dur (w)	% healing PGE_2	CIM (Ig)
Bardhan[52]	60	4 × 750 mcg	4	62	90

The duodenal ulcer healing rate obtained with trimethyl PGE_2, shown in Table VI, is low when compared with cimetidine.

Concluding remarks

The therapeutic applications of prostaglandins in gastrointestinal disease are still limited at present, but it is beyond doubt that these drugs can accelerate healing of gastric and duodenal ulcer. In several studies healing rates were similar to those obtained with cimetidine. In most of the studies, stool frequency increased in a substantial percentage of the patients. Another disadvantage of all prostaglandins of the E type is their capability of inducing contractions of the pregnant uterus. Their administration to women who are, or who may become pregnant is therefore prohibited. At present, trials are being conducted with arbaprostil in a dose of 10 μg q.i.d. which is cytoprotective only, or 25 μg q.i.d. which is predominantly cytoprotective and weakly anti-secretory. Results should indicate whether healing occurs comparable to the larger prostaglandin doses without increased bowel frequency.

The results of these trials have to be awaited before one can consider the prostaglandins as a first-line drug in the treatment of peptic ulcer disease. Theoretically, one certainly should consider prostaglandins for therapy, provided well tolerated and long-acting preparations become available, and provided it can be shown that these preparations are capable of improving the underlying inflammatory mucosal changes and thereby retard recurrence of peptic ulcer disease.

If it can be shown that peptic ulcer disease, especially gastric ulcer, is mainly related to a deficiency of endogenous prostaglandin production, repair of this deficiency by oral prostaglandins would be logical.

To answer these questions, investigators should study the degree and the extent of gastritis and the tissue concentrations of prostaglandins in patients with gastric ulcer, not only before, but also after therapy with anti-ulcer drugs. It is intriguing to note that there is a preliminary suggestion that the endogenous mucosal prostaglandin production seems to rise with treatment with sucralfate and colloidal bismuth subcitrate, two drugs which may retard ulcer recurrence in comparison with recurrence rates after histamine H_2-receptor antagonists.

Synthetic prostaglandins are being tested for therapeutic efficacy in other upper gastrointestinal tract disorders. One area of interest is the prevention of gastric mucosal damage after treatment with non-steroidal anti-imflammatory drugs in patients with rheumatoid arthritis. Another one is adjunctive therapy with prostaglandins in patients with upper gastrointestinal haemorrhage.

References

1. Robert A. Cytoprotection by prostaglandins. Gastroenterology 1979;77:761–7.
2. Tijtgat GN, Henzen-Logmans SC, van Minnen AJ. Human gastric mucosal changes after oral 15(R)-15 methyl prostaglandinE$_2$ (Pg) administration. Gastroenterology 1982;82:1200A.
3. Johansson C, Aly A, Kollberg B, Rubio C, Erikoinen T, Helander HF. In: Samuelson B, Paoletti R, Ramwell P (Eds). Advances in Prostaglandins, Thromboxane, and Leukotriene Research, Vol 12. New York, Raven Press 1982403–407.
4. Reinhart WH, Müller O, Halter F. Influence of long-term 16,16-dimethyl prostaglandin E$_2$ treatment on the rat gastrointestinal mucosa. Gastroenterology 1983;85:1003–1010.
5. Hart Hansen O, Pedersen T, Larsen JK. Gastric mucosal cell proliferation in duodenal ulcer patients. Gut 1975;16:23–7.
6. Willems G, Vansteenkiste Y, Verbenstel S. Autoradiographic study of cell renewal in fundic mucosa of fasting dogs. Acta Anat 1971;80:23–32.
7. Offerhaus GJA, Tijtgat GN, Samson G, Weinstein WM. Cell proliferation kinetics of the gastric mucosa after oral 15(R)-15-methyl prostaglandin E$_2$ (PG) administration. Gastroenterology 1984;86:1199A.
8. Tijtgat GNJ, Offerhaus GJA, van Minnen AJ, Everts V, Hensen-Logmans SC, Samson G. Influence of oral 15(R)-15-methyl PGE$_2$ on human gastric mucosa. A light – microscopic, cell-kinetic and ultrastructural study. Gastroenterology: to be published.
9. Robert A, Hanchar AJ, Lancaster C, Nezamis JE, Culp JW, Li LH. Prevention of cellular shedding as a mechanism of gastric cytoprotection by prostaglandins. Gastroenterology 1980;78:1244.
10. Ruppin H, Person B, Robert A, Domschke W. Gastric cytoprotection in man by prostaglandin E$_2$. Scand J Gastroenterol 1981;16:647–652.
11. Halter F, Meyrat P, Fritsche R, Müller O, Lentze MJ, Koelz HR. Both topical and systemic treatment with 16,16-dimethyl prostaglandin E$_2$ are trophic to rat gastric mucosa. Scand J Gastroenterology 1984a;19(Suppl 101):47–54.
12. Halter F, Reinhart WH, Koelz HR, Meyrat P, Lentze MJ, Müller O. 16,16-dimethyl prostaglandin E$_2$ stimulates growth and maturation of rat gastric and small intestinal mucosa. Scand J Gastroenteroly 1984b;19(Suppl 92):178–183.
13. Ramwell PW. Biologic importance of arachidonic acid. Arch Intern Med 1981; 14:275.
14. Ahlquist DA, Duenes JA, Madson TH et al. Prostaglandin generation from gastroduodenal mucosa: Regional and species differences. Prostaglandins 1982; 24:115.

15. Johansson C, Kollberg B. Stimulation by itnragastrically administered E_2 prostaglandins of human gastric mucus output. Eur J Clin Invest 1979;9:229.

16. Robert A, Nezamis JE, Lancaster C et al. Cytoprotection by prostaglandins in rats: prevention of gastric necrosis produced by alcohol, HCl, NaOH, hypertonic NaCl and thermal injury. Gastroenterology 1979;77:433.

17. Allen A, Garner A. Mucus and bicarbonate secretion in the stomach and their possible role in mucosal protection. Gut 1980;21:249.

18. Konturek SJ, Brzozowski T, Piastucki I et al. Role of locally generated prostaglandins in adaptive gastric cytoprotection. Dig Dis Sci 1982;27:967.

19. Sharon P, Zifroni A, Ligumsky M. Prostanoid synthesis by cultered gastric and duodenal mucosa: Possible role in the pathogenesis of duodenal ulcer. Scand J Gastroenterology 1983;18:1045 – 9.

20. Ahlquist DA, Dozius RR, Zinsmeister AR et al. Duodenal prostaglandin synthesis and acid load in health and in duodenal ulcer disease. Gastroenterology 1983;85:522.

21. Wright JP, Young GO, Klaff LJ et al. Gastric mucosal prostaglandin E levels in patients with gastric ulcer disease and carcinoma. Gastroenterology 1982; 82:263.

22. Reele GB, Bohan D. Oral antisecretory activity of prostaglandin E_2 in man. Dig Dis Sci 1984;29:390 – 393.

23. Samuelsson B, Grantstrom E, Green K, Hamberg M. Metabolism of prostaglandins. Ann NY Acad Sci 1971;180:139 – 161.

24. Magerlein BJ, Ducharme DW, Magee WE, Miller WL, Robert A, Weeks JR. Synthesis and biological properties of 16-alkylprostaglandins. Prostaglandins 1973;4(1):143 – 144.

25. Karim SMM, Carter DC, Bhana D, Ganesan PA. Effect of orally administered prostaglandin E_2 and its 15-methyl analogues on gastric secretion. Brit Med J 1973;1:143 – 146.

26. Salmon JA, Karim SMM, Carter DC, Adaikan PG, Bhana D. Effect of 15(R) 15-methyl PGE_2 methylester on basal and pentagastrin stimulated pepsin secretion in men. Int Res Comm Syst (Medical Science) 1975;3:83.

27. Konturek SJ, Kwiecien N, Swierczek J, Oleksy J, Sito E, Robert A. Comparison of methylated prostaglandin E_2 analogues given orally in the inhibition of gastric responses to pentagastrin and peptone meal in man. Gastroenterology 1976;70:683 – 687.

28. Robert A, Schultz JR, Nezamis JE, Lancaster C. Gastric antisecretory and antiulcer properties of PGE_2, 15-methyl PGE_2 and 16,16 dimethyl PGE_2. Gastroenterology 1976;70:359 – 370.

29. Fung WP, Lee SK, Karim SMM. Effect of prostaglandin 15(R) 15-methyl-E_2-methyl ester on the gastric mucosa in patients with peptic ulceration. An endoscopic and histological study. Prostaglandin 1974;5:465 – 472.

30. Kollberg B, Slezak P. The effect of prostaglandin E_2 on duodenal ulcer healing. Prostaglandins 1982:24:527.

31. Dajani EZ, Driskill D, Bianchi R, Collins P, Pappo R. Sc 29333: A potent inhibitor of canine gastric secretion. Am J Dig 1976;21:1049 – 1057.

32. Colton DG, Driskill DR, Phillips EL, Poy P, Dajani EZ. Effect of SC 29333 an inhibitor of gastric secretion, on canine gastric mucosal blood flow and serum gastrin levels. Arch Int Pharmacodyn Ther 1978;236:86 – 95.

33. Ramage JK, Denton A, Williams JG. Duration of action of Misoprostol, an orally active synthetic E_1 analogue of prostaglandin. Gut 1983;24:A973.

34. Larsen KR, Jensen NF, Davis EK, Jensen JC, Moody FG. The cytoprotective effects of (+)-15-deoxy-16-methyl PGE_1 methyl ester (SC 29333) versus aspirin

153

on shock gastric ulcerogenesis in the dog. Prostaglandin 1981;21(Suppl): 119–124.

35. Cohen MM, Clark L, Armstrong L, D'Sousa J. Reduced aspirin fecal blood loss with simultaneous administration of misoprostol (PGE$_1$, methyl analogue). Gastroenterology 1983;84:1126.
36. Gullikson G, Anglin C, Kessler L, Smeach S, Crowder S, Bauer R, Dajani EZ. Misoprostol prevents aspirin-induced damage in canine Heidenhain pouches. Gastroenterology 1983;84:1176.
37. Hunt JN, Smith JL, Jiang CL, Kessler L. Effect of synthesic prostaglandin E$_1$-analogue on aspirin-induced gastric bleeding and secretion. Dig Dis Sci 1983;28:897–902.
38. Bianchi RG, Casler JJ, Dajani EZ. Gastric antisecretory and antiulcer activity of SC 29333: A synthetic E-prostaglandin analogue. Pharmacologist 1981;23:121.
39. Tijtgat GN. Therapeutic use of prostaglandins in gastrointestinal disease. In: van Maercke YMF, van Moer EMJ, Pelckmans PAR (Eds). Stomach Diseases. Current status. Excerpta Medica, Amsterdam – Oxford – Princeton 1981: 49 – 54.
40. Fung WP, Karim SMM, Tye CY. Effect of 15(R) 15-methyl-prostaglandin E$_2$ methyl ester on healing of gastric ulcers. Lancet 1974;2:10–12.
41. Fung WP, Karim SMM. Effect of prostaglandin E$_2$ on the healing of gastric ulcers: A double-blind endoscopic trial. Aust N Z J Med 1976;6:121–122.
42. Gibinski K, Rybicka J, Mikós E, Nowak A. Double-blind clinical trial on gastroduodenal ulcer healing with prostaglandin E$_2$ analogues. Gut 1977;18:636–639.
43. Rybicka J, Gibinsky K. Methyl-prostaglandin analogues for healing of gastroduodenal ulcers. Scand J Gastroenterology 1978;13:155–159.
44. Chen F et al. Effect of prostaglandin E$_2$ and 15(R)-15-methyl PGE$_2$ on duodenal ulcer. Singapore Med J 1980;21:596.
45. Tijtgat GNJ, Huibregtse K. A double-blind trial with 15(R)-15-methyl PGE$_2$ in duodenal ulcer. Data on file Upjohn Company Kalamozoo, USA 1982.
46. Vantrappen G, Jansen J, Popiela J, Kulig J, Tijtgat GN, Huibregtse K, Lambert R, Pauchard JP, Robert A. Effect of 15(R)-15-methyl prostaglandin E$_2$ (Arbaprostil) on the healing of duodenal ulcers. A double-blind multicentre study. Gastroenterology 1982;83:357–363.
47. Brand D et al. Misoprostol, a prostaglandin E$_1$ analogue, is effective in healing duodenal ulcers: Results of a multi-center controlled trial. Gastroenterology 1984;86:1034.
48. Arvanitakis C et al. A comparative clinical trial of cimetidine and misoprostol (methyl PGE$_1$) in the treatment of duodenal ulcer. Gastroenterology 1984;86:1017.
49. Simon B et al. Misoprostol and cimetidine in a short-term treatment of duodenal ulcer. A double-blind, randomized multi-center study in Germany. Gastroenterology 1984;86:1253.
50. Nicholson PA. On behalf of an International Study Group. A multi-center international contolled comparison of two dosage regimes of misoprostol and cimetidine in the treatment of duodenal ulcer in out patients. To be published.
51. Shield MJ. Interim results of a multi-center international comparison of misoprostol and cimetidine in the treatment of outpatients with benign gastric ulcers. To be published.
52. Bardhan K et al. Trimoprostil vs. cimetidine in duodenal ulcer. Gut 1983;24:A580.

12. Discussion II

Rees:
Could I ask dr Pounder or dr Misiewicz whether they feel that there is any role at all for combination therapy. Obviously we are dealing with a very small proportion of patients, but it is my experience that there are some types of patients that do not respond to a single agent. If we change the treatment from an anti-secretory agent to a mucosal protective, again a proportion will heal but we are left with some that do not respond to that second line drug. Do you think that in this sort of patients there is any advantage in combination therapy? Pirenzipine when added to a histamine H_2-receptor antagonist may produce an additive effect, or potentiation, bearing in mind that there may well be some interaction between agents which reduce acid secretion and agents which act on the mucosa, such as sucralfate and the bismuth preparations.

Pounder:
There are two types of combinations. One is that one can add pirenzipine, atropine or another anti-cholinergic agent to an histamine H_2-receptor antagonist. Most studies show that some addition, even perhaps synergy, between the two agents develops. That has not been translated into clinical trials; there are very few people who can do these studies for only a small proportion of patients fail with an histamine H_2-receptor antagonist. Again there is no evidence that mixing either sucralfate, or bismuth with an histamine H_2-receptor antagonist provides more healing. The trouble with both of the mucosal protectors, sucralfate and bismuth, is that we have no idea how they work. If they work like a bandage or elastoplast, then certainly optimal precipitation of bismuth does occur at a pH of about 2.4. Shifting the intragastric pH from 1.4 to 2.4 with an histamine H_2-receptor antagonist might even improve precipitation of mucosal protective agents. I frankly do not believe they work by precipitation, so I think

156

it is attractive to mix two modes of treatment, but this has never been tested.

Misiewicz:

Just a word of caution in interpreting these various trials of patients who have failed to respond to histamine H_2-receptor antagonists. If you follow the patients long enough, some ulcers will heal spontaneously and if you follow them even for longer 8.4% of them will relapse each month. These are very interesting results, but remember the numbers are small and before they are accepted, one ought to think very carefully what these small numbers mean. If you go on and treat an ulcer for long enough, something will happen to it, even if the drug is not acting.

Tijtgat:

Can I follow that line? There must be ulcers where there is so much scarring in the bulb and collagen deposition and where the blood perfusion is so bad, that re-epithelialization is virtually impossible. If you send such patients to the surgeon as fully intractable, what can you really expect from surgery in that type of patients with a completely scarred bulb?

Misiewicz:

There are very few surgical studies that are followed up by endoscopy to show ulcer healing, they are assessed by Visick grading but there is not a great deal of endoscopic proof.

Tijtgat:

We are beginning to examine the quality of the epithelium that re-epithelializes the ulcer crater. There are lesions that re-epithelialize, but they are so fragile, so poorly vascularized that even with a minimal trauma, they will break open again. There are some animal data suggesting that if there is enough scarring and devascularization, you might retard epithelialization. In intractable ulcer the Japanese core out the ulcer, get rid of the true avascular zone, to get ingrowing new capillaries. Some of the gastric ulcers, which were resistant to any form of therapy for at least a year, healed with this approach.

Soll:

When we are talking about healing seen endoscopically, possibly we are only looking at a layer of intact epithelium over a granulation base. What we sometimes call a rapid recurrence after complete healing, will actually be a re-expression of an uncompletely healed ulcer. We need to assess what healing really is.

Misiewicz:

I take dr Soll's comment very seriously. I once went to a very heavy meeting and the start of a multicenter clinical trial, where a lot of people tried to define: What is a duodenal ulcer. (Not even: What is a healed duodenal ulcer.) We ended up by saying, all of us: 'Duodenal ulcer is what I say it is' and that was the best definition we could find. I think your point about healing is very well taken. May I also remind you of the observation that has been brought to people's attention many times before by dr Baron, dr Wormsley and by others. You can take multiple biopsies from the duodenal mucosa adjacent to a duodenal ulcer and these biopsy holes will heal, but the ulcer does not heal. There is something special about the location of the ulcer.

Tijtgat:

Dr Pounder, why are linear ulcer so difficult to heal? Does an excessive amount of scarring set the stage for an ulcer to be linear, or is there another factor which determines that healing is less easy for a linear ulcer? How do you differentiate between scarring and remaining linear ulcer? This can be very difficult in practice. Do you use special staining procedures? How are you sure it is a true re-epithelialized scar, or just a remaining ulcer?

Pounder:

I merely perform routine endoscopy without staining, or other specialized techniques. It might be that I will occasionally take a linear ulcer for a scar or vice versa. In practice I do not perform follow-up endoscopy if a duodenal ulcer patient has a satisfactory symptomatic response to treatment, unless the patient is part of a clinical trial.

Festen:

Coming back to the everyday situation: what are we treating, are we treating ulcers or are we treating symptoms? Usually in every day practice we are not going to re-endoscope patients after they have been treated and most probably a lot of these patients have asymptomatic ulcers. The key question is whether an ulcer which shows a tendency to heal can still give rise to complications.

Imburg (Groningen):

Scarring could be a problem in peptic ulcer disease. Is there any evidence that with medical treatment ulcers heal with less scarring? If so, this would be a major argument against on-demand treatment, because that form of treatment heals ulcer quickly, but does not prevent ulceration; so it will not prevent its complications.

Pounder:

The trouble is that scarring is very difficult to define endoscopically. We do not know what is happening to people with asymptomatic ulceration, whether they represent mild duodenal ulcer disease, or the kind of disease that is going to progress to a severely damaged duodenum. I have no doubt that if one wants to eliminate ulceration one has to do 'something' continuously. And that 'something' caneither be a surgical procedure that will alter the person's ability to make acid for the rest of their lives, or a tablet which affects the acidity for as long as they need it. The question is: Does asymptomatic ulceration reallly matter? I don't think we know.

Tijtgat:

But if we really want to prevent medical intractibility because of scarring and outlet obstruction, is there any other way apart from maintenance treatment? Every time patients have a breach in their mucosa, it will stimulate granulation tissue and connective tissue formation. To me this does not seem a reasonable policy. If we can prevent this by putting the patients on maintenance therapy, why should we put them on on-demand therapy, or only treat symptoms.

Tijtgat:

If that is not the case it is because we did not do a good job. It is because we did not treat the right patients with the right medication for the right amount of time. That was one of my questions: On the one hand there are data demonstrating that the perforation rate is decreasing, but on the other hand the incidence of surgery for complications of peptic ulcer disease was about the same in Bardhan's study. What is the actual situation: Is the incidence of surgery for complications decreasing, or is it the same as before?

Pounder:

Histamine H_2-receptor antagonists have been available now for 7 or 8 years. Do you think that has resulted in severe ulcers becoming less common? One would hope that people receiving fairly prompt and effective treatment, will suffer from less complications.

Johnson:

Could I answer that? Asymptomatic ulcers are important, because most of the patients admitted with perforations are asymptomatic before they perforate. We are observing an incrase in perforation rate, particularly in older people. I therefore think these asymptomatic ulcers do matter clinically. The very great majority of these patients have very few symptoms and may not even have sought medical attention. If I may just comment on the referral for elective procedures: this depends entirely on the philosophy of the physician. If he is doing a trial with a drug, he keeps his patients because he wants them for his next trial.

Soll:

With all the hundreds of million dollars that have been spent on clinical trials, we still not know whether we are decreasing the complication rate of the patients on maintenance treatment versus untreated controls.

Misiewicz:

The reason for this is, that in reality the numbers of patients undergoing very close surveillance in clincial trials is very small and the incidence of complications of peptic ulcer is relatively low. Most trials are short-term trials and there are not many maintenance trials around. So you don't collect enough patient/ulcer/years to acquire complications. I would say it is very dangerous to make statements about complication rates and treatment at the moment.

Tijtgat:

The results of the 5-year cimetidine trial, of which 4 years have passed now show a very low incidence rate of complications, certainly of major complications.

Pounder:

Seven hundred people were enrolled in the original Burland one-year European study of cimetidine versus placebo. In that population of 700 people watched over twelve months, one person had a GI haemorrhage, while a third of the study population or more were on placebo. There are many environmental changes, which necessitate a new collection of all the data on complications. We ought to have a modern, prospective study of people coming to hospital with either haemorrhage or perforation, and find out what was happened. Such a study must provide answers to the following questions: Are complicated ulcers often asymptomatic? Did the patient visit their doctor for upper abdominal complaints? Were patients treated effectively? What was the incidence of self-mediation? How many of the people who actually are threatened by their peptic ulcer are known to have had a peptic ulcer?

Amdrup:

Eight to ten years ago pyloric stenosis was nearly eliminated in the Danishh population. During recent years an increasing number of patients are coming to surgery for pyloric stenosis. The history is always the same: either a patient directed to on-demand treatment, or poorly controlled maintenance treatment. We are putting the patient in an unfavourable position if we have to postpone surgery to the time when the patient has got pyloric stenosis. How do we avoid that? How well should we control the patients, when we take the very serious decision to put the patient on maintenance treatment?

Misiewicz:

Dr Amdrup may I ask you, with respect, what are the figures on the increase of incidence of pyloric stenosis? Is that an impression of yours which we would take very seriously, or do you have a statistical perspective for that statement?

Amdrup:

I cannot give you exact figures, but I can tell you that in the seventies we would have 2 or 3 cases of real fibrous pyloric stenosis per year in our department. The last 2 or 3 years we have had between 15 and 20 cases.

Misiewicz:

You do not think that is an effect of your reputation – people are referring more difficult cases to you.

Wormsley:

The decision to undergo surgery is more serious than the decision to undertake maintenance treatment. To answer dr Soll's question: complications during *no* treatment are much more serious than the complications of recurrences *during* maintenance treatment. Patients suffering from chronic peptic ulcer usually have symptomatic recurrences and are seldom asymptomatic. Patients with asymptomatic complicated peptic ulcers have frequently been treated with nonsteroidal anti-inflammatory drugs. Those drugs are not only correlated with a high complication rate, but also with asymptomaticity. Another point is the resistance to treatment of the highly scarred ulcers. We have had 6 patients who after treatment with ranitidine for 9 months did not heal and they healed with omeprazole after four weeks. The interesting thing is that maintenance treatment with ordinary doses of ranitidine has kept these ulcers healed.

Tijtgat:

We have treated resistant ulcers with omeprazole and surprisingly, they heal. But as soon as we discontinued the therapy and switched back to maximal ranitidine plus pirenzepine therapy, the ulcers recurred extremely rapidly, at least ours did.

Boevé:

What is the risk of enteric infections during the use of potent gastrtic acid secretion inhibiting drugs?

Festen:

I think the risk is very low. There have been some reports, usually anecdotal, on systemic infections, candidiasis and bacterial infections associated with cimetidine treatment. But we know that in the anacidic patients with pernicious anaemia these infections don't usually occur. So the risk of general infections is not serious.

Soll:

It seems that medical disasters from drug therapy occur usually in a small number of patients, so small that we usually don't pick them up. Omeprazole is an exciting drug, but I am disturbed that it has such great potentials for trouble in inducing severe hypochlorhydria, or achlorhydria and the potentially dangerous effects on enterochromaffin cells in rats. Obviously we don't know if that applies to humans and one of my concerns is whether we are going to find out before marketing. I am concerned about the studies showing that a 20 mg dose in some patients has very little effect while in others has profound effects in inhibiting acid secretion. If that type of variability in responsiveness is true and if achlorhydria is going to be the mediator of complications in these patients, then does not that mean that every patient who is treated with omeprazole has to be monitored for pH. And does not it mean we have to look at all of the complication rates over a prolonged period of time, examining every individual patient and not looking at means, because the big trouble may come in the 2 or 3% of the patients who are tremendously sensitive and may develop profound achlorhydria, or may be responsive to other factors, or have endocrine-like cells that are very responsive to the effects. I am extremely concerned and I wonder whether the studies that have been considered to furhter evaluate this exciting drug are going to deal adequately with these problems.

Festen:

Omeprazole is a very safe drug, but it is the first drug which confronts us with the sequelae of almost complete suppression of acid secretion. The enterochromaffine like cell problem is a problem secondary to acid inhibition and not related to omeprazole itself. Of course, that does not make it less important. Most probably in short term use there are no serious problems. Omeprazole could prove to be very useful for intractable duodenal ulcers in the acute stage. Long-term use is still a problem. This could be solved if we could establish that suppression of acid secretion for just a part of the week would be enough to prevent recurrences. Alternatively another preparation should be found which gives more reproducible blood levels and a more stable acid inhibition.

Soll:

If omeprazole is used by doctors who are educated with these compounds and know the literature, maybe all this reasoning will be true. But if we look at the years of cimetidine and ranitidine: how many people that prescribe it have read the literature? In the United States 80% of the prescriptions are not for indicated use following indicated guidelines. How many patients will use it unauthorized? So I wonder whether we can really risk the consequences of a drug with such profound effect as omeprazole has. Even if we can plan how it should be used, we can not guarantee that it will be used in that way.

Festen:
There are many drugs that are toxic in doses above the advised dose. With proper management and proper instruction a drug of this kind could be very usable indeed.

Tijtgat:
To me the most exciting thing is the fact that it is apparently sufficient to decrease nocturnal acid secretion to some extent in order to heal the lesion in the duodenal bulb and keep it healed. The question is: What should we aim for? Should we aim for a minimal disturbance of physiology, just enough to heal most ulcers, or should we be on the safe side and choose a drug and a dose which will heal practically all ulcers?

Pounder:
As compliance is a big problem, a once-a-day regimen should be chosen. We should probably give the strongest drug during the acute phase, in order to heal 99% of ulcers. The side-effects of those drugs, like omeprazole, will not be a great worry if given for only very short periods. After healing we can switch to the mildest drug that is effective in maintenance treatment. I thought the mildest thing that worked was cimetidine, but as we have seen maybe cimetidine is just a bit too mild and perhaps ranitidine would be a reasonable compromise.

One of the other things I would like to hear this afternoon is: What is surgery doing to gastrin? Surgery, by causing a life-long 24-hours-a-day action, actually causes an upregulation of gastrin and one must wonder what happens to ECL cells in people who have had an effective gastric operation.

Van der Vegt:
In pernicious anaemia patients there is an increased risk of gastrinoma's, but these are not malignant. The cells in pernicious anaemia-associated gastrinoma's are always euploid, while cells in malignant gastrinoma's are often aneuploid.

Tijtgat:
There are at least 50 cases in the world literature of carcinoidosis of the stomach in patients with pernicious anaemia and quite a percentage of these patients had metastases to other organs. The majority had infiltration of all layers up to the serosal layer, so there is a

potential for metastases from gastrinoma's in patients with pernicious anaemia.

Festen:

Of course there is paid much attention to these carcinoids and ECL'oma's following omeprazole treatment. But I want to stress that these are only observed in female rats. And a rat is a completely different animal from other species as far as ECL cells are concerned. The density of ECL cells in the gastric mucosa of the rat is much higher than it is in human beings. The exceedingly high serum gastrin levels following omeprazole administration to the rat are never met with in humans. Although ECL-oma's have been described in humans with long-standing achlorhydria and very high serum gastrin levels, it remains a very rare tumor.

Johnston:

I would like to respond to dr Pounder's point about the possible long-term harmful effects of effective surgery. I think the point is that modern surgery does not create anything like achlorhydria and HSV will reduce MAO from 40 to 20 mmol/hr. So the intragastric pH through the day is going to be pretty acid. There aren't any, as yet, long-term deleterious effects, there is no evidence of any increased risk of long-term carcinoma.

Tijtgat:

Omeprazole decreases pentagastrin-stimulated acid by approximately 60%, but if you measure intra-gastric acidity over 24 hours, there is nearly total anacidity. So we need values of 24 hours intra-gastric pH rather than the maximal acid output.

Johnston:

These date are available from the studies by dr Hunt (Portsmouth) and dr Pounder. We know that during the day there is quite a lot of acid around.

Pounder:

The effect is cimetidine-like. There is a greater effect during the night than during the day. If the treatment is a shift in acid, there will also be a reciprocal rise in gastrin, but I am not aware of published data.

Johnston:

There is a rise in gastrin after vagotomy. It is a modest, but a significant increase: about 2-3 fold.

Pounder:

The full dose of omeprazole causes a 4-fold rise, so surgery and omeprazole are in the same range. Omeprazole one might take for 4 weeks, whereas surgery is for life, and these are grounds for concern.

Kennedy:

Yes, gastrin levels do rise after gastric surgery, after vagotomy, but nowhere near as much as 2 or 3-fold. We have studied gastrin levels in many hundreds of patients before and after vagotomy and found an increase of about 50%. But with regard to what David Johnston has just said about cancer following vagotomy: if your are going to get cancer following operations, it is going to occur many years later and this year is the 15th anniversary of the HSV operation and 15 years is not yet long enough for us to know whether there will be an increased risk. I don't believe there will be an increased risk after HSV, but what we do know is that after other forms of gastric surgery, not only gastrectomy, but also after truncal or selective vagotomy with drainage, there is an increased incidence of cancer after 15-25 years.

Guth:

I would like to ask dr Festen about the carcinogenic potential of omeprazole. You showed in one of your slides an increase in the intragastric concentration of nitrosamines, nitrates and bacteria. Those working in the field of gastric carcinoma might then expect to see adenoma's and gastric carcinoma's not carcinoids or ECL-oma's.

So, there has been no evidence of adenomatous and adenocarcinomatous growth in these rats, as there has been with tiotidine. Are we really talking about the same thing? What is the difference between carcinogenic potential and carcinoid-like tumors?

Festen:

These are completely different lesions. The ECL cell abnormalities observed in female rats with omeprazole have nothing to do with the adenocarcinoma's observed with tiotidine or SKF 93479. On the other hand, there has been much concern about the significance of nitrosamines, but it has never been shown that these nitrosamine concentrations have really produced cancer. In pernicious anaemia you could have a firm discussion whether gastric cancer is increased in pernicious anaemia or not. If so, it is only to a very low extent. As we saw from dr Pounder's data, there were just a few patients who had a significant increase in nitrosamine concentration, but there were a lot of patients where the increase was not significant at all. Moreover, these potent drugs will probably be given for short treatment courses and carcinogenesis will need a very long exposure time.

Misiewicz:

You know, if alcohol was invented to-morrow, it would never be marketed, it would be too dangerous. Drugs like omeprazole are paying the price of progress. I don't agree with the statement, that it is a very safe drug. I don't think we know, because the clinical experience with omeprazole is minimal. We don't know what side-effects might come from the drug itself. It may be a safe drug. It is a highly selective animal subpopulation of female rats that develops the ECL hyperplasia. But once they are there they cannot be ignored and they put the whole question of long-term therapy with omeprazole in a very serious situation. As dr Pounder pointed out: in the short-term omeprazole may be acceptable, but in the long-term, I wonder. If one is going to give omeprazole in lower doses to produce not complete anacidity, but only partial control of gastric secretion, what is the advantage over currently available histamine H_2-receptor antagonists, or vagotomy?

Pounder:

The data relating to adenocarcinoma associated with histamine H_2-receptor antagonists in animals are now being reviewed again, to decide whether they are carcinomas, or whether they are endocrine tumors. The rumour has it that in fact some of them are now being reclassified, because ECL cells in rats can resemble closely poorly differentiated carcinoma cells. Even in humans with pernicious anaemia there is doubt whether all tumors classified as carcinoma's could actually be endocrine tumors.

Busman (Leeuwarden):

We also documented a rise in fasting serum gastrin levels after HSV. In patients who had ever been treated with cimetidine prior to

HSV the post-operative increase in serum gastrin was consistently higher than in patients never treated with cimetidine before.

Festen:

We did a study on serum gastrin levels in gastric and duodenal ulcer patients treated with histamine H_2-receptor antagonist and we could find hardly any rise in serum gastrin levels during treatment. Three days after discontinuation of cimetidine the serum gastrin levels returned to pre-treatment levels in all patients. So there is no explanation whatsoever for the observation you have made.

Tijtgat:

We followed our patients on cimetidine maintenance treatment and there is only a very minor rise after 4 years in serum gastrin levels. These still are well in the normal range, but significantly different from the pre-treatment and 1 and 2 years values.

Van Blankenstein:

It is quite conceivable that patients who have once been exposed to the delights of cimetidine may go back to it after surgery. That might be the reason why mr Busman's ex-cimetidine patients have higher levels of serum-gastrin.

Wormsley:

Just one point about gastrin levels. Don't be mesmerized by high gastrin levels with omeprazole because there has recently been a report that the ECL cells release gastrin-releasing peptide. Now it may well be that the gastrin levels are secondary to the ECL cell hyperplasia and not primary.

Festen:

No, it is not a secondary phenomenon. In gastric biopsies of humans treated with omeprazole hyperplasia of ECL cells is not seen, while there is a definite increase in serum gastrin levels.

Tijtgat:

What dr Wormsley is saying is that perhaps the gastrin rise is secondary to stimulation of a gastric-releasing factor from the endo-crine cells.

168

Festen:

That is possible indeed.

Busman (Leeuwarden):

It has been documented in the surgical literature that the rise in gastrin is not directly related to the decrease in acid secretion. Serum gastrin levels could also rise if an inhibitor of gastrin secretion is abolished by HSV. This has recently been suggested by Dekkers in the American Journal of Surgery.

After vagotomy serum gastrin levels rise immediately and that rise is independent from the reduction in acid secretion. Even when the antrum is titrated to a fixed pH, the gastrin will rise. I am not aware of similar data after inhibition of gastric acid secretion by drugs.

Pounder:

There is more to gastrin than meets the eye. You can see all sorts of different reasons why different types of gastric surgery will have different effects on serum gastrin levels. Antrectomy removes the main source of gastrin production. People who have undergone pyloroplasty may develop antral gastritis which again may effect gastrin release, whereas people after HSV have an intact mucosa, which may protect their G-cells and results in normal or raised levels of serum gastrin.

It is fascinating that the discovery of omeprazole's problem has opened a whole new area of questions that need to be asked about cimetidine, ranitidine and surgery, as well as about omeprazole.

Van Blankenstein:

Is there any evidence that proglumide, a gastrin-receptor blocking drug, might be useful in preventing the development of ECL-oma's after omeprazole treatment?

Festen:

It was already mentioned by dr Soll that proglumide is an anti-gastrinic, but effective only in very high doses and even then its effect is very weak. I have reviewed all the literature about proglumide, but there is no indication whatsoever that proglumide inhibits acid secretion and it does not have any effect on ulcer healing rate. That does not exactly answer your question, but clinically, I think that proglumide is not effective.

Van Blankenstein:

It has not been looked at in those female rats?

Festen:

No. You might hypothesize that proglumide binds on a gastrin receptor, but if so, the binding is very weak.

Tijtgat:

Does anybody know whether gastrin receptors are present on the ECL cells?

Soll:

I cannot provide any direct evidence. In rats, these studies have not been done. There is only indirect suggestion that gastrin remodulates histamine-formation, which should be present in the ECL cell. And yet, when we are talking about ECL cells, I don't believe these have been typed very well. ECL cells are only identified by silver staining and I don't think we know whether they produce peptides or whether they contain DOPA-decarboxylase, or serotonin, or one of the other markers of endocrine, or endocrine-like cells. The only information we have in dogs would suggest that at least using serotonin and DOPA-decarboxylase as a marker, gastrin-receptors on ECL cells can not be demonstrated by our techniques. This not only highlights the fascinating area for study, but also shows our ignorance of these cells, what regulates them and what they do.

Allgöwer:

Would it be possible to change over to prostaglandins for a second. I have a very tactless question to Dr Tijtgat: You have shown that there is a medical treatment which combines the disadvantages of surgical and medical treatment by causing diarrhoea.

Tijtgat:

Not diarrhoea, but increased bowel frequency.

Allgöwer:

Well, anyhow enough to make people unable to work. It may be very interesting pathophysiologically what prostaglandins do to the pyloric mechanism, because it looks as if you are committing a medical crime against the pylorus as we have done it in surgery.

Tijtgat:

I don't think gastric motility, or gastric emptying is influenced by prostaglandin therapy. It is mainly a stimulation of small intestinal motility and enteric pooling of water and electrolytes which by itself stimulates propulsive motility.

Van de Ende (Den Haàg):

I would like to come back to dr Pounder's remarks on the 800 mg cimetidine tablet. The volume of that tablet is about 15% more than the volume of the 400 mg tablet. To facilitate swallowing the shape of the tablet has been adjusted.

De Vries (Tilburg):

We have charged gastrin with very horrible facts, but maybe gastrin has advantageous effects. It has important trophic effects on the upper gastrointestinal tract and it may work together with the epidermal growth factor, healing gastric and duodenal ulcers. What is your opinion?

Misiewicz:

Very interesting hypothesis, but I can't throw any factual light on it.

Festen:

I don't know. I am not aware of anyone studying the healing effect of gastrin in peptic ulcers.

Tijtgat:

I have a couple of burning questions: Dr Pounder, for how many years should we prescribe drugs for maintenance therapy?

Pounder:

That is a very difficult question. I think at worst one has to accept that one may be offering it for life. The traditional wisdom is that people grow out of their duodenal ulcers after 10 or 15 years. I am not sure that is true and I think it is quite possible that people need it for much longer.

Tijtgat:

I am sure peptic ulcer patients should be advised not to smoke. The only clue we have was identified by dr Wormsley, that there seems to be a degree of resistance to histamine H_2-receptor antagonists of people who smoke. But the mechanism, I think remains unclear.

Festen:

May I make a short comment on that? The only thing that is proven about smoking is that it reduces bicarbonate secretion by the pancreas. But I think nobody knows if it is smoking, or the smoker which causes histamine H_2-receptor antagonist ineffectiveness. You can overcome these effects by increasing the dose, as dr Pounder showed really.

Pounder:

Yes, the corrolally of that study is that the investigation was upon people who were either non-smokers or smokers and I don't think a comparable study has been done where smokers have converted to non-smokers. There are many other things which go along with smoking, like drinking and so on.

Tijtgat:

I am always a bit uneasy when I see the figures of the relapse rates for gastric ulcer. What percentage of gastric ulcer is iatrogenic, drug-induced, and do these ulcers relapse if the insulting drug is discontinued?

Misiewicz:

I can't show any relapse figures for gastric ulcer, because I don't know what they are. I have a very strong clinical impression that the use of non-steroidal anti-inflammatory drugs make gastric ulcers worse. But if you stop them, which you never can because the patients usually take them for very good reasons, I would suppose the outcome for gastric ulcer would be very much better. The outcome for gastric ulcer generally is not as bad as people believe. There is one study from England which showed that many years later over 60% of the patients remained healed on medical treatment.

Spencer:

I suggest we congratulate my Dutch collegues on persuading the Medical Officer from the Department of Welfare that drug treatment of peptic ulcer is really saving money, something like a 140 million guilders a year. We found that cimetidine and other agents just delay the time at which an operation is performed. Meanwhile the patient who is not admitted to hospital, is replaced in that bed by somebody else on whom the Government spends money. I would like comments from the panel on the overall costs of medical and surgical treatment.

Festen:

This is a very long subject to discuss, but I completely disagree with you. There are several studies which have shown that surgery for gastric and duodenal ulcer has decreased and especially since cimetidine was marketed. There has been a survey in Britain published by Wyllie, who showed the same figures. There is no doubt that the hospitalization rate for peptic ulcer has gone down since the introduction of histamine H_2-receptor antagonists.

Spencer:

The point I'm making is that somebody else fills those beds and the money in the hospital is still spent, meanwhile the ulcer patient is at home on an expensive drug. And what Wyllie and others have shown is that there was in the early days of cimetidine a dramatic decrease in the number of operations, which has been steadily increasing after these first few years.

13. Genetic aspects of peptic ulcer

J. KREUNING, M.D.

Department of Gastroenterology, University Hospital, Leiden, The Netherlands

Like other chronic diseases, peptic ulcer develops as a result of the interaction of a genetic component with environmental factors. Genetic factors are considered important as promoting susceptibility to peptic ulcer. This view is based primarily on three lines of evidence: 1. family studies; 2. twin studies; and 3. gene marker associations.

Family studies

Familial aggregation was already noted even before 1900, but the first studies had no control data and no distinction was made between gastric and duodenal ulcers. The first really informative data were collected 34 years ago in the Central Middlesex Hospital. Doll and Buch,[1] who studied the incidence of gastric and duodenal ulcer in the siblings of such patients, found that gastric ulcer occurred 1.8 times and duodenal ulcer 2.6 times more frequently among the living sibs of ulcer patients than among comparable groups in the general population. (Tabel I) Furthermore, there were indications pointing to a tendency for sibs to have ulcers at the same site as the affected sib. Doll and Kellock[2] studied 109 families and found that the relatives of gastric ulcer patients tend to have gastric ulcers and the relatives of duodenal ulcer patients tend to have duodenal ulcers. They also used population incidence figures to calculate the expected numbers of gastric and duodenal ulcers and compared the results with the observed numbers. The excess of ulcers in siblings was almost entirely due to an excess of ulcers at the same site as in the propositi. This led the authors to conclude that gastric and duodenal ulcers were inherited independently. (Table II) One endoscopic study performed in Finland confirmed earlier radiological findings concerning a familial predisposition to peptic ulcer disease.[3] Endoscopic evidence of present or past duodenal or pyloric ulcer was found in 20 (13%) of the

Table I. Observed and expected prevalence of peptic ulcer in siblings of propositi. (Modified from Doll & Buch, 1950)

	n	Observed	Expected
Brothers			
all ages	521	60*	28.3
14 – 64 years	459	56*	24.7
Sisters			
all ages	543	15[+]	5.7
14 – 64 years	483	14[+]	5.7

* p <0.00001
+ p <0.001

Table II. Comparison between the number of relatives observed and expected to have gastric or duodenal ulcer. (Doll & Kellock, 1951)

Propositus	Sex	Observed		Expected		Excess	
		S	D	S	D	S	D
Stomach	male	21	13	6.8	12.1	+ 14.2	+ 0.9
Duodenum		10	42	6.5	13.5	+ 3.5	+ 28.5
Stomach	female	9	3	2.2	3.1	+ 5.4	− 0.1
Duodenum		5	6	2.2	2.0	+ 2.8	+ 4.0

duodenal ulcer relatives, as against only 6 (3.9%) of the control relatives and this difference is statistically significant (p <0.01).

Twin studies

The frequency of peptic ulcer has been studied in concordant monozygotic twins and compared with that in dizygotic twins. There are no reports on gastric ulcer in these groups and only a few reports on duodenal ulcer. In Denmark, all twins born between 1870 and 1910 were located and followed up. In 1958, Harwald and Hauge[4] found 181 pairs in whom a duodenal ulcer had occurred. These authors found a low concordance rate of 18.2% in monozygotic twins, and a rate of 12.9% in dizygotic pairs of the same sex. However, with 10 more years of follow-up, the concordance rate had risen to 52.6% and 35.7%.[4,5] This difference between the concordance rates is significant. The finding of a higher concordance between monozygotic than dizygotic twins supports the concept that hereditary factors are important for the expression of duodenal ulcer disease.

Gene marker associations

ABO blood groups

Aird and his colleagues[6] were the first to discover the relationship between blood group 0 and peptic ulcer. People with blood group 0 were about 35% more likely to develop a peptic ulcer than were people with blood groups A, B, and AB. This held more strongly for duodenal than for gastric ulcer. Clark et al[7] confirmed the high frequency of blood group 0 in duodenal ulcers, and reported that the blood group distribution did not differ significantly between patients with gastric ulcer and the control population. Among duodenal ulcer patients blood group 0 was present in 56.5%, among gastric ulcer patients in 52.4% and among controls in 45.8%.

When the gastric ulcer data was broken down according to the site of the ulcer, a similarly high frequency of blood group 0 was found among patients with ulcers in the antrum and pre-pyloric region and patients with localization in the duodenum.[8]

The blood group genes seem able to influence the severity of peptic ulcer disease. Langman and Doll[9] analyzed their peptic ulcer data and found a higher incidence of blood group 0 in patients with bleeding duodenal ulcers (59.3%) than in non-bleeding ulcers (52.3%). This relationship was confirmed by other investigators. Later, it was also reported that the frequency of blood group 0 was higher among patients with a perforated ulcer and that the incidence of blood group 0 in perforated ulcers was in the same range as in patients with bleeding ulcers.[10,11] The incidence of blood group 0 in perforated ulcer was 56.9% in Evans' series and 58.7% in Langman's series, compared to 50.6% and 52.9% respectively in uncomplicated ulcers.

Secretor status

Secretors are persons who secrete blood group substances into their saliva and gastrointestinal fluids; those who do not are called non-secretors. An association with peptic ulcer and non-secretor status has been found and this is most marked for duodenal ulcer. Only a slight increase of non-secretor frequency has been found in gastric ulcer, but the number of gastric ulcer patients tested was small and no differentiation was made according to the site of the ulcer. The relative risk that a person who is non-secretor will develop a duodenal ulcer is 1.5. Unlike the blood group 0 association, no relationship was found between non-secretor status and the severity of the ulcer. It seems, therefore, that the secretor genes influence susceptibility to duodenal ulcer. The relative risk for secretors with blood group 0 is 1.3 but for individuals who are both blood group 0 and non-secretor, the relative risk of developing a duodenal ulcer is 2.5.[4]

Alpha-1-antitrypsin deficiency

Alpha-1-antitrypsin is the main protease inhibitor whose lack is a well-known cause of pulmonary emphysema. On the other hand, an association between pulmonary emphysema and peptic ulcer has been reported and this suggested an association between alpha-1-antitrypsin deficiency and peptic ulcer. Four studies have been published on this association in the present context.[12-15] In two, a positive association was found.[13,15] In a recent study done in Leiden we found no relationship between any of the alpha-1-antitrypsin phenotypes and duodenal ulcer disease.

HLA antigens

Several studies have dealt with the distribution of HLA antigens in patients with duodenal ulcer disease. Positive associations with HLA-B5, HLA-B12, and HLA-Bw35 have been described.[16-18] Of special interest with respect to the HLA-Bw35 association was that these patients had a lower acid secretion than other patients. No associations were found in four other studies.[19-22] A study done in Leiden[23] in Dutch duodenal ulcer patients also showed no association between HLA antigens and duodenal ulcer in general, but when age was taken into account the HLA distribution was found to differ between the younger (≤ 30 years) and the older (> 30 years) age groups. HLA-Bw35 was not found in the younger age group, whereas the frequency of HLA-Bw35 was higher in the older age group than in the controls (20.3% as against 15.9%). The difference between the younger and the older patient group was significant ($P = 0.015$ in Fisher's exact test), but the difference between patients over 30 years of age and normal controls did not reach significance.

This difference in the distribution of HLA-Bw35 might be explained by the existence of two kinds of duodenal ulcer disease.

Hyperpepsinogenaemia I

Pepsinogen is the inactive precursor of pepsin and together with hydrochloric acid is one of the main secretory products of the gastric mucosa. Pepsinogen has been shown to comprise two immunochemically distinct groups differing with mucosal distribution. Pepsinogen I, which consists of five electrophoretically distinct fractions (Pg1 – Pg5), is found in serum and urine. Pepsinogen II, which consists of two electrophoretically distinct fractions (Pg6 and Pg7), is found in serum and seminal fluid, but not in urine. The mechanism by which pepsinogen is transferred from the gastroduodenal mucosa to the circulation is not known.

Immunohistochemical studies have shown the existence of five types of peptic cells in man.[24-26] Two types, the chief cell and the mucus neck cell, are located in the fundic gland mucosa and produce PG I and PG II; the remaining three cell types are clear-staining cells of the cardiac glands in the cardia, the pyloric glands in the antrum, and the Brunner's glands in the proximal duodenum, and produce only PG II. Pepsinogen I and II can be measured by radioimmunoassay or ELISA (enzyme-linked immunosorbent assay).[27,28] Since Samloff found that the serum group I pepsinogen is produced only in the acid secretory part of the stomach, several studies have been published on the positive relationship between serum PG I and gastric acid secretion.[29,30] A study done in Leiden[31] showed rather poor correlation between serum PG I levels and gastric peak acid output. (Table III) The accumulated data indicate that serum PG I concentration cannot be used to predict gastric acid output on an individual basis, except that a low level is highly specific for marked hypoacidity or anacidity. A survey of duodenal ulcer patients and healthy controls showed that serum PG I concentration of ulcer patients were significantly higher than those of controls, and that the

Table III. Relationship between basal serum pepsinogen I and peak acid output, corrected for body weight. (From: Goedhard et al, 1984)

PG I		Peak acid output (mmol/hr)					
µg/l	n	< 10		10 – 40		> 40	
< 50	40	29	(73%)	11	(27%)	0	
50 – 150	180	34	(19%)	127	(71%)	19	(10%)
> 150	39	6	(16%)	22	(56%)	11	(28%)

PG I concentration in duodenal ulcer patients were bimodally distributed.[32] (fig. 1) Measurement of serum PG I concentration in two
large families with duodenal ulcer suggested that elevated concentration are transmitted in an autosomal dominant mode of inheritance.[33] A study of 123 duodenal ulcer sibships showed hyperpepsinogenaemia I in about half of the duodenal ulcer patients and normopepsinogenaemia I in the remainder.[34] Approximately 50% of the
offspring of relatives with an elevated PG I had an elevated PG I and
all offspring of relatives with a normal PG I had a normal PG I. Both
forms of duodenal ulcer were accompanied by an increased risk for
sibs of duodenal ulcer patients compared with control groups. Some
20% of the sibs were affected, which means that about 40% of the
relatives with an elevated pepsinogen I concentration have a clinical

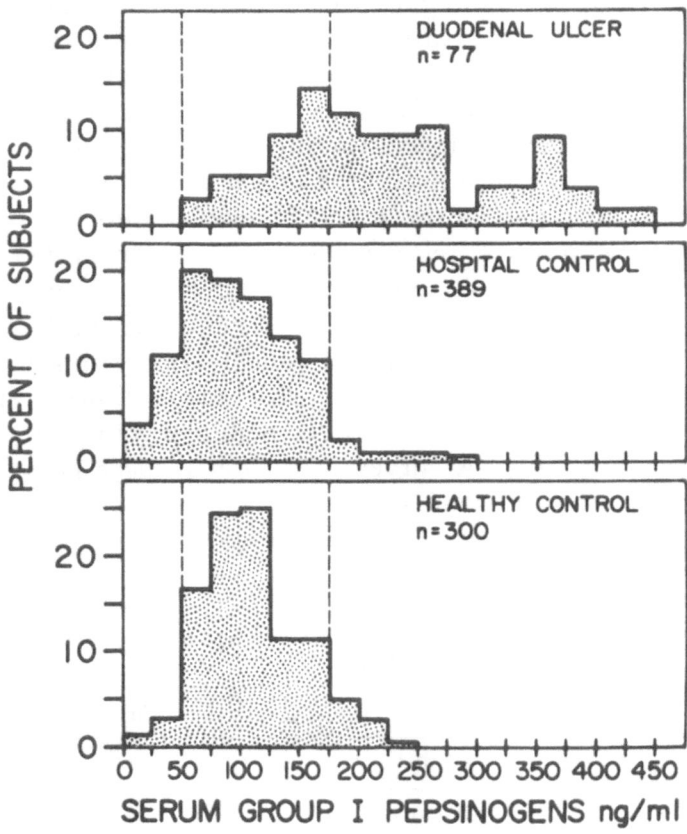

Figure 1. Serum group I pepsinogens in control subjects and patients with peptic ulcer.

duodenal ulcer. Hyperpepsinogenaemia I can be used as a subclinical marker, but there are enough data suggesting that the influence of additional factors is needed for the development of duodenal ulcer in the presence of high level of pepsinogen I.

At present results suggest that there are at least two forms of duodenal ulcer. The use of other subclinical markers might make it possible to subdivide these groups further. An exaggerated serum gastrin response to a protein meal (antral G cell hyperfunction) is associated with hyperpepsinogenaemia I. In the normopepsinogenaemia I duodenal ulcer patients a subgroup with rapid gastric emptying has been identified, both on a familial basis.[35,36]

Conclusion

There is evidence indicating clinical and genetic heterogeneity in peptic ulcer disease. We hope that the study of subclinical markers will help to elucidate the effect of environment on the expression of the disease.

Acknowledgement

The figure has been reproduced with permission of dr I.M. Samloff and the Editor of Gastroenterology from: Samloff IM, Liebman WM, Panitch NM. Serum group I pepsinogens by radioimmunoassay in control subjects and patients with peptic ulcer. Gastroenterology 1975;69:83 – 90.

References

1. Doll R, Buch J. Heriditary factors in peptic ulcer. Ann Eugen (London) 1950;15:135 – 46.
2. Doll R, Kellock TD. The separate inheritance of gastric and duodenal ulcers. Ann Eugen (London) 1951;16:231 – 40.
3. Tarpila S, Samloff IM, Pikkarainen P, Vuoristo M, Thamäki T. Endoscopic and clincical findings in fist-degree relatives of duodenal ulcer in patients and control subjects. Scand J Gastroenterol 1982;17:503 – 6.
4. McConnell RB. The genetics of gastro-intestinal disorders. London Oxford University Press, 1966.
5. Jensen KG. Genetics of peptic ulcer. Scand J Gastroenterol 1980;15:S63, 11 – 5.

180

6. Aird I, Bentall HH, Mehigan JA, Roberts JAF. The blood groups in relation to peptic ulceration and carcinoma of colon, rectum, breast and bronchus. Brit Med J 1965;II:315-21.
7. Clarke CA, Cowan WK, Edwards JW, Howel-Evans AW, McConnell RB, Woodrow JL, Sheppard PM. The relationship of the blood groups to duodenal and gastric ulceration. Birt Med J 1955;II:643-6.
8. Johnson D. Gastric ulcer: Classification, blood group characteristics, secretion patterns and pathogenesis. Ann Surg 1965;162:996-1004.
9. Langman MJS, Doll R. ABO blood groups and secretor status in relation to clinical characteristics of peptic ulcers. Gut 1965;6:270-3.
10. Evans DAP, Horwich L, McConnell RB, Bullen MF. The influence of the ABO blood groups and secretor status on bleeding and on perforation of duodenal ulcers. Gut 1968;9:319-22.
11. Langman MJS, Doll R, Saracci R. ABO blood group and secretor status in stomal ulcer. Gut 1967;8:128-32.
12. Lieberman J. Heterozygous and homozygous alpha-1-antitrypsin deficiency in patients with pulmonary emphysema. New Engl J Med 1969;281:279-84.
13. André F, André C, Lambert R, Descos F. Prevalence of alpha-1-antitrypsin deficiency in patients with gastric or duodenal ulcer. Biomedicine 1974;21:222-24.
14. Blenkinsopp WK. Alpha-1-antitrypsin antibodies, PiZ phenotype, and peptic ulcer. Gut 1978;19:157-8.
15. Fuente A de la, Millan J, Molina LM, Garcia Forero R, Gallego JL. Variaciones del poder antitripsico del suero en los enfermos con Ulcus Gastro-duodenal. Rev Esp Engerm Apar Dig 1978;54:253-58.
16. Rotter JI, Rimoin DL, Gursky JM, Terasaki P, Sturdevant RAL. HLA-B5 associated with duodenal ulcer. Gastroenterology 1977;73:438-40.
17. Ellis A, Woodrow JC, HLA and duodenal ulcer. Gut 1979;20:760-2.
18. Gough MJ, Rajah SM, Giles GR. HLA antigens in relationship to duodenal ulceration, gastric acid secretion and clinical results following vagotomy. Brit J Surg 1982;69:105-7.
19. Heschl R, Tilz GP. Untersuchungen über die Verteilung der HLA Antigene bei Patienten mit Zwölffingerdarmgeschwüren. Acta Med Austriaca 1976;3:80-2.
20. O'Brien BD, Thomson ABR, Dossetor JB. HLA and peptic ulcer. Dig Dis Sci 1979;24:314-5.
21. Kang JY, Doran T, Crampton R, McClenchan W, Piper DW. HLA antigens and peptic ulcer disease. Digestion 1983;26:99-104.
22. Hetzel DJ, Gabb BW, Bennett GD, Hay J, Shearman DJC. Is there an HLA antigen association with duodenal ulcer? Digestion 1982;25:252-7.
23. Goedhard JG, Biemond I, Peña AS, Kreuning J, Schreuder GMTh, van Rood JJ. HLA and duodenal ulcer in The Netherlands. Tissue Antigens 1983; 22:213-8.
24. Samloff IM. Cellular localization of group I pepsinogens in human gastric mucosa by immunofluorenscence. Gastroenterology 1971;22:213-8.
25. Samloff IM, Liebman WM. Cellular localization of the group II pepsinogens in human stomach and duodenum by immunofluorescence. Gastroenterology 1973;65:36-42.
26. Weinstein WM, Lechago J, Samloff IM, Bowes KL. Pepsinogens in human gastric, cardiac and esophageal glands. Clin Res 1977;25:690A.
27. Samloff IM. Pepsinogens I and II: Purification from gastric mucosa and radio-immunoassay in serum. Gastroenterology 1982;82:26-33.

28. Biemond I, Pals G, Giliams JP, Kreuning J, Peña AS. Enzyme linked immunosorbent assay of pepsinogen I. In: Kreuning J, Samloff IM, Rotter JI, Eriksson A (Eds). Pepsinogens in man. Clinical and genetic advances. New York, Alan R Liss 1985:55 – 66.

29. Samloff IM, Secrist DM, Passaro E Jr. A study of the relationship between serum group I pepsinogen levels and gastric acid secretion. Gastroenterology 1975;69:1196 – 1200.

30. Waldum HL, Burhol PG, Straume BK. Serum group I pepsinogen and gastrin in relation to gastric H$^+$ and pepsin outputs before and after subcutaneous injection of pentagastrin. Scand J Gastroenterol 1978;13:943 – 6.

31. Goedhard JG, Biemond I, Giliams JP, Pals G, Kreuning J. Serum pepsinogen I levels: Assessment of gastric acid secretion. In: Kreuning J, Samloff IM, Rotter JI, Eriksson A (Eds). Pepsinogens in man. Clinical and genetic advances. New York, Alan R Liss 1985:139 – 46.

32. Samloff IM, Liebman WM, Panitch NM. Serum group I pepsinogens by radioimmunoassay in control subjects and patients with peptic ulcer. Gastroenterology 1975;69:83 – 90.

33. Rotter JI, Sones JQ, Samloff IM, Richardson CT, Gursky JM, Walsh JH, Rimoin DL. Duodenal-ulcer disease associated with elevated serum pepsinogen I. An inherited autosomal dominant disorder. N Engl J Med 1979;300:63 – 6.

34. Rotter JI, Petersen G, Samloff IM, McConnell RN, Ellis A, Spence MA, Rimoin DL. Genetic heterogeneity of hyperpepsinogenaemic I and normopepsinogenimic I duodenal ulcer disease. Ann Int Med 1979;91:372 – 7.

35. Taylor IL, Calam J, Rotter JI, Vaillant C, Samloff IM, Cooke A, Simkin E, Dockray GH. Family studies of hypergastinemic, hyperpepsinogenemic I duodenal ulcer. Ann Int Med 1981;95:421 – 5.

36. Rotter JI, Rubin R, Meyer JH, Samloff IM, Taylor IL. Inherited rapid gastric emptying and duodenal ulcer disease. Clin Research 1982;30:293A.

14. Possibilities of surgical treatment of peptic ulcer

M. ALLGÖWER, D. LIEBERMANN-MEFFERT,
S. MARTINOLI, C. MÜLLER

Decrease, or elimination of vagally stimulated gastric secretion, particularly during the night – by whatever means – is followed by healing of gastric and duodenal ulcers and is very effective in preventing recurrence. This would appear an important clue to one crucial pathogenic factor in gastroduodenal ulcer disease. 'Vagal autosabotage' – particularly at night – appears to be the final link in the chain of events leading to the disease and its tendency to recurrence.

This does not explain the whole 'pathogenic cascade' with its likely psychosomatic origin. It does not explain either why different ulcer types may be induced by the same triggering mechanism. Individual anatomical and histological variations at the level of the stomach and duodenum may lead to these various ulcer types.

Eliminating the vagal autosabotage – knowingly or unknowingly – has led to very successful medical and surgical treatments of the acute disease and also to successful prevention of recurrence, if vagal stimulation of gastric activity remains restricted to moderate 'demand-secretion' induced by food.

The known modes of treatment are all symptomatic and address themselves to the end organ of acid and enzyme secretion. There are three main possibilities of treatment:

1. Medical treatment – which is dealt with by other speakers.
2. Surgical treatment – by more or less exentisive decrease of acid secreting parietal cell mass and elimination of the gastrin producing antrum: Billroth I and Billroth II type resections.
3. Surgical treatment by various modes of eliminating or decreasing the vagal influence on the stomach, its most 'physiological' form being *proximal selective vagotomy* (PSV), also called selective proximal vagotomy (SPV), or highly selective vagotomy (HSV).

The evaluation of any treatment has to be in the light of four criteria:
1. Effectiveness of ulcer healing;
2. Recurrence;
3. Morbidity;
4. Mortality.

Medical treatment – to summarize it very briefly – has become very effective, but on stopping the medication the recurrence rate is very high. Medical treatment has practically no morbidity and no mortality.

Gastric resection is very effective and has a very low recurrence rate, if resection is carried out correctly and rather extensively. The recurrence rate, however, continues to increase slowly over the years.

Morbidity is relatively high in terms of impaired gastrointestinal absorption and there is a fairly high incidence of dumping and diarrhoea.

Mortality rate is the highest of all the treatment modes: in experienced hands it may be 1%, but the average mortality is more likely to be between 2 and 5%.

Proximal selective vagotomy is very effectrive and gives permanent inhibition of acid secretion independent of patient's compliance. Recurrence rate depends very much on the ulcer type on the one hand and on completeness of vagotomy on the other. It can be influenced by appropriate intra-operative controls for completeness of vagotomy.

Morbidity is very low. There is hardly ever any dumping and only mild diarrhoea in a small percentage of patients – in contrast to the combination of vagotomy with any of the drainage operations.

Mortality is below 1% in any of the published series, including multicentre trials.

Before going into details, it seems appropriate to first define the types of gastroduodenal ulcers we are dealing with and which make it impossible to recommend one operation for all ulcer types. The following ulcer types should be distinguished – the symbols will be used throughout this paper:

DU   Duodenal ulcer (0.5 cm distal from centre of pylorus);
PU   Pyloric ulcers (± 0.5 cm from centre of pylorus);
PPU   Pre-pyloric ulcers – within 2.5 cm from centre of pylorus (gastric ulcer type II);
GU   Gastric ulcers – more than 2.5 cm from pylorus (gastric ulcer type I)
DGU Combined gastric and duodenal ulcers (gastric ulcer type II).

My contribution to this symposium relates primarily to two studies from the Basel group. Firstly a multicentre trail of PSV on 717 ulcer patients, all treated within 15 months and followed now for 10 years was done. I will, however, have to restric myself to the five year results, because the ten year evaluation is not yet complete. The second study is probably of some relevance to this symposium, because it concerns the structure and histology of the gastric antrum in gastroduodenal ulcer disease. For the first study credit goes primarily to my colleagues Claude Müller and Sebastiano Martinoli, for the second to Doris Liebermann-Meffert.[6,7]

The multicentre study include five German, one French and three Swiss surgical departments and has recently been extensively published by Müller and Martinoli.[8]

Table I. Patients in the study.

	DU	PU	PPU	GU	DGU	Total
Number	524	58	36	71	28	717
Elective	508	54	34	67	28	691
Emergencies	16	4	2	4	0	26
Mortality rate	1	0	0	0	0	1(0.14%)

DU: Duodenal ulcers.PU: Pyloric ulcers (± 0.5 cm). PPU: Pre-pyloric ulcers (within 2.5 cm of pylorus). GU: Gastric ulcers. DGU: Combined gastric and duodenal ulcers.

Table I shows the number of patients with the various ulcer types treated within this study and shows that there was only one death. Table II illustrates that only a very small percentage of duodenal and pyloric ulcers had an additional drainage operation.

Table II. Drainage operations.

	DU	PU	PPU	GU	DGU	Total
With drainage	31	23	4	–	–	58
Without drainage	493	35	32	71	28	659
Total	524	58	36	71	28	717

DU: Duodenal ulcers.PU: Pyloric ulcers (± 0.5 cm). PPU: Pre-pyloric ulcers (within 2.5 cm of pylorus). GU: Gastric ulcers. DGU: Combined gastric and duodenal ulcers.

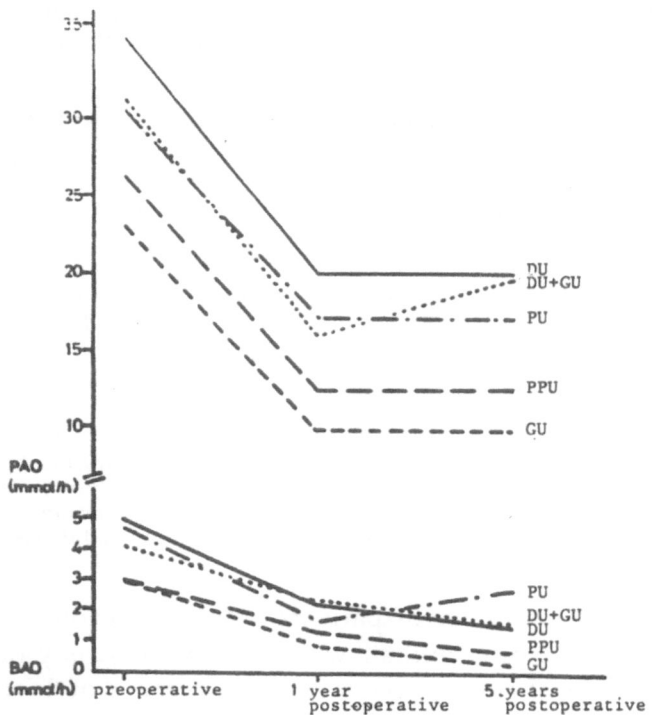

Figure 1. BAO and PAO$_{Pg}$ pre-operatively, 1 and 5 years after HSV for various ulcer types.

Table III. Clinical and total (actuarial) recurrence rate of multicentre study for various ulcer types after HSV.

Ulcer type	n	Clinical recurrence rate (%)	Total recurrence rate after HSV
DU	524	5.6 (40%)	13.9 (60%)
PU	58	9.2 (38%)	24.3 (62%)
PPU	36	15.9 (56%)	28.5 (44%)
GU	71	7.9 (45%)	17.5 (55%)

DU: Duodenal ulcers. PU: Pyloric ulcers ($\pm$ 0.5 cm). PPU: Pre-pyloric ulcers (within 2.5 cm of pylorus). GU: Gastric ulcers. DGU: Combined gastric and duodenal ulcers.

Figure 1 illustrates that the reduction in BAO and PAO_{pg}, at one and five years are practically identical. We observed only three cases of patients after a complete vagotomy going back to fairly high acid output. In these three cases regeneration of some of the innervation may have occurred.

Table III gives the crucial data of the recurrence rate. A high percentage of the five year controls were studied also endoscopically (62% of the initial number of patients) and an additional 10% at least agreed to have a radiological control, which gives a total of some 72% five year control. From these late endoscopic controls we learned the interesting fact that most recurrent ulcers are without symptoms, so that we have to distinguish between clinical and total recurrence rates. (figs 2 and 3)

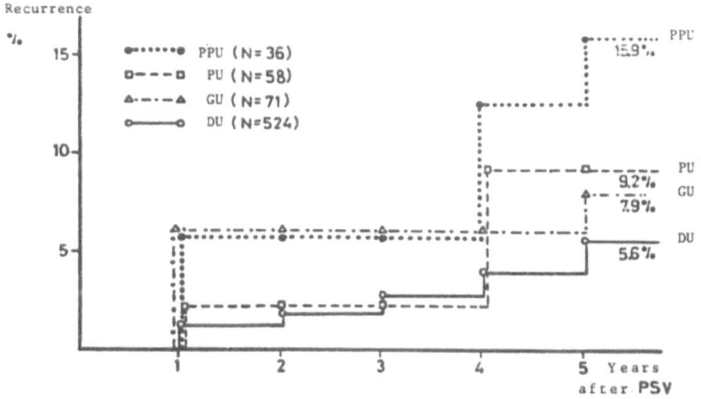

Figure 2. Cumulative clinical recurrence rate during 5 years.

Table IV. Clinical and total recurrence rate at 5 years re-operation rate for various ulcer types.

Ulcer type	n	5 years recurrence rate		Re-operations
		clinical (%)	total (%)	(%)
DU	524	5.6	13.9	2.3
PU	58	9.2	24.3	–
PPU	36	15.9	28.5	5.6
GU	71	7.9	17.5	5.6
DGU	28	8.2	20.3	3.6

DU: Duodenal ulcers. PU: Pyloric ulcers (± 0.5 cm). PPU: Pre-pyloric ulcers (within 2.5 cm of pylorus). GU: Gastric ulcers. DGU: Combined gastric and duodenal ulcers.

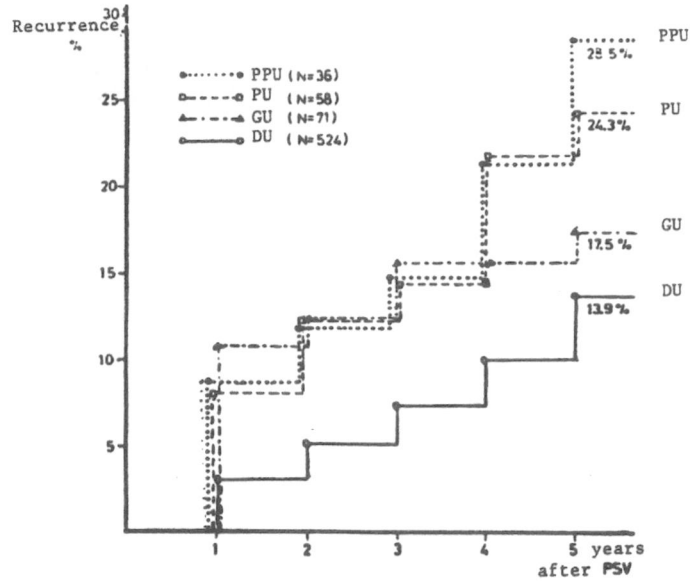

Figure 3. Cumulative total recurrence rate during 5 years.

Table IV shows in addition, that the re-operation rate – the really crucial figure – is considerably lower than the clinical recurrence rate, because conservative management of the recurrent ulceration after HSV is successful in at least half of the patients.

Figure 4 illustrates one of the important findings of this multicentre study: that a carefully done intra-operative vagomotor electrotest[1,2,9] correlates very significantly with the five year recurrence rate. The total recurrence rate where the vagomotor electrotest showed slight incompleteness is almost 19%, compared to 5.5% in those with wholly negative intra-operative vagomotor electrotest. Secretion studies at one and five years after HSV show, that the decrease in motor activity elicited by the vagomotor electrotest parallels the decrease in BAO

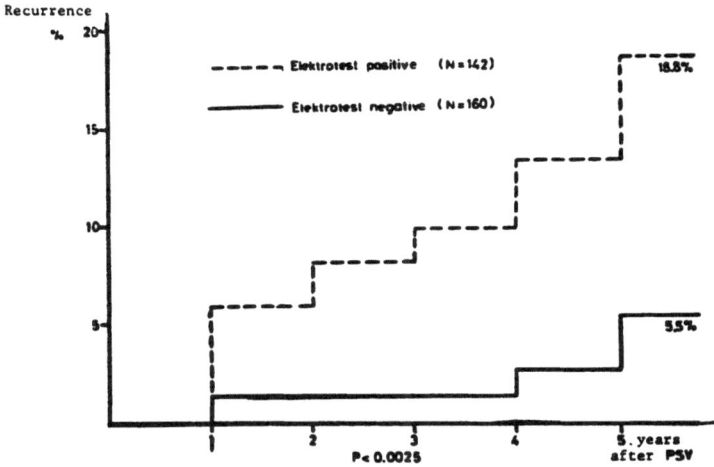

Figure 4. Recurrence rate in relation to results of intra-operative vagomotor electrotest.

and PAO_{Pg}. It is unfortunate that surgeons do not regularly take advantage of this technique of intra-operative quality control. It is useful in learning to do a careful HSV. Even the experienced vagotomist will find 10 to 20% of his anatomical dissections incomplete when carrying out the test. 89 Surgeons were taking part in the multicentre study. In more than 40% the first intra-operative test remained positive. The test discovered some residual vagal innervation of the proximal stomach which would have been missed if tests had not been done. After three evaluations, only 4% remained incomplete; that is, the anatomical cause of incompleteness could not be detected. This test, therefore, shows a very high sensitivity for incompleteness and appears clinically very useful. *

The other possibilities of intra-operative quality control, such as leucomethylenblue (Lee), congo red painting and intra-gastric pH-mapping were not as effective in our hands.

* The Vagorec 5 produced by Institute Straumann, CH 4437 Waldenburg, was used.

190

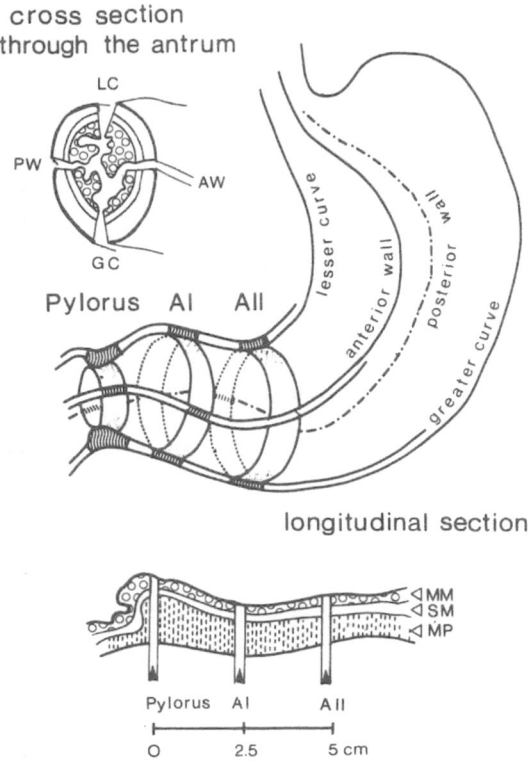

Figure 5. Longitudinal sections were taken along the lesser (LC) and greater curves (GC), the anterior (AW) and posterior walls (PW). Tissue for histology was taken from these sections at the pylorus, 2.5 cm (AI) and 5 cm (AII) proximal to the pylorus. the thickness of the mucosa (MM), submucosa (SM) and muscularis propria (MP) were measured at these sites.

The second study of the Basel group concerned the gastric antrum of resection specimens in gastric ulcer, duodenal ulcer and controls taken from kidney donors and autopsies. Ulcer formation in gastroduodenal ulcer disease is a symptom of a generalized disease of the stomach – as already pointed out by Konjetzny in 1947.[5] Careful histomorphological analysis, first of the gastric ulcer stomach compared with controls,[6] and later on also in resection specimens of duodenal ulcer patients, have revealed generalized disease of the antrum. Patients with gastric ulcer invariably had an irregularly thickened antral wall. Figure 5 shows the investigations done on three

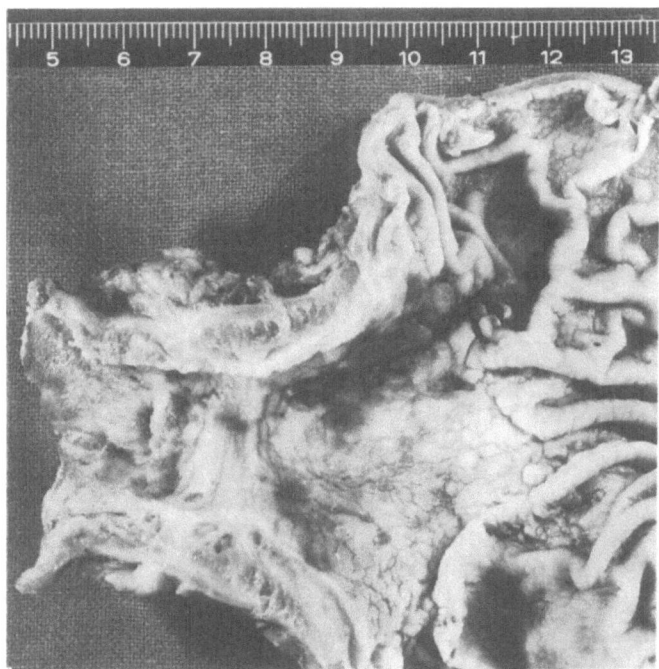

Figure 6. Gastric ulcer specimen with two ulcers at 3 cm from pylorus with marked antral wall thickening and muscular fibrosis.

segments of the gastric outflow tract. Figure 6 represents a resection specimen with two gastric ulcers with focal hypertrophy of the antral and pyloric musculature, the ulcerations being at 3 cm from the pylorus. Figure 7 shows various specimens with focal hypertrophy of either pylorus, or the antral wall, compared with a normal specimen of the human antrum.

Figure 8 compares the human antrum and its wall thickness in gastric ulcers (type I), in duodenal ulcers and in control stomachs taken from organ donors and autopsy specimens. Compared with controls, the duodenal ulcer patients has a significantly thickened antral wall ($p < 0.02$), whereas the thickening in gastric ulcer patients is more marked ($p < 0.001$). Figure 9 shows that all layers of the antral wall are thickened, illustrating the point that ulcer formation is a symptom of a generalized gastric and mostly antral disease.

Studies on peristaltic response of stomachs with gastric and duodenal ulcers to the vagomotor electrotest revealed the surprising fact, that gastric ulcer stomachs compared with stomachs in duodenal ulcer patients showed stronger and more prolonged motor responses to the stimulus.[7] This appears somewhat paradoxical in the light of the fact

192

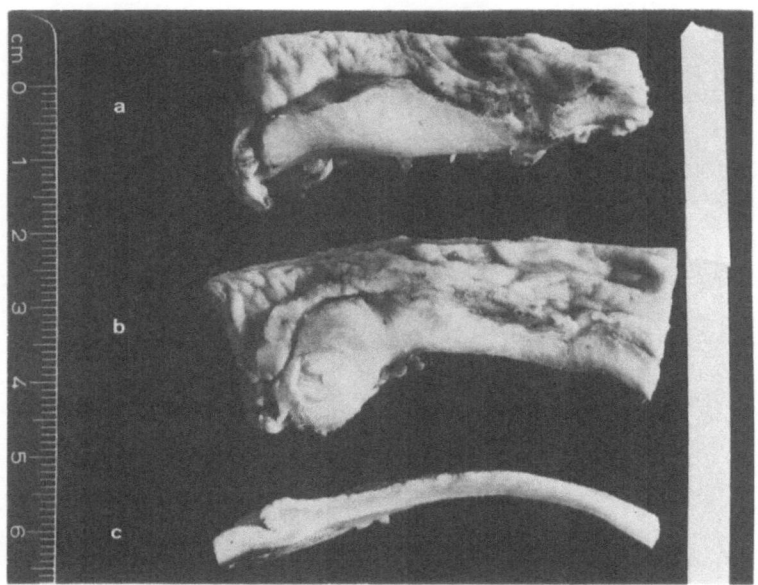

Figure 7. a. Focal muscular hypertrophy in gastric antrum and b. in pylorus in specimens of gastric ulcer stomachs, c. normal antral wall in organ donor.

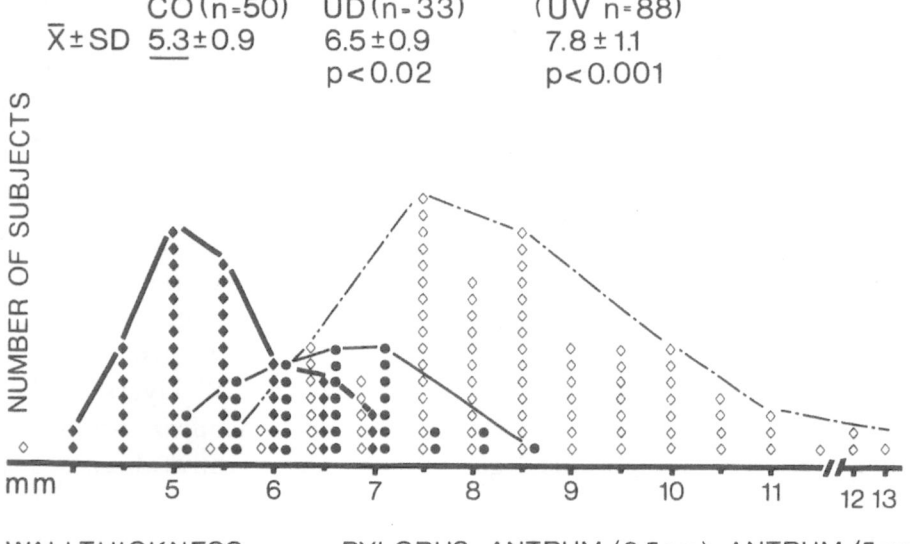

Figure 8. Average outflow tract thickening at 12 measuring points of pylorus, 2.5 and 5 cm from pylorus in controls (closed diamonds) in duodenal ulcer specimens (closed circles) and in gastric ulcer specimens (open diamonds).

TISSUE THICKNESS

Muscular + Submucosa + Mucosa

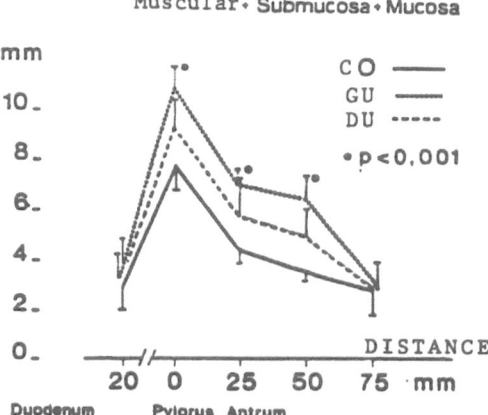

Figure 9. Average thickening of the various layers of the gastric outflow tract. CO control
——————, GU gastric ulcer ...., DU duodenal ulcer – – – – .

that gastric ulcer patients very often have delayed gastric emptying. Histology of the gastric antrum with its focal muscular hypertrophy, its damaged muscular nucleoid and its vacuolized Auerbach's plexus would indicate, that co-ordinated peristalsis may be disturbed, thus explaining delayed emptying. The histological changes of the antrum in 'duodenal ulcer stomachs' – although somewhat similar to 'gastric stomachs' – are distinctly less pronounced than in the latter.

The pathogenic significance of increased motor responses in the fact of delayed gastric emptying has not been appreciated as yet. Observing such stomachs during contraction – most marked on the lesser curvature – reveals completely white, non-perfused gastric wall areas, resolving only very slowly.

These findings are not without significance for our choice of operative methods. The histological appearance of the musculature and of the Auerbach's plexus would suggest reversibility of the changes up to a certain point. If, however, antral disease is very marked, changes appear to be irreversible.

This then leads to the following practical conclusions in surgical management of gastroduodenal ulcer:

GU: Gastric ulcer type I   – HSV + excision of ulcer for precise histology
  – in rare cases Billroth I resection if marked antral disease is present

DGU: Gastric ulcer type II – treatment will be carried out according to which ulcer appears to be 'dominant'

PPU:Gastric ulcer type III

  – HSV + drainage operation, or preferably restricted antrectomy

PU: Pyloric ulcer   – HSV + anterior pylorectomy or pyloroplasty

DU: Duodenal ulcer   – HSV most of the time without any 'crime against the pylorus', if no clinical stenosis is present. If clinical stenosis is present and located in the first duodenal part, a duodenoplasty and not a pyloroplasty is recommended

In summary, it may be stated that most gastric and duodenal ulcers will do well after highly selective vagotomy, a small proportion of cases needing either antrectomy or pyloroplasty. Whenever highly selective vagotomy is carried out, there is general agreement about the importance of complete vagal denervation of the parietal cell mass. Therefore intra-operative control of the completeness of vagotomy would appear mandatory.

There has been controversy concerning the practical effectiveness of such intra-operative controls[3] as staining of vagal fibres by methylenblue, detecting acid secreting areas of the stomach by congo red painting, or mapping of the stomach with the pH-electrode, or by carrying out the electrotest originally devised by Burge and Vane.[4] The multicentre study[8] involving 89 surgeons has provided good evidence that the testing of the remaining motor activity in the proximal stomach, if carried out according to strict rules, permits incompleteness of vagotomy to be corrected during operation in many cases. Evidence has been quite clear that this approach to the problem of completeness of vagotomy significantly reduces recurrence rates. The histomorphological study of the stomach as a whole and particularly of the gastric antrum has shown that in some cases antral disease is too far advanced to be amenable to highly selective vagotomy only. In these cases antrectomy or pyloroplasty must be added to the HSV.

References

1. Allgöwer M, Schultheiss HR, Meine J, Perren SM. Intraoperative Prüfung der Mageninnervation. MMW 1969;III:767.
2. Allgöwer M, Perren SM. Comments concerning intraoperative Electrotest for Completeness of Vagotomy. Prog Surg 1970;8:69– .
3. Baron JH, Alexander-Williams J, Allgöwer M, Müller C, Spencer J. Vagotomy in Modern Surgical Practice. Butterworths & Co 1982.
4. Burge H, Vane JR. Methods of Testing for complete Nerve Section during Vagotomy. Br Med J 1958;I:615.
5. Konjetzny CE. Die Geschwulstbildung im Magen, Duodenum and Jejunum. Enke, Stuttgart 1947.
6. Libermann-Meffert D, Allgöwer M. The Morphology of the Antrum and Pylorus in Gastric Ulcer Disease. Prog Surg 1977;15:109.
7. Liebermann-Meffert D, Müller C, Allgöwer M. Gastric Hypermotility and Antropyloric Dysfunction in Gastric Ulcer Patients. Br J Surg 1982;69:11.
8. Müller C, Martinoli S. Die proximal-selektive Vagotomie. Springer-Verlag, Stuttgart 1985.
9. Schultheiss HR, Perren SM. Allgöwer M. Elektrische Reizung der Vagusäste und intragastrische Druckmessungen beim Hund. Helv Chir Acta 1969; 36:328.

15. Discussion III

Johnston:

Mr. Allgöwer, you demonstrated an 8% recurrence rate for gastric ulcers at 5 years and my data are comparable. You reported a 5–6% symptomatic recurrence rate for duodenal ulcer at 5 years and the over-all figures for our unit in Leeds are about 8%. So I fully support your opinion on the unifying concept of gastric and duodenal ulcer with the similar kind of operative approach with, of course, taking enourmous care that the gastric ulcers are benign.

We cannot talk about recurrence rates unless there is some kind of quality control, whether intra-operative or post-operative, otherwise we do not exactly know what we are talking about.

Johnson:

Mr. Allgöwer, you had one death in 700 patients: what was the cause of death? Could you also give us the world wide death rate for HSV? If we have identified the surgical death rate we can compare it with death rates in patients treated medically. The last trial I saw with histamine H_2-receptor antagonists had three coronary deaths.

Allgöwer:

Our death was due to pulmonary embolism which was related to the operative procedure. I calculated a hypothetical mortality of 0.5% to 1.5%. the highest death rate I have come across in a large study of vagotomy was 1.5%.

Johnston:

We had one death out of 600 elective HSV procedure for duodenal ulcer, also a pulmonary embolus. This patient had not received pro-phylactic low-dose heparin therapy, which we give routinely in patients over 40 years of age.

Amdrup:

Neither surgeons, nor physicians can make use of the mortality figures from the pre-cimetidine era and compare them to the present day figures. Before cimetidine was available we had to operate on all sorts of patients, the elderly, the obese and those with pulmonary and cardiac disease. We do not have to operate on these high risk patients now and we as surgeons nowadays owe the physicians the present mortality rates, which can be very close to zero.

Kennedy:

Mr. Allgöwer, you included ulcers 0.5 cm distal to the pylorus in your pyloric ulcer group, which have a higher recurrence rate in your and other's hands. Most of us would include these ulcers in the duodenal ulcer group. If you would do that, your duodenal ulcer recurrence rate would be considerably higher.

Allgöwer:

That is the reason we exclude them!

Kennedy:

The other point I would like to make concerns the Burge test. The Burge test really indicates that the recurrences are due to small accessory nerve fibres. Rosetti in Italy has drawn attention to the nerve branches coming up from the distal stomach. The Burge test tests the proximal fibres, but we hardly pay attention to the distal nerves.

Allgöwer:

The major cause of imcomplete HSV in earlier studies was due to inadequate denervation of the distal oesophagus. The Rosetti problem of the crawfoot is rare, I have only one documented case where we had to go down to the greater curve. There have been descriptions of persisting positive congo red tests until the greater curve was dissected, but clinically it is not that important if the proximal denervation has been done meticulously.

Johnston:

The Rosetti nerve is relatively unimportant. Matheson, who has a very low recurrence rate of one out of 70 patients with a 5 year follow up, does not pay attention to the Rosetti nerve. Neither do I, and my recurrence rate is low. Proper denervation of the oesophagus is the most important point in prevention of recurrences.

Tijtgat:

What percentage of surgeons rely on intra-operative testing?

Allgöwer:

That depends. In Germany 15 – 20% of the surgeons do intra-operative tests. I always use intra-operative testing during an HSV. It prolongs the operation by 30 minutes on average.

Tijtgat:

Quite a few patients have dyspeptic symptoms starting approximately 6 months after HSV. These complaints are difficult to interpret and treat. I do not know what the mechanism of this discomfort is, May it be related to delayed gastric emptying?

Allgöwer:

It could be due to antral denervation. Extending the vagotomy at the distal end can seriously affect gastric emptying.

Amdrup:

With intra-operative testing the device is placed round the oesophagus, but the nerves to the left and on the back of the oesophagus are missed.

Allgöwer:

We have not had problems in including the posterior nerve fibres in our measurements.

Wormsley:

Mr. Allgöwer, the postoperative peak acid output in your group of patients with a low recurrence rate (5 %) was 6 mmol/hr and in the group with a high recurrence rate (18%) 9 mmol/hr. Why do you consider this difference to be important and how do you relate it to the observation that in the non-operated patient duodenal ulcers do not recur if gastric secretion is below 15 mmol/hr?

Allgöwer:

I cannot answer your question, I just showed you the facts. There is still much work to be done.

16. The surgical treatment of gastric ulcer

J. SPENCER, M.S., F.R.C.S.

Department of Surgery, Royal Postgraduate Medical School, Hammersmith Hospital, London, United Kingdom

With the advent of histamine H_2-receptor antagonists and other agents, it seemed possible a few years ago that surgical management of gastric ulcer would have disappeared by the 1980s. Studies from several countries however, including The Netherlands,[1] have indicated that gastric ulcer (GU) disease has not fallen in incidence as has duodenal ulcer, and admissions to hospital for its treatment have declined only slightly. It remains possible that 'traditional' gastric ulcers are disappearing and being replaced by a different form. For example, GU associated with the use of non-steroidal anti-inflammatory drugs seems to be increasing in frequency, one informal report in the United Kingdom stating that 36% of GU patients seen were on such medication. It is a clinical impression, worthy of further investigation, that these ulcers are more aggressive and resistant to treatment, whether medical or surgical.

The typical gastric ulcer lies on the lesser curve of the stomach. In the large Veterans Administration trial of 637 ulcers published in 1971,[2] seven were in the fundus, 357 (56%) in the body, and 273 (43%) in the 'antrum'. The latter allocation was probably not strictly accurate, as it is known that the histologically defined antrum usually extends up the lesser curve to include the ulcer.

The patient with gastric ulcer

It was been a clinical impression and teaching of mine for many years that the patient with a GU is 10 kg lighter and 10 years older than the patient with a duodenal ulcer (DU). This turns out to be nearly true in a randomly selected group of our own patients, (Tables I and II) the differences in mean weights being 6.9 kg and in mean ages

2.7 years. Because of the age factor smoking has been of longer duration in most cases, and arguably in dose/kg terms more damaging.
Pulmonary problems therefore become more likely after operation, as
do other complications such as cardio-vascular and thrombo-embolic
disease.

The pylorus and gastric ulcer

The aetiology of GU has been discussed in detail earlier. I have however been sufficiently impressed by data concerning duodeno-gastric
reflux to make one observation here. Reflux of barium from the duodenum during the test described years ago by Capper, Airth and
Kilby[3] was often directed along the lesser curve, sometimes into an
ulcer crater. On doing similar tests I was struck by the possible
importance of this factor in the localization of ulcers. This observation, plus the more general acceptance of pyloric malfunction in GU
disease, makes it possibly unwise to preserve the pylorus when operating for GU. However, interpretations of data available to date are
not clear-cut on this issue.

Possible operations

When Rydygier reported in 1882[4] the first gastrectomy for benign
GU (done the year before), his paper was abstracted in another journal, whose editor expressed the hope that it would be the last operation of its kind.[5] Fortunately this was not the case, and the Billroth I
partial gastrectomy has been used for GU ever since. It has remained
the yard-stick against which other operations for GU are measured.
Billroth II (Polya) partial gastrectomy is known to give even better
results in terms of recurrence. Mr Norman Tanner used to say that
in his vast experience he rarely, if ever, saw a recurrent GU after a
Polya operation. However, the incidence of bile-reflux and nutri-
tional problems is higher, and the operation has never been accepted
as a standard procedure for GU, at least in the United Kingdom.
    A high lesser-curve ulcer makes a Billroth I operation more diffi-
cult, but not impossible. The extension of resection up to lesser curve,
around the ulcer, was described by many surgeons. Not least among
them was mr H. Daintree Johnson from my own institution. He gave

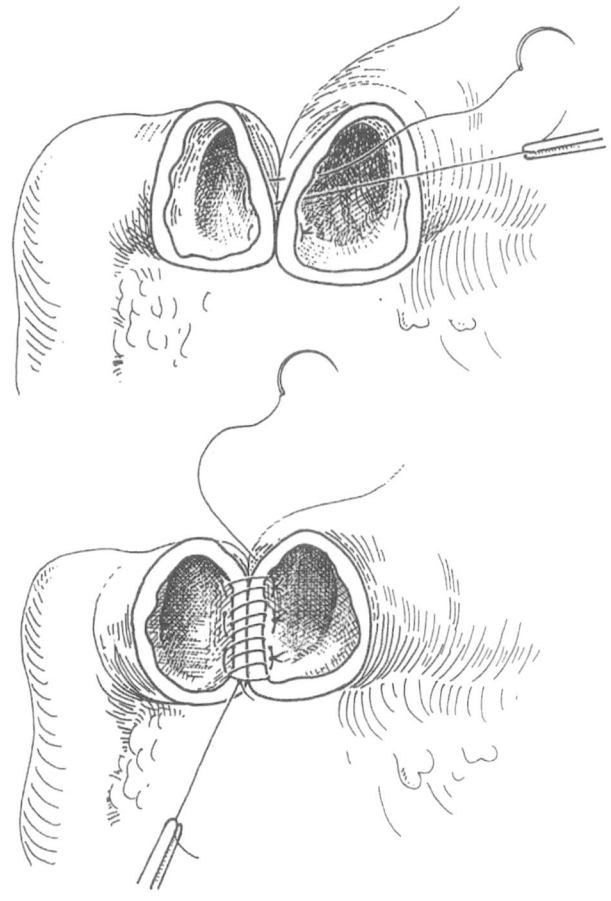

Figure 1. Technique of Billroth I anastomosis using mattress sutures posteriorly.

an excellent account of what Tanner used to call a 'rotation' gastrectomy, in 1954.[6]

Every surgeon has his own technical tricks for performing a Billroth I gastrectomy. I will mention but two. During anastomosis, I have always used three through-and-through mattress sutures to oppose the stomach and duodenum, instead of the traditional posterior line of sutures. These are quick, and give excellent positioning of the lumens for commencement of the inner layer of sutures. (fig. 1) There are many ways of constructing the new lesser curve, and it is now fashionable, but expensive, to use automatic stapling devices. A much cheaper but equally helpful instrument is the furniss clamp

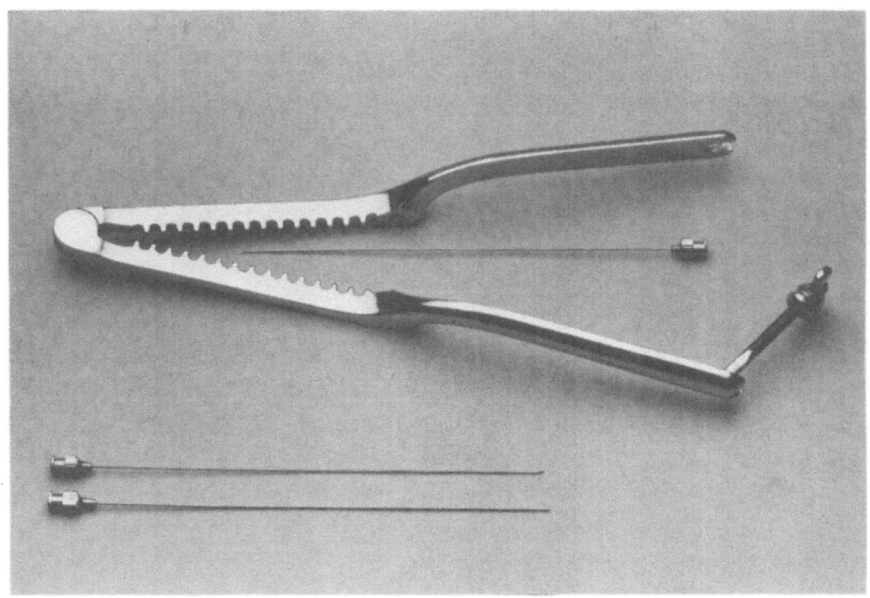

Figure 2. The Furniss clamp. Each jaw is grooved and interdigitates with its partner. The grooves then form a hole through which a needle is passed to transfix the crimped 'lesser curve' along its length.

illustrated in figure 2. After clamping, inserting a needle, and removing the clamp, the new lesser curve is found plicated along the needle. It is cleanly and rapidly oversewn before the needle is withdrawn. (fig. 3)

Truncal (TV), selective (SV) or proximal gastric (highly selective, PGV) vagotomy are also possible procedures. All must be combined with ulcer excision to avoid missing a carcinoma, which is a real risk. Excision may be performed through a gastrostomy, and if this is combined with a PGV then a transverse rather than a longitudinal incision should be used. This minimises interruption of blood supply to the lesser curve, which is compromised to a variable degree by this operation. (fig. 4)

It is often asked why vagotomy may be used for GU when acid secretion is normal. The answer is that secretion is *inappropriately* high for a patient with a diminished mucosal resistance. Reduction of acid, either medically or surgically, permits healing.

Segmental gastrectomies of many kinds have been attempted over the years, an early description being that of Riedel in 1909.[7] The most successful and carefully method studied is that of Maki[8] which

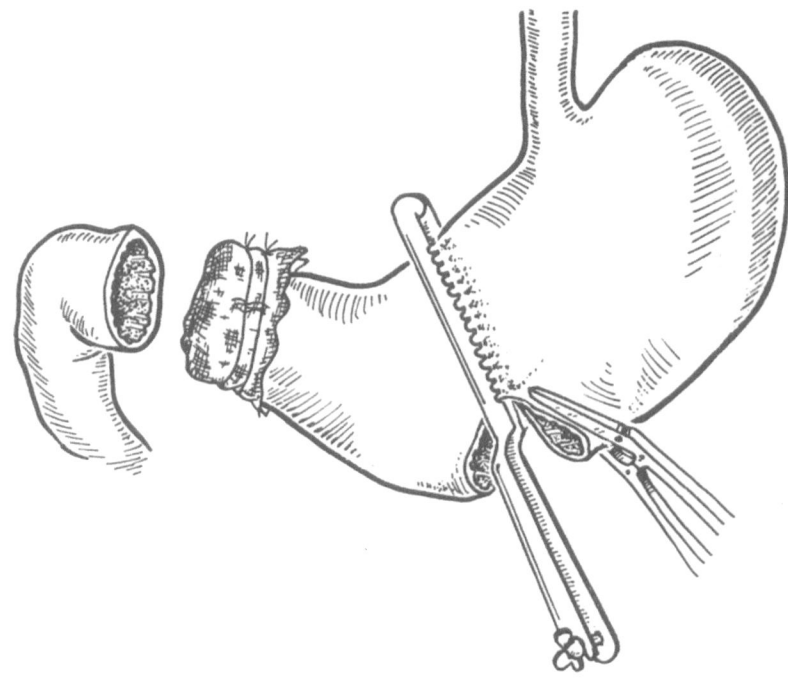

Figure 3. The Furniss clamp in use on the stomach during a Billroth I resection.

consists of a resection similar to a Billroth I but with division and anastomosis 1.5 cm orad to the pylorus, in an attempt to preserve normal pyloric function. (fig. 5)

Mucosal antrectomy is theoretically attractive, but has been used in man (association with vagotomy) more for DU than for GU. It is a more complex operation, which in more general use would almost certainly carry a higher morbidity and mortality than a standard resection.

Types of ulcer

The question of the homogeneity of a GU population has implications for therapy. Are all ulcers the same, or if different do they demand different treatment? This topic has once again come to the foreground as newer operations have been used, sometimes with unpredicted results.

206

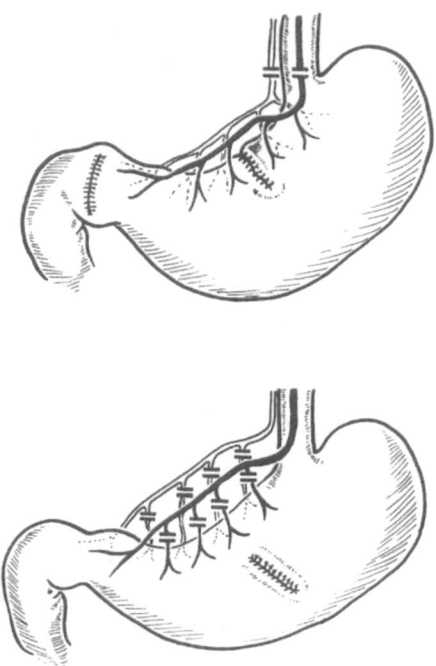

Figure 4. Truncal vagotomy (above) and proximal gastric vagotomy (below) with ulcer excision. A transverge gastrotomy during proximal gastric vagotomy gives access to the ulcer for mucosal excision, while not compromising the blood supply to the lesser curve.

My one-time senior colleague and friend, H. Daintree Johnson, first described three types of GU in 1957[9]:
– Type I is the 'common' lesser curve GU.
– Type II is a similar ulcer associated with an active or healed duodenal ulcer.
– Type III is a prepyloric peptic ulcer (PPU), living within 2 cm of the pylorus.
Johnson indicated that Type II and III ulcers had the nocturnal acid secretion pattern of duodenal ulcer, whereas Type I behaved like normal control subjects. (fig. 6)

He produced other supporting evidence (blood group, secretor status) for this heterogeneity, which has been broadly accepted since that time as a guide to treatment. The inherent assumptions however have been recently challenged. Venables[10] has found that in terms of basal and stimulated output (pentagastrin or insulin) Type III ulcer did not

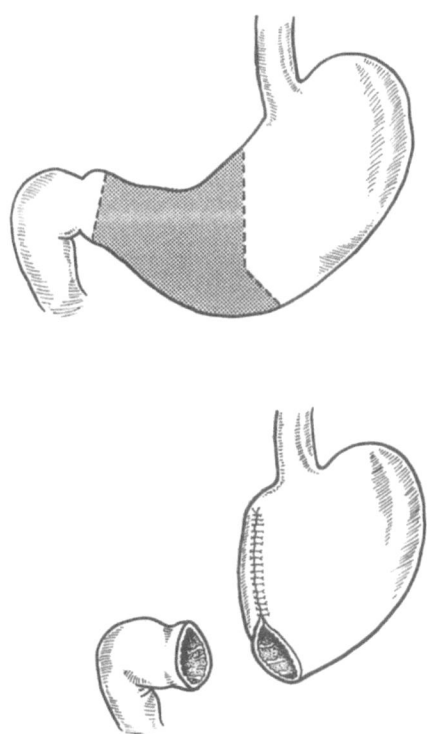

Figure 5. Maki pre-pyloric gastrectomy. the distal resection line and subsequent anastomosis lie 1.5 cm orad to the pylorus.

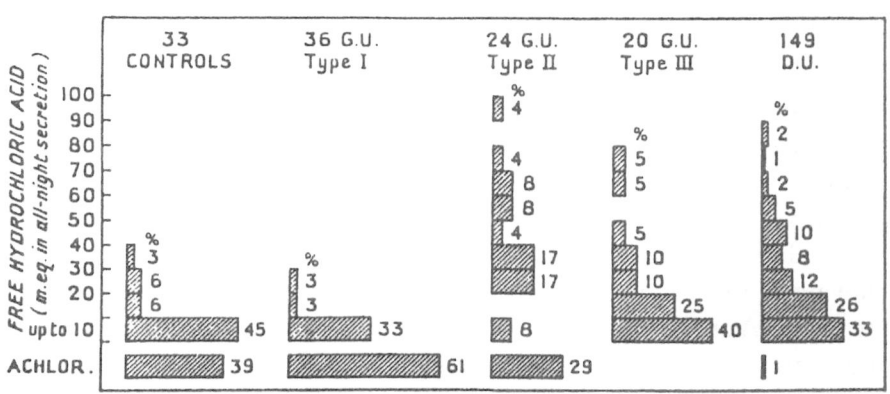

Nocturnal secretion of acid by healthy people and peptic-ulcer patients.

Figure 6.

differ from Type I. Type II ulcers secrete more, but in his opinion the overlap is so great that the difference cannot be accepted as a guide to treatment. It is possible that ulcers differ in different places and probably over the years also. On the basis of body weight and age, our PPU patients certainly resemble GU patients and differ statistically from DU patients. (Tables I and II)

Table I. Peptic ulcer – body weight kg.

Ulcer	n	x̄	SD	P	SEM
Duodenal	92	67.0	± 10.7	} <0.01	1.11
Prepyloric	9	58.6	± 6.8	} >0.5	2.26
Gastric	18	60.1	± 13.3		3.13

Table II. Peptic ulcer – age (years).

Ulcer	n	x̄	SD	P	SEM
Duodenal	92	46.2	± 12.6	} <0.05	1.31
Prepyloric	9	54.8	± 9.6	} >0.3	3.2
Gastric	18	58.9	± 9.2		2.17

Results of surgery

One of the most important factors in surgery is safety. If the GU patient, as I have presented him, is somewhat loaded with inherent risks, then there seems a good case for conservative, non-resecting operations for GU. In practice however, it seems that for elective operations the mortalities of vagotomy and gastrectomy do not differ markedly. No large-scale control data pertaining to this topic exist and available data may well reflect a policy of reserving vagotomy for sicker patients. Taking this into consideration, it is interesting to note that in the Ann Arbor series quoted by Kraft[11] the mortalities of 449 vagotomies and 2,152 gastrectomies for GU were 2.0 and 1.6% respectively. Data collected from several other series gives a similar figure. (Table III) Nielsen et al from Denmark reviewing 354 operations for GU reported an overall mortality rate of 5% and a mortality of 2% in elective cases.[12] Thomas has reported a series of 144 Billroth I resections from Bristol with a zero mortality in elective cases and a 0.7% overall mortality.[13] (Table IV) The recurrence rate after a Billroth I resection is low. (Table III) In the Bristol series it was 3%[13] and in Denmark[12] rather higher at 5% after gastrectomy. Many other series could be mentioned giving similar results.

Table III. Results of surgery for GU: Collected data.

| | n | Percentage | |
		Mortality	Recurrence
Billroth I	1309	4	2
TV and pyloroplasty	495	2	10
PGV	182	2	6

Table IV. Percentage mortality (†) and recurrence rates for Billroth I partial gastrectomy.

Author	Year	n	†	† in elective cases	Recurrences
Nielsen	1973	354	5	2	11
Thomas	1982	144	0,7	0	3

If resection is safe and prevents recurrence, are its long-term effects too serious? Once again, long-term follow-up has indicated that they need not be so. In particular Thomas[13] has found in his long-term follow-up that Visick gradings are good, with 88% of patients being in Grades I and II. Body weights were maintained in that series also, 59.7 kg pre-operatively, and 64.05 kg post-operatively, and anaemia was not a serious problem. This contrasts with what we were expecting some years ago, and I suspect that social changes, with the population as a whole enjoying a much higher standard of living, has had an effect. We must not exclude the chance that a few problems will appear; remembering the resection is then the clue to diagnosis. The worst post-gastrectomy osteomalacia I have seen followed a Billroth I gastrectomy twelve years previously.

Truncal vagotomy can give good results also, as indicated in Table V.[14,15,16] Symptomatic relief is achieved in most patients, but there is considerable discrepancy in the reported incidence of recurrence. Early assessment may suggest a low recurrence rate, but Eastmann and Gear[16] found that an 8% recurrence increased to 22% on subsequent follow-up. Similarly, Kraft reported a 5% recurrence at one

Table V. Truncal vagotomy for GU.

| Authors | Year | n | Percentage | |
			Recurrence	Good/ satisfactory
Farris and Smith	1973	33	0	90
Cade and Allan	1979	58	2	96
Eastmann and Gear	1979	80	8 → 22	83

year, increasing to 11% at ten years, after 135 elective operations (including some selective vagotomies[11]).

Madsen et al[17] compared TV and pyloroplasty with Billroth I gastrectomy in a prospective randomized trial. Of 45 patients, 22 had a resection (one dying of a pulmonary embolus) and 23 a TV. Two TV patients developed a documented recurrence and a third, who was on a non-steroidal anti-inflammatory drug, developed a gastrocolic fistula, presumably due to recurrence, and died. At three years the survivors were not different as regards overall symptom grades. However, 6/23 in the vagotomy group and 3/21 in the resected group had diarrhoea.

Resection has also been compared with PGV combined with excision of the ulcer. Emas and Hammarberg at the Karolinska Institute randomized 30 patients.[18] There were two recurrences at three years after PGV, and one after gastrectomy. Post-prandial fullness was more common after gastrectomy, but overall gradings were very similar and in both groups 6 patients were classified Visick III – IV.

Reid and Duthie et al[19] performed a larger similar trial, with 26 PGV and 29 gastrectomy patients followed up for about 8 years. There were 4 'unrelated' deaths in each group, and 6 and 5 recurrences respectively. There were significantly fewer overall symptoms at follow up in the PGV group. Pooling the data of these two similar trials gives a recurrence rate of 15% after PGV and 7% after resection, which is suggestive but not significant different.

If one examins all the comparative and other data availble on conservative operations for GU and compares them with data on gastrectomy, it would appear that resection has an overall mortality about twice as high as vagotomy – though as mentioned earlier there are large series that do not show this difference. Vagotomy seems to be followed by an overall ulcer recurrence rate about five times as high

Table VI. Type II GU (combined ulcers): Incidence.

Author	Year	Place	Percentage
Lee	1982	Auckland	15
Welch and Burke	1969	Boston	15
Henley and Bowers	1965	Memphis	19
Angel, Giacobine and Jordan	1967	Houston	30
Kraft	1984	Ann Arbor	36
Duhamel, Block and Haubrich	1963	Detroit	50

Table VII. Type II GU: Results of surgery.

Author	n	Operation	Percentage recurrence
Pichlmayer et al	16	BI	7
Kronborg	16	TVP	0
Douglas and Duthie	39	TVP	0
Johnston et al	25	BGV	0
Pichlmayer et al	5	PGV	20

as gastrectomy. Whichever operation is employed, it must be remembered that about 5% of gastric ulcers unexpectedly turn out to be malignant[20] making ulcer excision mandatory.

Type II ulcers are not always easy to define. Perhaps this explains the huge variation in incidence reported from different centres, ranging from 15 to 50%.[11,21-25] (Table VI) If considered to be secondary to (rather than just associated with) DU disease, then conservative operations might be expected to give good results. On the whole, this approach is justified by the general results obtained, which are illustrated in Table VIII.[26-29] There is a clear discrepancy concerning the incidence of recurrence after PGV, and further data on this are awaited with interest. Douglas and Duthie[28] compared the results of truncal vagotomy and pyloroplasty for Types II and I GU, in 39 and 44 patients respectively. 'Good' results were found in 83% and 54% respectively, and 'poor' ones in 3% and 21%, indicating that Type II ulcers tend to do far better than Type I when treated by vagal section.

Type III ulcers have been suggested to represent really 'ectopic' DUs, which happen to lie on the wrong side of the pylorus. As mentioned earlier, this view may be challenged. Pragmatically, it has been a surprise to find very high recurrence rates in PPUs treated by PGV,

Table VIII. Type III GU: Results of surgery.

Author	n	Operation	Percentage recurrence
Pichlmayr et al	15	BI	0
Kronborg	78	TVP	6
Anderson et al	59	PGV	22
Becker and Siewert	40	PGV	20
Pichlmayr et al	32	PGV	25

these being as high as 35 – 40% at 5 – 6 years. Results are better after resection, but data are hard to evaluate because in earlier series PPU was not always defined. Pichlmayer[26] treated 15 by Billroth I gastrectomy with no recurrence. Kronborg[28] treated 78 by TV with pyloroplasty with 6% recurrence. However, after PGV, Anderson et al[30] had 22% recurrence in 59 patients, Becker and Siewert 20% in 40[31], and Pichlmayer 25% in 32.[26] It seems therefore that PGV should not be used for PPU. A Billroth I resection or vagotomy and antrectomy is to be preferred. Controlled trials may be indicated, but few of us now see enough such ulcers to compare procedures adequately.[26-29] (Table VIII)

On balance it appears that Billroth I partial gastrectomy remains the best choice for most gastric ulcers, with the Type II ulcer possibly being treated by truncal, or selective vagotomy and drainage. If resection is to be used extensively, is there a place for preserving the pylorus?

The *Maki gastrectomy* certainly maintains nearly normal gastric emptying as noted by Sekine et al.[33] The same workers found a zero recurrence rate in 60 patients, but others, notably Teigan et al[33] have found recurrence to be a significant problem (1.6% of 47 patients). In general, it has been found that this procedure prevents dumping, but occasionally gives problems with gastric retention, which, together with a higher recurrence rate, suggests that Billroth gastrectomy is to be preferred.

Complicated ulcers

It is not within the scope of this paper to give a full review of ulcer complications and their management, but a few comments are appropriate.

It is important to recognize that bleeding and perforation carry a significant mortality. Kraft[11] reported from Ann Arbor that in patients undergoing an emergency operation there was an overall mortality of 8% after vagotomy in 561 patients, and 9.4% after 1,647 gastrectomies. These figures cannot be compared in any meaningful way, but they tally well with most published results.

Mortality from *bleeding GU* is dependent on the severity of bleeding, increasing dramatically in those needing six or more units of blood. At operation, this is seen to be associated with haemorrhage from an atheromatous non-contractile left gastric artery which is clearly not going to stop bleeding without intervention. Although photocoagulation is now possible in some of these patients, most will need resection. Under-running of the ulcer is less practical and effective than in DU, but remains a possible treatment, with vagotomy in some subjects. Age is the other most important factor, almost all death occurring in those over 50 years of age and the mortality increasing steeply with age.

These factors have encouraged an 'early surgery' policy for bleeding, especially in the elderly. In the Birmingham study comparing early with more conservative indications for operation, mortality in the over-60 population was 2% in the early group and 13% in the remainder.[34] Although criticism of that study has been directed mainly at the lack of stratification for several important factors, the data are very suggestive. Similar support for a more surgically agressive policy can also be found. For example Hunt, Hansky et al from Melbourne have increased their operation rate from 27% to 42%, with a fall in overall mortality from 18% to 10%.[35] This study has all the defects of a sequential assessment, but the current results achieved are good. There certainly seems a need to overcome reluctance to operate on elderly patients with bleeding GU.[34] (Table IX)

Table IX. Early surgery in bleeding PU. From: Birmingham data, BMJ 1984;288:1277.

	n	Percentage operation	'Over 60' mortality	Percentage GU
Early	71	59	2	0
Conservative	71	21	13	24
	142	40	10	12

Perforated GU remains a problem. A recent Scottish study indicated an increasing incidence in females, as others have noted.[36] The overall perforated GU incidence remained constant at 2.5/100,000 and carried an overall mortality of 17% in 288 patients. All the deaths were in patients more than 65 years old, this groups representing a third of the whole. There are conflicting data concerning the results of different forms of management. In one recent series,[37] an 18.2% mortality in 22 patients whose ulcer was oversewn compared poorly with no deaths in six resections. In the much larger Scottish series oversewing gave a mortality of 8.2% and there was an overall mortality of 10.1%. Most patients with a perforated GU need a laparotomy, and choice of operation must be made according to the findings and circumstances. In contrast to DU, there seems little argument for adding vagotomy to the treatment of a perforated GU, if resection is performed.

References

1. Bulthuis R, Laing WA. Cost effectiveness of cimetidine. Lancet 1982;2:828–9.
2. Sun DCH, Stempien SJ. The site and size of the ulcer as determinants of outcome. Gastroenterology 1971;61:576–84.
3. Capper WM, Airth GR, Kilby JO. A test of pyloric regurgitation. Lancet 1966;2:621–3.
4. Rygidier L. Exstirpation des carcinomatösen Pylorus. Tod nach 12 Stunden. Deutsche Ztschr Chir 1880;14(3)4:252.
5. Zentralbl Chir 1882;9:198–199.
6. Johnson HD, Orr IM. Selective surgery for peptic ulcer. Surg Gynecol Obstet 1954;98:425–432.
7. Riedel B. Entfernung des mittleren Abschnittes vom Magen wegen Geschwür. Dtsch Med Wochenschr 1909;35:17–54.
8. Maki T, Shiratori T, Sugawara K. Pylorus-preservering gastrectomy as an improved operation for gastric ulcer. Surgery 1967;61:838–45.
9. Johnson HD. The pathogenesis of peptic ulcers. Lancet 1957;2:515–517.
10. Venables CW. Chronic peptic ulcer: Surgical treatment. In: Bouchier IAD et al (Eds). Textbook of Gastroenterology. London, Bailliere Tindall 1984:156–64.
11. Kraft RO. Long-term results of vagotomy and pyloroplasty in the treatment of gastric ulcer disease. Surgery 1984;95:460–6.
12. Nielsen JE, Amdrup E, Christiansen P, Fenger C, Jensen H-E, Lindskov J, Damgaard Nielsen SA. Gastric ulcer II. Surgical treatment. Acta Chir Scand 1973;139:460–5.
13. Thomas WEG, Thompson MH, Williamson RCN. The long-term outcome of Billroth I partial gastrectomy for benign gastric ulcer. Ann Surg 1982;195:189–95.
14. Farris JM, Smith GK. Long-term appraisal of the treatment of gastric ulcer in situ by vagotomy and pyloroplasty with a note on the Jaboulay procedure. Am J Surg 1973;126:292–9.
15. Cade D, Allen D. Long-term follow-up of patients with gastric ulcers treated by vagotomy, pyloroplasty and ulcerectomy. Br J Surg 1979;66:46–7.
16. Eastmann MC, Gear MWL. Vagotomy and pyloroplasty for gastric ulcers. Br J Surg 1979;66:238–41.

17. Madsen P, Kronborg O, Hart Hansen O, Petersen T. Billroth I gastric resection versus truncal vagotomy and pyloroplasty in the treatment of gastric ulcer. Acta Chir Scand 1976;142:151 – 3.
18. Emas S, Hammarberg C. Prospective, randomised trial of selective proximal vagotomy with ulcer excision and partial gastrectomy in the treatment of corporeal gastric ulcer. Am J Surg 1983;146:631 – 4.
19. Reid DA, Duthi HL, Bransom CJ, Johnson AG. Late follow-up of highly selective vagotomy with excision of the ulcer compared with Billroth I gastrectomy for treatment of benign gastric ulcer. Br J Surg 1982;69:605 – 607.
20. Editorial. Conservative operations for gastric ulcers. Lancet 1979;2:80 – 1.
21. Lee SP. Rising female incidence of gastric ulcer. Br Med J 1982;285:853 – 4.
22. Welch CE, Burke SF. Gastric ulcer reappraisal. Surgery 1969;65:708 – 16.
23. Henley WH, Bowers RF. Observations of surgical therapy for gastric ulcer. Arch Surg 1965;90:205 – 8.
24. Angel RT, Giacobine JW, Jordan GL. A current evaluation of the problem of gastric ulcer. Am J Surg 1967;114:730 – 5.
25. Duhamel PA, Block MA, Haubrich WS. Are benign gastric ulcers really benign? Arch Surg 1963;87:391 – 5.
26. Pichlmayr R, Lohlein D, Kujat R. Vagotomy or partial gastric resection as elective treatment for gastric ulcer. In: Baron JH et al (Eds). Vagotomy in Modern Surgical Practice. London, Butterworths 1982:205 – 12.
27. Kronborg O. Truncal vagotomy and drainage for gastric ulcer. In: Baron JH et al (Eds). Vagotomy in Modern Surgical Practice. London, Butterworths 1982:195 – 6.
28. Douglas MC, Duthie HL. Vagotomy for gastric ulcer combined with duodenal ulcer. Br J Surg 1971;58:721 – 4.
29. Johnston D, MacDonald RC, Axon ATR. Highly selective vagotomy with ulcer excision. In: Baron JH et al (Eds). Vagotomy in Modern Surgical Practice. London, Butterworths 1982:197 – 201.
30. Anderson D, Høstrup H, Amdrup E. Aarhus County Vagotomy Trial II: An interim report on reduction in acid secretion and ulcer recurrence following parietal cell vagotomy and selective gastric vagotomy. World J Surg 1978;2: 91 – 100.
31. Becker HD, Siewert JR. Advances in ulcer disease. In: Holtermuller KH, Malagelada JR (Eds). Advances in ulcer disease. Amsterdam-Oxford-Princeton Excerpta Medica 1981:512 – 26.
32. Sekine T, Sato T, Maki T, Shiratori T. Pylorus-preserving gastrectomy for gastric ulcer: One to nine year follow-up study. Surgery 1975;77:92 – 9.
33. Teigan T, Liavag I, Rowland M. Pylorus preserving gastric resection for gastric ulcer. A 5 – 7 year follow-up. Acta Chir Scand 1978;144:249 – 53.
34. Morris DL, Hawker PC, Brearley S, Simms M, Dykes PW, Keighley MRB. Optimal timing of operation for bleeding peptic ulcer: Prospective randomised trial. Br Med J 1984;288:1277 – 80.
35. Hunt PS, Hansky J, Gorman MG, Francis JK, Marshall RD, McCann W. The management of bleeding gastric ulcer: A prospective study. Aust NZ J Surg 1980;50:41 – 1.
36. Dark JH, MacArthur. Perforated peptic ulcer in South-West Scotland. J Roy Coll Surg Ed 1983;28:19 – 23.
37. Coutsoftides T, Himal HS. Perforated gastroduodenal ulcers. Factors affecting morbidity and mortality and the role of definitive surgery. Am J Surg 1976;132:575 – 6.

17. Long term results of highly selective vagotomy for duodenal ulcer and gastric ulcer

D. JOHNSTON, M.D., Ch.M., F.R.C.S.

University Department of Surgery, The General Infirmary, Leeds

Introduction

Highly selective vagotomy (HSV) is still regarded as 'experimental' in most centres in the United States, on the ground that follow-up is too short and incidences of recurrent ulceration too high. In fact, HSV has been used extensively in Europe for 15 years, long-term results are available, and, as I will show, incidences of recurrence of 1 – 5 % at 5 years' follow-up are quite common, when appropriate surgical expertise is available and some form of quality control is employed.

The original hypotheses advanced by Amdrup and Jensen, and by Wilkinson and myself in 1969 were that the pyloric sphincter could be left intact if the vagal nerve supply to the gastric antrum were preserved, and that preservation of an intact antro-pyloro-duodenal segment would permit normal 'grinding' of solid food, regulate gastric emptying and eliminate dumping and diarrhoea as major side effects of gastric surgery: also, reflux of 'bile' into the stomach would be minimized, and this would eliminate bilious vomiting, gastritis and perhaps gastric carcinoma as sequelae of surgery for peptic ulcer.

It is well known by now that HSV is the safest operation for a patient who requires elective surgery for duodenal ulcer, and that its use has indeed virtually eliminated dumping, diarrhoea and bilious vomiting as side effects of surgery for peptic ulcer. What is causing concern, however, is the incidence of recurrent ulceration, which has been reported to be as low as 1.4% at 5 years, or as high as 30%. I will therefore devote much of this paper to that important topic. I will describe our own results over a 16-year period in Leeds, and also the results of several excellent prospective controlled trials from other centres.

First, however, I would like to say a few words about the changes that take place in man's gastrointestinal physiological functions after HSV and after truncal vagotomy with a drainage procedure (TV + D).

Physiological considerations: The changes in man after HSV and TV + D

Serum gastrin levels are no higher after HSV than after TV + D. Both types of vagotomy lead to a modest increase in gastrin levels. Hence, it is not logical to deprive the antral mill of its motor nerve supply, nor is it logical to destroy or bypass the pyloric sphincter, because clinical and experimental work alike has shown that gastric emptying is not impaired after HSV. Gastric emptying of fluids is faster than normal after HSV (because of impaired accommodation to distension in the fundus and body of the stomach), and gastric emptying of solids is normal. The accelerated emptying of liquids after HSV does not amount to the 'gastric incontinence' that is observed after TV + D, but is nevertheless responsible for a 6% incidence of mild dumping in the first two years after HSV, which diminishes to about 3% (always mild) on longer follow-up.

The much better-regulated pattern of gastric emptying after HSV than after TV + D also leads to a more normal pattern of intestinal transit, and this, together with preservation of various integrative reflexes (antro-cholecystic, antro-pancreatic) eliminates the problem of severe 'post-vagotomy' diarrhoea that is such a curse to perhaps 2 – 4% of patients who undergo truncal vagotomy.

Preservation of the extra-gastric vagi as in HSV permits the pancreas to secrete normally in response to food in man, whereas after TV + D pancreatic enzyme output is reduced by about 50%, as Malagelada and McGregor have shown. Truncal vagotomy predisposes to gallstone formation, whereas HSV probably does not. Truncal vagotomy and drainage leads to a doubling of faecal fat output, such that 40% of patients have steatorrhoea (> 6 g fat per day), whereas after HSV faecal fat output is unaltered.

Duodeno-gastric reflux of bile salts into the stomach is reduced significantly after HSV (because of the continuation of an intact pylorus mechanism and raised intra-gastric pressure), whereas TV + D, vagotomy and antrectomy (V + A), or partial gastrectomy (PG) all lead to increased duodeno-gastric reflux. Such reflux may be harmful in causing a 'chronic gastric mucosal reaction' (Lawson, du Plessis) and, perhaps, in the long term, cancer.

Highly selective vagotomy for uncomplicated duodenal ulcer indications

The indications for surgical treatment for duodenal ulcer remain:
- failure of medical treatment;
- the occurrence of severe complications;

Medical treatment is much more effective today than previously, with the advent of cimetidine, ranitidine, bismuth subcitrate etc., and most patients with DU can be treated successfully medically, without the need for operation. However, in about 10% of patients the ulcer does not heal, and when treatment is stopped after ulcer healing, about 80% of patients suffer recurrence of ulceration within one year. Even if maintenance treatment is used, 'breakthrough' recurrent ulceration occurs in 15 – 20% of patients within a year. When the ulcer fails to heal, or if frequent recurrence takes place, surgical treatment should be strongly considered. It must be borne in mind that long-continued medical treatment allows the pathology to develop, and it must be recognized clearly that pyloric stenosis, haemorrhage and perforation may threaten the lives of patients who are on long-term medical treatment for peptic ulcer. Since the mean operative mortality of *elective* HSV is about 0.2 – 0.3%, whereas the mean operative mortality for severe haemorrhage is 10% – and nearer 20% in the elderly – the desirability of timely, planned elective surgery in certain patients is obvious. Thus patients who would be at special risk if ulcer complications were to develop, such as patients over 55 years of age, those with cardio-respiratory disease, and perhaps those who travel a lot to places with poor surgical services, should all be seriously considered as candidates for surgical treatment.

To sum up, unplanned, emergency surgery often implies a surgeon who is not of one's choice (and who may be alarmingly junior), an operative procedure that may be less than optimal (truncal vagotomy, perhaps, or partial gastrectomy), and a relatively high operative mortality of 5 – 30%, depending on the patient's age and general condition and the surgeon's skill. Planned, elective surgery, in contrast, today in Europe implies the use of HSV, almost no mortality and minimal side effects.

It must also be emphasized that, compared with the best modern medical treatment, surgical treatment for duodenal ulcer is significantly more effective and, surprising as it may seem, more specific. Histamine H_2-receptor antagonists, for example, are present not only in the stomach, but also in the brain, the heart, the liver and the male genital tract. Hence, although the incidence of clinical side effects is relatively low, cimetidine is an anti-androgen, may provide changes in liver enzymes, and can lead to mental confusion in the elderly. In contrast, surgical treatment in the form of HSV, though cruder in its mode of access, is confined to the parietal cell area of the stomach. With regard to effectiveness, a recurrence rate of 20% at one year would be regarded as very successful medical treatment, whereas after any form of surgical treatment, the incidence of recurrence at one year ranges from 0% to 3%.

Another important point is that, if the histamine H_2-receptor antagonists are to achieve their full therapeutic effect, the patient must not smoke, drink alcohol or ingest anti-rheumatic drugs. Thus it is only under 'ideal' and somewhat unreal conditions that incidences of healing of over 90% can be achieved by medical therapy over a period of 6 – 12 months. In the real world, at least in Britain, most patients with duodenal ulcer are young or middle aged men. Their social life often revolves around the pub, where apart from drinking a few beers, they also tend to smoke. If you say to such men 'either you give up this type of lifestyle, take pills for years, and even then you may not guaranteed to be free from ulcer trouble, or else you can have an operation that is unpleasant, but safe, produces few side effects, and cures 90% of patients permanently' – many often will choose surgery, simply because they want to 'eat, drink and be merry', in accord with the 'gaudeamus igitur' philosophy. Otherwise, the ulcer is apt to dominate their lives, and in some places, it is also an expensive possession, because some physicians seem obsessed by the need for repeated endoscopies.

Clinical results of highly selective vagotomy for duodenal ulcer

Operative mortality

In my Department at the Leeds General Infirmary, there has been one death after about 600 elective HSV procedures, an operative mortality of 0.17%. In a collected series that I published in the British Medical Journal in 1975, the mortality was 0.3% in over 500 cases, and today the mean mortality is about 0.2%. The single death in our own series was 'non-specific', from pulmonary embolism. We have had one case of lesser curve necrosis, which fortunately was not fatal.

Post-operative morbidity

Post-operative morbidity has been very low in our experience, though of course the patients are not immune from the usual complications of laparotomy and aneasthesia. In uncomplicated cases, I nurse patients who have undergone HSV without an intravenous drip and without a nasogastric tube.

Side effects of operation

The incidence of various symptoms 10 years after HSV are shown in Table I. Note that dumping, diarrhoea and bilious vomiting are virtually absent as clinical problems. This significant advantage for HSV as compared with TV + D is well illustrated by the results of prospective randomized trials, as shown in Table II.

Table I. 'Morbidity' after elective HSV for duodenal ulcer. (Symptoms of alimentary dysfunction in 100 patients 10–16 years after operation)

Symptom	Percentage
Dumping (mild)	2
Diarrhoea (mild)	3
Bile vomiting	2
Dysphagia	3
Heartburn/reflux	17
Fullness after meals	21
Pain (non-ulcer)	6

Not all symptoms experienced by patients *after* operation are *due* to the operation: 'post hoc, ergo propter hoc?' As Muller, Salaman et al and Kennedy have shown, not all 'normal' people are in Visick grade I, and indeed many suffer from symptoms such as mild heartburn, post-cibal satiety and mild episodic diarrhoea. Thus, Salaman, Harvey and Duthie showed that the Visick grades and the symptoms of patient who had undergone HSV did not differ significantly from those of patients who had a herniorrhaphy.

Table II. Patients with troublesome symptoms 4 to 8 years after operation. (From: Stoddard, Johnson and Duthie, 1984)

	HSV	TV + P	p
Dumping (early + late)	1%	8%	<0.05
Diarrhoea	3%	12%	<0.05
Post prandial distension	3%	8%	
Flatulence	9%	14%	
Bile vomiting	1%	5%	
Food vomiting	1%	4%	
Heartburn	4%	11%	
Dysphagia	0%	1%	

Long term sequelae

Compared both with their ideal body weight-for-height and with their best recalled weight, patients lose about 5 kg on average after PG or V + A and about 2 – 3 kg after TV + D. After HSV, we found that they returned on average to their 'best' weight, and remained at that weight for up to 15 years. We have found no case of gastric carcinoma, one case only of tuberculosis, no bone disease, and no megaloblastic anaemia among patients after HSV. Likewise, the few cases found to have iron-deficiency anaemia were all explicable on other grounds, such as menorrhagia or carcinoma of colon.

Recurrent ulceration

As mentioned previously, it is this subject that has led to so much controversy over the merits of HSV. Let us first define our terms. I will discuss only *symptomatic* recurrence, diagnosed by endoscopy or re-operation. In Leeds, we have not endoscoped asymptomatic patients, but fully accept the data of Muhe, Muller and Allgöwer and others that there is a considerable incidence of 'silent' recurrence – though such 'silent' ulcers also exist in the general population, and after other procedures for peptic ulcer.

Symptomatic recurrence may be further divided into true recurrence – that is, pyloroduodenal – and new gastric ulceration, which may be pre-pyloric or more proximal in the stomach. We do not regard recurrence as *absent* until we have a *minimum* period of follow-up of five years.

Recurrence: Author's personal series

The influence of recurrence was 2% at 5 years, and 4% at 10 years, among the first consecutive 100 patients followed up. Fifteen per cent of patients were lost to follow-up. The explanation for this low incidence of recurrence is undoubtedly the low incidence of incomplete vagotomy, only 4% of the first 100 consecutive patients having a positive Hollander test one week after operation. Among the patients with *no* response to insulin one week after HSV, the incidence of recurrent ulceration was 0% after 5 years' follow-up and 1% after 10 years follow-up.

Thus, under conditions of good 'quality control', which may be achieved by simple surgical technique, or with the aid of intra-operative tests such as the Grassi test or Burge electrotest, HSV may be associated with very low incidences of recurrent ulceration. For example, in Matheson's series from Aberdeen, there was one recurrent ulcer among 68 patients followed up for 5 years after HSV (1.4% recurrence), and in Narbona's large series in Valencia, patients who had a negative intra-operative Grassi test also had an incidence of recurrent ulceration of about 1%. Similar results from Giuseppe Grassi's series in Rome have been reported by Giovanni Grassi. In the Basel multicentre study, patients with a negative intra-operative Burge test had an incidence of recurrence of 5% after 5 years of follow-up.

From these data, it is clear that a high incidence of recurrent ulceration is not an intrinsic or specific feature of HSV. When expertly performed, the incidence of recurrent ulceration at 5 years after HSV is in the range 1–5%, which is little higher than the incidence of recurrent ulceration after PG or V + A, which are both easier operative procedures to standardize.

Recurrent ulceration: Total experience in the University Department of Surgery, Leeds General Infirmary

The *overall* experience is not so felicitous, partly because differing operative techniques have been used, because junior surgeons had a 'learning curve' and, perhaps, because more senior people went on using faulty technique.

The incidence of recurrent ulceration for all surgeons is 7% at 5 years and 11% at 10 years. If calculated by the life-table method, the

incidence of recurrent ulceration after 12 years' follow-up is 13%.
These mean figures conceal the most interesting feature, however,
which is the wide *range* of recurrent ulceration, depending on the
surgeon who operated.

Inter-surgeon variation

The wide range of recurrent ulceration, ranging from 2% to more
than 20%, is illustrated in Table III. The two experienced surgeons
(C and D) had widely differing results (significantly different at 10
years), while the two more junior surgeons (A and B) both had recurrence rates of about 30%. It should be emphasized, however, that
some quite senior surgeons also had high recurrence rates, and some
surgeons in training quickly learned a good technique and achieved
low incidences of reucrrent ulceration.

Table III. Recurrence and the individual surgeon after elective HSV for duodenal ulcer*

Surgeon	Number of patients	Recurrent ulceration			
		at 5 years		at 10 years	
		n	(%)	n	(%)
A	14	4	(29)	4	(29)
B	22	7	(32)	7	(32)
C	86	7	(8)	13	(16)
D	119	2	(2)	4	(4)
Total	241	20	(8)	28	(12)

* Symptomatic recurrence: true recurrence and new GU included.
(A + B) vs C and (A + B) vs D statistically significant.

Recurrence: Pre-operative and post-opeartive acid secretion

No correlation was found between pre-operative BAO or MAO, and
long-term recurrence after HSV. This finding is in agreement with
the findings of Amdrup, Jensen and Kronborg.

With post-operative acid secretion the correlation was significant. For
example, 86 of the first 100 HSV procedures that I performed were
evaluated by a technically valid insulin test about one week after
operation: 83 tests were Hollander-negative and three were positive.
Only one of the 83 'negatieve' patients developed recurrent ulceration,

whereas two of the three 'possitive' patients developed recurrence. Over many hundreds of tests, the chances of a patient developing a recurrent ulcer were 4% if the Hollander test was negative, whereas 41% of patients with positive Hollander tests one week after HSV subsequently developed recurrence.

The lesson is clear. The parietal cell vagotomy must be complete: if it is complete, the incidence of recurrent ulceration is low (1 – 5% at 5 years and 4 – 8% at 10 years).

How to achieve a complete parietal cell vagotomy

Oesophageal dissection The oesophagus must be fully mobilized and cleared of all fibres over a distance of 5 – 7 cm. This may take a long time, up to 40 minutes in an obese patient.

Distal dissection At least one major terminal branch of the nerve of Latarjet should be identified and preserved, anteriorly and posterior-ly. This usually means leaving about 5 – 6 cm of pre-pyloric stomach innervated. Following Goligher's paper in the British Journal of Surgery (1974), there was a vogue among some surgeons for leaving 8 – 10 cm of distal stomach innervated, but this is too much, because the antrum is small in patients with duodenal ulcer, and such a prac-tice leaves the distal parietal cell mass innervated in 20 – 30% of patients: it doubles the incidence of recurrent ulceration.

Clinical aspects of recurrent ulceration after highly selective vagotomy for duodenal ulcer

Site Of 50 recurrences in this Department, 40 were pyloro-duodenal and 12 were gastric (two patients had DU + GU).

Presentation One patient presented with perforation, nine with haemorrhage and 45 with pain. The mean interval between the operation and recurrence was 3.7 years, and GU's tended to present later than DU's.

Mortality There was no mortality.

Treatment Thirteen patients have been treated by re-operation in the form of PG or re-V + A, with no mortality, but with very good clini-cal results (Visick grades I & II) in only half of them.

In contrast, of the 45 patients who were treated medically, with histamine H_2-receptor antagonists and other measures, most did well and 70% are currently in Visick grades I & II.

Perforated duodenal ulcer

We have treated 65 *selected* patients with perforated DU by HSV, with no mortality, and mostly good long-term results, though 13% of patients have developed recurrent ulceration. Selective – both of patient and of surgeon – is important, if HSV is to be used. The ulcer should be a troublesome, chronic one, the interval between perforation and operation relatively short (usually less than 12 hours), the patient 'fit' to withstand anaesthesia and a more lengthy operative procedure, and of course the surgeon himself must be experienced in the use of HSV. Charlo's group in Sevilla has treated more than 100 patients with perforation in this way, with a 1% mortality, and PH Jordan Jr, about 70, again with only one operative death. A perforated ulcer is a vicious ulcer, and to treat it merely by simple closure is inadequate, leaving the ulcer process untreated, and the patient exposed to serious risk of re-perforation, massive haemorrhage from a 'kissing' posterior wall ulcer, gastric outlet obstruction or subsequent recurrent ulceration.

Haemorrhage from peptic ulcer

Again, selection of operative procedure, and of surgeon to suit the circumstances, is vital. In general, we prefer vagotomy and underrunning of the bleeding vessel to partial gastrectomy, both for DU and GU, though in the case of GU we excise the ulcer if possible, or leave its base on an adjacent organ, usually the pancreas. In high-risk elderly patients, in those with ischaemic heart disease or those in severe shock, truncal vagotomy and pyloroplasty is preferred, because it can be performed quickly, but when considerations of time are not so pressing, HSV is used, combined either with duodenotomy or gastrotomy to gain access to the ulcer. The duodenotomy is then closed longitudinally, without pyloroplasty. About 30 – 40% of patients are treated by HSV, and the remainder by TV + P. Operative mortality has been 0% after 45 HSV procedures (in which mean blood replacement has been 10 units), 6% after TV + P and 25% after PG, in this Department.

Pyloric stenosis: Results of HSV plus dilatation

Unlike the good results of HSV described above, HSV combined with either digital or Hegar's dilatation for DU with pyloric stenosis has yielded disappointing results in the long term. First and foremost, there were two 'avoidable' deaths among the 80 patients so treated: avoidable in that mortality was due to sepsis and haemorrhage occasioned by leakage from the duodenum, caused by the dilatation of unyielding fibrous tissue. Overall operative mortality was 4%. Furthermore, gastric outlet obstruction recurred in 10% of patients, and in 17% of patients the operation failed because of re-stenosis, recurrence or both these factors.

Currently, we think that mild cases of pyloric stenosis should be treated by HSV combined with gentle dilatation with Hegar's dilators, that cases with post-pyloric stricture are best treated by 'Kocherising' the duodenal loop and performing a duodenoplasty and HSV, while severe pyloric stenosis in the presence of a large active ulcer is best treated by HSV combined with gastroenterostomy. HSV is still preferred to TV, however, because its advantages are not solely due to preservation of the pylorus.

Gastric ulcer

Like duodenal ulceration, uncomplicated benign gastric ulceration should be treated medically at first. *Benign* is the operative word, however, for it is tragic error to treat an eminently curable ulcer-cancer medically, until advancing disease makes the diagnosis only too obvious. Thus endoscopy with multiple (7 – 10) biopsies is essential. Moreover, since ulcer-cancers may heal temporarily on medical treatment, re-endoscopy and further biopsy of the ulcer or of the residual scar should be performed 8 – 12 weeks after the initial examination. Even gastric ulcers in the presence of concomitant duodenal ulceration may be malignant, and so too may pre-pyloric ulcers. If treated by timely radical gastrectomy, we have found a corrected 5-year survival of 67% in patients with ulcer-cancer.

Indications for surgical treatment

These do not differ much from the indications for surgery for duodenal ulcer. However, patients with gastric ulcer are on average ten years older than patients with duodenal ulcer, and are less fit generally. Hence if severe haemorrhage or perforation should occur the mortality is about double that found in patients with such complications of duodenal ulcer. Hence it is all the more important to avoid emergency operations in these patients, which implies that the 'threshold' for advising elective operation should be lower than in patients with duodenal ulcer.

Choice of surgical procedure for gastric ulcer

Billroth I partial gastrectomy has been the operation of choice for 100 years, whereas vagotomy has supplanted PG in the surgical treatment of duodenal ulcer. Prospective clinical trials have geared the progress of surgery for duodenal ulcer, but in gastric ulceration such trials have been rare, no doubt because of the difficulty of obtaining enough patients to allow such a trial to be performed.

The advocates of Billroth I PG cite its 'acceptable' operative mortality (2%), low incidence of recurrent ulceration and good long-term results. There is no doubt that the results of Billroth I PG are good, but the question in 1985 is whether an operation that preserves the entire stomach and the pylorus might not yield even better results, particularly in thin elderly patients. Before discussing the use of HSV for gastric ulcer, however, a brief note about other surgical options is required.

Pylorus-preserving partial gastrectomy (Maki)

This is like a Billroth I PG, except that the pylorus and 1 – 2 cm of pre-pyloric stomach are preserved. In the hands of its originators Maki, Sekine and others in Japan, the clinical results have been good and dumping in particular has been eliminated. However, a careful study by Teigan, Liavag and Roland in Oslo found a 17% incidence of failure among 50 patients, mainly because of gastric stasis and/or recurrent ulceration in the short pre-pyloric remnant of antrum: the remaining patients had excellent functional results and did not experience dumping. Thus the place of the Maki PG remains unclear, and further careful evaluation of it seems desirable.

Polya partial gastrectomy

Simulate any medical student or F.R.C.S. candidate with a question on the surgical treatment of gastric ulcer, and you elicit the reflex response – Billroth I PG! And yet, there is really little hard evidence that the long-term clinical results of Billroth I PG are significantly better than the results of Polya or Billroth II for gastric ulcer. Indeed, the operative mortality of Billroth II PG procedure may be slightly less than that of Billroth I PG, maybe because of less tension at the anastomosis, and the incidence of recurrent ulceration may also be less. With both Billroth I and Polya PG for *gastric* ulcer, the extent of the gastric resection should be modest, only 40 – 50% of the stomach being removed, compared with the 60 – 70% excision used in the course of Polya PG for duodenal ulcer. De Miguel of Valladolid has suggested that excision of only the distal 6 cm or so of the stomach, with the pylorus, and the ulcer, is sufficient, because after using this procedure in a large series of cases he has had a very low incidence (1 – 2%) or recurrent ulceration.

Truncal vagotomy and pyloroplasty or gastrojejunostomy (TV + P/GJ)

It is important to remember that TV + P cures 90% of type I (lesser-curve) gastric ulcers. For example, in the large series reported by Madsen en Schousen from Copenhagen, the operative mortality was 2% and the incidence of recurrent ulceration, 8%. However, prospective trials by Duthie et al and by Madsen et al showed that Billroth I PG yielded slightly superior results to those of TV + P, though the difference was not statistically significant. Hence TV + P (plus excision) may be a useful option when one has to operate for severe haemorrhage from a gastric ulcer, or for a difficult high lesser curve ulcer in an unfit patient.

Highly selective vagotomy with excision of the ulcer (HSV-E)

In Leeds, we have treated 85 patients with uncomplicated type I gastric ulcer by HSV(E), with one operative death (1.1%) and a 10% incidence of recurrent ulceration on follow-up ranging from 1 to 15 years. The functional results in most patients have been very good; just as good, in fact, as the results of HSV for duodenal ulcer.

The rationale for the use of HSV(E) in gastric ulcer is as follows: the ulcer is peptic, and the defect in the gastric mucosa is created by the corrosive action of acid and pepsin. It is a fallacy that acid output is low in these patients; it is normal, for their age and weight. Duodeno-gastric reflux is excessive in some patients with gastric ulcer. HSV greatly reduces acid-peptic 'attack', and at the same time it reduces duodeno-gastric reflux of 'malevolent gall', as Paxton Dewar and collegues have shown. These effects of HSV should be sufficient to cure most gastric ulcers. Excision of the ulcer (not as a 'wedge' from the lesser curve, but trans-gastrically from a gastrotomy on the greater curve) may also be of therapeutic value by eliminating a vulnerable area, as well as providing pathological material for final confirmation that the ulcer is benign.

Trial of HSV(E) and Billroth I PG for gastric ulcer

The results of a prospective randomized trial of HSV and Billroth I PG in the treatment of type I GU were published recently from Sheffield. Follow-up averaged 8 years. As shown in Table IV, side effects of operation were significantly worse after Billroth I PG than after HSV. Recurrent ulceration was surprisingly common after both procedures (23% after HSV, 17% after Billroth I PG), but patients with recurrence after HSV fared well on cimetidine or after re-operation, whereas patients with recurrence after Billroth I PG fared badly, one dying of haemorrhage and another of myocardial infarction some weeks after melaena. Thus in the end, 95% of patients who had undergone HSV obtained good clinical results, whereas only 60% of patients who had undergone Billroth I PG obtained good long-term results. These findings, taken in conjunction with our own uncontrolled patients, constitute strong evidence that HSV(E) is a better option than Billroth I PG in the surgical treatment of gastric ulcer.

Combined gastric and duodenal ulceration

The gastric ulcer must be proved to be benign. If it is, this condition can be treated as for DU alone.

Table IV. Incidence of various symptoms 8 years after operation for gastric ulcer (type I).*
(From: Reid, Duthie, Johnson. British Journal of Surgery 1982)

	HSV(E) (%)	Billroth I (%)
Ulcer pain	0	20
Nausea	0	25
Vomiting		
bile	0	15
food	0	20
Dumping	0	25
Diarrhoea		
mild	13	35
severe	0	10
Epigastric fullness	13	55
Reflux	7	30
Dysphagia	0	10

* excluding patients with recurrent ulcer.

Table V. Prospective randomized trial of operations for GU alone (type I).* (From: Reid, Duthie, Johnson. British Journal of Surgery 1982)

	HSV(E)		Billroth I	
n	26		30	
Traced	26		30	
Operative mortality	0		0	
Subsequent deaths	4		4	
Recurrent ulceration	6	(23%)	5	(17%)
Good clinical result	20	(95%)	15	(60%)

* Follow-up was 8 years (5–12 year).

Pre-pyloric gastric ulcer

Again, one must check that the ulcer is benign. Most surgeons who have employed HSV in the treatment of these ulcers, including our group, have experienced poor results, with an incidence of recurrent ulceration of 20–30%. We found that patients with combined pre-pyloric ulcer and duodenal ulcer faired particularly badly after HSV, roughly half of them developing recurrent ulceration. H-E Jensen of Copenhagen, however, reports that recurrent ulceration after HSV for these ulcers was no more common than after HSV for DU. What then should be done for these patients? The only honest answer must be that we do not know for sure: vagotomy with antrectomy will virtually guarantee freedom from recurrence, but the price in terms of operative risk and side effect is probably too high. Perhaps some form of vagotomy combined with a drainage procedure might be the best compromise.

18. Discussion IV

Boevé:

Dr. Kreuning, you presented evidence for a genetic predisposition in a proportion of the peptic ulcer patients. Will the risk of an ulcer diminish for these people if they migrate from a high risk area for peptic ulcer to a low risk area?

Kreuning:

I can only speculate, as epidemiological data to answer this question are absent. The expression of genetic factors into the actual disease probably needs one, or more environmental factors in addition. These environmental factors have not all been identified, but probably smoking and eating habits are among them. Some of these environmental factors are related to personality and some may be related to certain geographical areas and hence change with migration. The balance of these factors will probably determine the final outcome.

Johnson:

Is there any evidence that ulcer patients with a positive family history or with hyperpepsinogenaemia I are more likely to respond poorly to medical treatment?

Kreuning:

Only one study showed an increased risk of complications and early recurrences in patients with familiar hyperpepsinogenaemia I. Perhaps these patients should be operated at an earlier stage, but there is no convincing evidence.

Tijtgat:

I agree that patients with a positive family history have a more agressive ulcer disease, but they respond as well to medical treatment as patients with a negative family history.

Boevé:

Could mr Johnston and Spencer explain the differences between Type I, II and III gastric ulcers.

Johnston:

I find this gastric ulcer typing confusing and not useful. The main point in gastric ulcer is malignancy, which is not always easy to demonstrate. There is a tremendous responsibility on the endoscopist to inspect and biopsy the ulcer thoroughly and re-examine the patient after medical treatment. Early gastric cancer is curable if we operate soon, so to me that is the top priority in the management of gastric ulcer. Exact endoscopic localization of gastric ulcers is important, as the ulcer should be excised at operation. However, it can be very difficult to localize the juxta-pyloric ulcer precisely as immediately pre-pyloric, or post-pyloric. Gastric ulcers, or gastric ulcers combined with duodenal ulcers seem to do quite well in most cases with an HSV, provided that they are not pre-pyloric and that gastric stasis is abstent.

Spencer:

Lesser curve ulcers should be treated by either HSV or Billroth I resection, but for pre-pyloric ulcers, I would favour selective vagotomy and drainage, and not HSV.

Kennedy:

I would like to suggest a type IV gastric ulcer in addition. There is a small group of patients who have a very high lesser curve ulcer, within one or two cm from the cardia, combined with gastric hyperacidity. Those patients do not have the characteristic extension of the antrum running up the lesser curve, which is normally seen in gastric ulcer. These ulcers are difficult to treat surgically. Proximal partial gastrectomy has been advocated for these ulcers, but is difficult to do and carries some mortality. Perhaps continuous medical treatment is best for these patients.

Johnston:

I agree with mr Kennedy, but proximal partial gastrectomy does not carry a higher mortality than Billroth I or II partial gastrectomy.

Tijtgat:

Why do pre-pyloric ulcers heal so poorly with HSV? Did the 25% recurrences have an abnormal insulin response, or gastric distension and problems with emptying?

Johnston:

Recurrence is not related to incompleteness of vagotomy, but it has something to do with the anatomical location of the ulcer. Emptying rates have not been analysed.

Guth:

Perhaps as many as one in five patients on aspirin, or non-steroidal anti-inflammatory drugs have an asymptomatic ulcer. Have you analysed your patients with pre-pyloric ulcer to see whether they are on such agents?

Johnston:

I think you are right. I strongly suspect that from my own population, but it has not been scientifically analysed.

Guth:

You suggested that the early detection of malignancy in a gastric ulcer means curable disease. However, most surgeons in the USA and the surgeons I spoke at this meeting said exactly the opposite. When they look at their five year cure rate, no matter when they pick up the malignancy, the results are very discouraging.

Johnston:

We just completed a survey on the last 16 years of gastric cancer in my department: between 300 and 400 cases. Early gastric cancer, though not very many patients, had no operative mortality and a 90% five year survival. Malginant ulcer of less than 2.5 cm diameter had a five year survival of 66%: certainly are doing significantly better than the average gastric cancer, even better than the average gastric cancer after curative resection. I think it is important not just to do a Billroth I resection in these cases. We have to do quite a radical operation for these small lesions. We take both omenta and the lymph nodes along the lesser and greater curve out and try to do a dissection along the hepatic artery. I cannot prove that this kind of rather agressive lymphadenectomy is the cause of our better survival rates, but the figures are getting better when we are more radical.

236

Kreuning:

Did you ever see gastric cancer after an HSV for a gastric ulcer with benign appearance on endoscopy?

Johnston:

When I advocated this policy in 1972 in the British Journal of Surgery, I knew that this would be the biggest danger. But given the formal policy of ulcer excision combined with many biopsies pre-operatively we have not had a case of cancer.

Tijtgat:

Mr Spencer, you favour Billroth I partial gastrectomy for gastric ulcer, but I have got the impression that most surgeons in The Netherlands do a Billroth II resection at present.

Spencer:

Quite a lot of evidence indicates that Billroth I gastrectomy is to be preferred. In my hands patients undergoing Billroth I partial gastrectomy for gastric ulcer do much better than patients under-going vagotomy and antrectomy for duodenal ulcer in terms of reflux gastritis and bile vomiting. There is reasonable evidence from our trials that people after Billroth I partial gastrectomy do much better nutritionally than might be expected, but people do better after HSV than after any form of gastrectomy. The results are better after Bill-roth I resection than after Billroth II resection, except in terms of recurrence.

Tijtgat:

Dr Wormsley and dr Pounder stressed repeatedly that the results of medical treatment are independent on the prescriber, whereas the results of surgery are highly dependent on the quality of the indi-vidual surgeon. How do you handle this individual variability in practice and in training?

Johnston:

Every unit has its own quality control I don't rely on testing during the operation as mr Allgöwer does, because it did not seem to have any impact on my own recurrence rate. But we stress the post-operative acid tests, which give a fairly good guide to the quality of the vagotomy. I admit that these tests do not help the individual patient who has an incomplete vagotomy, but it is a psychological pressure on the trainees to perform better next time.

Boevé:

That does mean that you teach your trainees to work very carefully and bloodlessly?

Johnston:

Yes, we try to. But it is not just a training problem, it concerns all surgeons. The good results of Billroth I partial gastrectomy compared to vagotomy and antrectomy is the absence of vagotomy in Billroth I resection. The innervated gastric remnant is probably more capable of expansion and receptive relaxation without rise in intra-gastric pressure. The best results with Billroth I partial gastrectomy came from surgeons who perform a rather limted resection.

Misiewicz:

Mr Johnston, you stated that there is a problem of the individual surgeon. Are there any initiatives to solve this problem, because HSV is falling into disrepute, not because it is a bad operation, but because it is not done properly.

Johnston:

The kind of initiatives that we have seen from Allgöwer's and Johnson's approach are going to give us good results and render us to expert surgeons who are prepared to take time to show their trainees how to perform HSV properly.

To the surgeon who is only doing a small number of operations for peptic ulcer a year I would suggest to choose the operation he or she has most experience with.

Spencer:

The medical treatment of peptic ulcer has, for he time being, reduced the number of patients treated surgically. That provides an important logistic problem in terms of training to do this kind of operation properly. I am interested in the Swiss data on the Burge test, because the figures are so impressive. I have used the Burge test and the Grassi test, but I did not find them helpful in improving the results.

Pounder:

How many HSV procedures should a trainee see before he does one independently and how many should he do under supervision before he is allowed to do them on his own?

Johnston:

If he is a surgeon he knows theoretically from the books what he is supposed to be doing. I think it helps him to see two or three operations done and then going on to operate under supervision.

Johnson:

The first thing the trainee sees is a film on HSV made in Sheffield, Leeds and Belfast. then it is a matter of time. I will help my trainees with their first five operations and subsequently looking over their shoulders for the next five and checking at the end of the operation by doing the Grassi test.

Rutten (Roermond):

I do not agree with my medical colleagues: if a benign gastric ulcer recurs after medical treatment, it should be surgically attacked by Billroth I partial gastrectomy.

Johnston:

I would have agreed with you a few years ago, but I have been very impressed by the results the physicians obtain in gastric ulcer. I am not very agressively inclined towards gastric ulcer and I think they need medical treatment first, provided it is not a complicated ulcer.

Festen:

Does any of the surgeons have experience in using a modified sham feeding test instead of the unpleasant and dangerous insulin test for evaluating the results of vagotomy?

Spencer:

We have now for some time abandoned the insulin test in favour of the sham feeding test, purely because of the safety factor.

Johnston:

Sham feeding is supposed to be a cleaner test for vagal activity, but it is not correlated to recurrence. The insulin test is not very dangerous, provided it is not used in elderly people, people with ischaemic heart disease and epileptic patients.

Misiewicz:

What do the surgeons feel about the way the results of surgical treatment are being analysed? As physicians we stress having an endoscopy done in all the patients to monitor recurrence of symptomatic, or asymptomatic ulcers. Your have a moving cohort of patients operated on for the past 15 years, so your follow-up time varies from 1 to 15 years.

Would you not feel that there should be some standards, for example that all patients should be endoscoped and the results analysed in an actuarial way by life table analysis?

Spencer:

In terms of follow-up we should indeed use life time analysis, but I do not think it is necessary to endoscope patients who are asymptomatic.

Johnston:

I do not agree that we should endoscope all patients, because it is an invasive and expensive examination. Even mr Allgöwer only succeeded in following up 85% of the operated patients and of those he managed to endoscope only 65%. I fully agree that I am talking about symptomatic recurrences only, that is to say I underestimate my true recurrence rate because I do not see the asymptomatic recurrences.

Kennedy:

We cannot possibly take dr Misiewicz's suggestion, that we are not following our patients properly. Surgeons just are not interested in the results inside one year, but in the results after 5 or 10 years. We are following the patients in terms of time, while the physicians follow them for a few weeks. Routine endoscopy in patients who are symptomless is really meddlesome and totally wrong.

Wormsley:

But we are talking about recurrence rate and now we hear that all surgical results are so excellent because it is unethical to do re-endoscopies. Dr Rösch should tell us about his follow-up data, because he has a more than 90% rate of endoscopy and he performed life table analysis as dr Misiewicz suggested.

Kennedy:

The interest of the physician is whether the ulcer is healed or not. We surgeons are interested in problems like dumping and post-operative diarrhoea and these cannot be diagnosed down an endoscope.

Wormsley:

If surgeons were interested in dumping and diarrhoea, they would give up gastric operations.

Rösch:

Our figures are included in the ones mr Allgöwer presented, but they are quite different from the collective data. We re-endoscoped more than 90% of the operated patients every year and we found a cumulative recurrence rate of 20.7% at 4 years and 46% at 5 years, of which 40% are asymptomatic.

Johnston:

This is not necessarily a description of the operation, but a description of the operation performed at your center by your surgeons.

19. Morphological changes in the stomach remnant after partial gastric resection

G.N.J. TIJTGAT, M.D.

Division of Gastroenterology-Hepatology, University of Amsterdam, Academic Medical Center, Amsterdam, The Netherlands

Gastric operations render the gastric mucosa abnormal.[1] Of special concern is the development of severe dysplasia and cancer in longstanding post-gastrectomy patients. Only screening of asymptomatic post-gastrectomy patients may allow detection of early malignancy. The yield of such endoscopic screening is probably too low and the technique is probably too invasive for widespread use, except in countries with a very high incidence of gastric malignancy. The low yield of endoscopic screening in asymptomatic patients, the average high age of the population at risk, and the high morbidity and mortality rates for total gastrectomy with increasing age, render the value of screening procedures doubtful.

The spectrum of histological abnormalities in endoscopic biopsies of the gastric remnant

Various histological abnormalities are commonly observed in endoscopic biopsies of post-gastrectomy patients. The frequency with which the histological abnormalities can be detected on screening asymptomatic longstanding post-gastrectomy subjects is summarized in Table I. As a rule, these histological abnormalities, including dysplasia and malignancy, are more frequently observed in biopsies from the stomal area than in those obtained along the lesser or greater curvature.[2,3] (Table II) Atrophic gastritis with foveolar hyperplasia and cystic changes and intestinal metaplasia are common findings in the gastric remnant. Various degrees of dysplasia[4] are also frequently observed and most biopsies show chronic active inflammation.

Table I. Histological abnormalities (%) in the stomal area of the gastric remnant approx. 20 years after resection.

Reference	v.d. Stadt [2,3]	Domellöf et al[44]	Ewerth et al[45]	Savage et al[46]	Geboes* et al[47]
No patients	564	214	106	63	56
No biopsies	4–10	6		4–5	
Atrophy	45	68	51	41	
Foveolar hyperplasia	49				36
Cystic changes	54	70		55	55
Intestinal metaplasia	35	33	54	34	39
Dysplasia grade I	20		18	34	21
grade II	2.6		5	19	7
grade III	1.1		1		1.8
Chronic active inflammation	75	97		73	90
Carcinoma	1.8	2.8	0	0	8.9
Normal mucosa	5			0	7

* includes symptomatic patients

Table II. Histological abnormalities (%) in the gastric remnant.

	Stomal area	Lesser curve	Greater curve
456 male patients			
atropy	45	27	24
intestinal metaplasia	35	31	21
chronic inflammation	24	19	17
chronic active inflammation	51	50	47
dysplasia (grade I–III)	20	3	0.8
carcinoma	1.3		
normal mucosa	4		
40 female patients			
atropy	40	30	19
intestinal metaplasia	49	12	12
chronic inflammation	28	26	21
chronic active inflammation	53	60	58
dysplasia (grade I–III)	23	4.7	2.3
carcinoma	2.1		
normal mucosa	5		

Malignancy in the gastric remnant

Carcinoma in patients with previous gastric surgery, has been recognized throughout the world, especially in recent years. The incidence has been subject of a large number of reports with contradictory findings. (Table III) The incidence differs in different parts of the world. The incidence is low in the USA and in Japan, but may be quite high in some Scandinavian countries, with values reaching 8.9%.

Table III. Incidence of malignancy in the post-gastrectomy stomach remnant.

	Year of publication	No operated patients followed up	No of death patients	Cancer observed No	(%)	No expected
Helsingen[48]	1956	222	38	11	(5)	5.2
Krause[49]	1958	361	210	28	(7.7)	11.3
Liaväg[50]	1962	616		9	(1.5)	9.6
Griesser et al[51]	1964	701	446	54	(7.7)	
Hilbe[52]	1968	371		30	(8.2)	5.4
Stalsberg et al[53]	1971		558	7	(8.7)	3.0
Peitsch et al[54]	1976	806	315	22	(7.0)	
Hakkiluoto[55]	1976	196		1	(0.5)	2.3
Clemençon et al[56]	1976	534		21	(3.9)	
Schmid et al[57]	1976	705		48	(6.8)	
Domellöf[44]	1977	676		12	(1.8)	4.7
Cheli et al[58]	1978	517		16	(3.1)	1.9
McLean Ross et al[33]	1982	779	360	8	(1.0)	10.4
Welvaart et al[59]	1982	257	130	5	(1.9)	
Offerhaus et al[7]	1983	2633	741	38	(5.1)	
Schafer et al[32]	1983	338	214	2	(0.6)	2.6
Fischer et al[11]	1983	1000	522	13	(1.3)	10.6
Pickford et al[12]	1984	307		9	(3.0)	3

All reports of cancer in patients with previous gastric surgery indicate the vulnerable period to be 10 to 25 years after the initial surgery, with the greatest risk between 20 and 25 years.[5-7]

Although not all studies are concordant, there is some evidence to support the hypothesis that the incidence of stump cancer is higher after gastrectomy for gastric ulcer, than for duodenal ulcer.[8-12] In the latter study, the risk of later development of carcinoma was 7% if gastrectomy was performed for gastric ulcer, which was significantly greater than that following operation for duodenal ulcer (1.6%).

It has also been thought that the type of anastomosis affects the cancer risk, with Billroth II being more predisposing to malignant transformation. This would fit with experiments in which the incidence of gastric carcinoma in rats was highest after gastroenterostomy (70%), intermediate after Billroth II (30%), and lowest after Billroth I resection (10%). Of importance was the observation that cancer risk in these animals could be abolished by diverting bile away from the stomach by means of a Roux-en-Y jejunostomy.[13,14] It appears therefore from such studies that the number of malignant neoplasms rises in proportion to the intensity of duodenogastric reflux. Recent studies, however, suggest that the enhanced risk of a Billroth II stomach may have been an artefact due to the greater prevalence of

Billroth II compared with Billroth I type resection. When a group of patients having had previous Billroth I surgery was examined, the incidence of gastric cancer was found to be as high as that in comparable patients with a Billroth II anastomosis, at least in a Scandinavian study.[15] As the enteroanastomosis is the site of the most marked proliferative changes, it is to be expected that carcinomata will usually arise at, or near, the anastomosis.[16]

The prognosis of gastric stump cancer, when detected in the symptomatic stage with complaints of weight loss, subxiphoid pain, anorexia or early satiety, is dismal. Five year survival of 162 patients with stump cancer from Amsterdam was 3.7%.[6,7]

Mechanism of carcinogenesis

Many hypotheses have been suggested to explain the premalignant character of a gastric remnant. Some authors have drawn a parallel between gastric resection and other gastric situations with impaired secretion such as pernicious anaemia and chronic atrophic gastritis.[18,18] According to this hypothesis, the decreased secretion of acid is thought to permit colonization of the stomach by bacteria, capable of reducing salivary and dietary nitrate to nitrite.[20] Subsequently the nitrite reacts with secondary, or tertiary amines or amides, or other peptides of gastric juice and food proteins, to form nitroso compounds which may be carcinogenic.[21] This hypothesized nitrosation, however, involves the formation of nitrous acid and nitrous anhydride from nitrite, a reaction which requires the presence of hydrogen ions, so that conditions associated with anacidity are unsatisfactory for the formation of nitroso compounds. Alternatively, nitrogen oxides may react with aliphatic and heterocyclic amines in a neutral or alkaline environment.[22] It is perhaps through this pathway that carcinogenic substances are formed in the hypoacidic gastric remnant.

An alternative hypothesis concentrates on the abnormalities of cellular proliferation and differentiation seen in pernicious anaemia, chronic atrophic gastritis and in the post-gastrectomy-stomach.[4,23-26]

It is generally accepted that proliferating tissues are more susceptible to carcinogens and that the effect of initiating carcinogens may be enhanced by inducing abnormal proliferation.[18] To what extend bile reflux is responsible for enhanced desquamation of epithelial cells with subsequent speeding up of proliferative activity, is unknown at present.

Endoscopic screening of the gastric remnant

The only hope of detecting malignancy in the gastric remnant in a curable state lies in its detection at an early phase of mucosal infiltration. Therefore several prospective screening studies, mostly of asymptomatic patients, have been done as summarized in Table IV. The yield of malignancies, of which approximately half are at a stage of early cancer, is quite variable. Early lesions are found only in asymptomatic patients, whereas virtually all symptomatic patients have advanced and usually unresectable disease.

Early gastric cancer has been described with the Billroth I and II anatomy.[27,28] The commonest appearance has been that of a small polypoid mass of type I, or IIa variety. Less commonly the endoscopist may recognize focal mucosal discolouration, or a depressed lesion.

Table IV. Prospective endoscopic screening of post-gastrectomy patients.

	Year of publication	No	No death	No death cancer	No endoscop.	No stump cancer	
Rehner et al[60]*	1974				160	4	(2.5%)
Domellöf et al[5]	1977	676	198	3	336	12	(3.6%)
Ewerth et al[45]	1978	569	238	2	111	0	(0.0%)
Savage and Jones[46]	1979	224			63	1	(1.6%)
Peitsch et al[10]	1979	1100	355	27	87	0	(0.0%)
Stokkeland et al[61]**	1981	421			108	4	(3.7%)
Graem et al[62]	1981				196	0	(0.0%)
Hiltz et al[63]	1982				66	4	(6.0%
Farrands et al[1]	1983				71	2	(2.8%)
Fisher et al[11]	1983	100	522	13	196	0	(0.0%)
Pop[6]	1983				181	5	(2.8%)
Offerhaus et al[7]	1984				504	10	(2.0%)

* Non-specific upper abdominal complaints.
** Total cancer incidence rises to 7, when 3 *in situ* carcinomata are added.

The erosive-ulcerative type of early gastric cancer is distinctly rare. Although early cancers may rise anywhere within the remnant and in some cases may be multicentric, the mucosa within 2 cm of the stoma is the commonest site. The endoscopist should realize that quite often early cancers are invisible to the naked eye. In order to discover such early lesions it is mandatory to take multiple biopsies, not only when the diagnosis is suspected, but also when no suspicious endoscopic changes are visible.

246

Most gastric remnant cancers are seen as advanced lesions with the appearance of a polypoid mass, or an infiltrating tumour, involving the stoma and extending for a variable distance into the remnant. Some patients present with a linitis plastica type appearance, involving the entire remnant and extending submucosally above the gastro-esophageal junction.

The Amsterdam prospective endoscopic screening study

A few years ago, 2633 consecutive patients on whom a gastric operation had been performed between 1931 and 1960 for benign reasons, were selected for a follow-up study. In 741 already deceased patients, mortality due to gastric cancer was 5.1%.

Agreement was obtained from 504 truly asymptomatic post-gastrectomy patients to take part in an endoscopic screening programme. Ten stump cancers have been detected (1.98%). Seven of the ten had a radical curative resection and are still alive. In five, the cancer was limited to the mucosa and not visible at endoscopy. Two patients were inoperable: one had a positive lymph node.[6,7] From these data cancer incidence in post-gastrectomy patients was estimated to be at least twice as high as in an age-matched Dutch control population with intact stomach. The risk depended on the post-operative interval and the age at which the initial operation was done. Patients from the age of 50 onwards, or at more than 10 to 15 years after initial surgery, were at risk.[6,7]

Another aspect of that study was the follow-up of patients with dysplastic changes, in order to delineate the importance of dysplasia as a pre-cancerous lesion. There still is some debate whether severe dysplasia is reversible or not. In a large follow-up study of dysplasia in the intact stomach, Oelert et al[29] found reversibility, persistence and worsening of even severe dysplasia. Four of 46 patients with severe dysplasia developed early cancer more than 3 years after the first biopsy.

In the Amsterdam study, gastric dysplasia was found in 70 patients. (Table V) Of the 31 patients with mild/moderate dysplasia on second endoscopy, on first endoscopy 22 had no dysplasia and 9 had mild/moderate dysplasia. Of the 5 patients with severe dysplasia on second endoscopy, on first endoscopy 1 had no dysplasia, 3 had mild/moderate dysplasia and 1 had severe dysplasia. On subsequent follow-up these five patients showed mild/moderate dysplasia in 1, unchanged severe dysplasia in 1 and in 3 patients with severe dysplasia, intramucosal carcinoma was detected during follow-up. In two it could be demonstrated that cancerous degeneration took place at the site of preceding severe dysplasia. True regression of severe dysplasia to normal mucosa could not be demonstrated.

Table V. Endoscopic follow-up of dysplasia in the gastric remnant.

	Endoscopy I	Endoscopy II	Further follow-up
No dysplasia	427	121	
Mild/moderate dysplasia	69	31	1
Severe dysplasia	1	5	1
Carcinoma	7		3

From the Amsterdam follow-up study and from the literature dealing with post-gastrectomy patients with and without dysplasia, it appears that dysplastic changes may be reversible, especially when mild or moderate. Severe dysplasia, however, tends to remain unchanged or to get worse. Apparent disappearance of severe dysplasia is probably due to sampling error. One should not accept regression of severe dysplasia, unless the biopsy site is precisely known and unless on several examinations severe dysplasia from that particular area can not be detected.

Cell proliferation kinetics in the gastric remnant

To further analyze the premalignant character of the gastric remnant mucosa, Offerhaus et al[26] performed extensive cell kinetic studies in 5 normal controls and 60 asymptomatic post-gastrectomy patients with a mean post-operative interval of 24.1 year (range 15–38 yr). Endoscopic forceps biopsies were taken from the gastric mucosa adjacent to the gastroenterostomy in the post-gastrectomy patients and from corresponding levels of the mid-corpus region in the normal controls. The biopsies were incubated with 25 μCi tritiated thymidine and after 1 hour of incubation fixed in formalin and embedded in paraffin. Serial sections were cut for histopathological examination and for radioautography.

The proliferative parameters were determined in each patient in at least 50 gastric pits at various sites of the biopsy specimen. All labelled cells per individual gastric pit were counted. The thymidine incorporation rate (TIR) was defined as the ratio between the number of labelled cells and the number of pits. The cell position of the labelled cells was determined taking as a reference position (R = 0) the limit between the last foveolar cell and the first specialized glandular cell. The individual cell position data were pooled and represented in a collective frequency histogram, the spatial distribution of the labelled cells being expressed in percentages of the total number of labelled cells. (fig. 1) The TIR is the parameter for cell proliferation and the

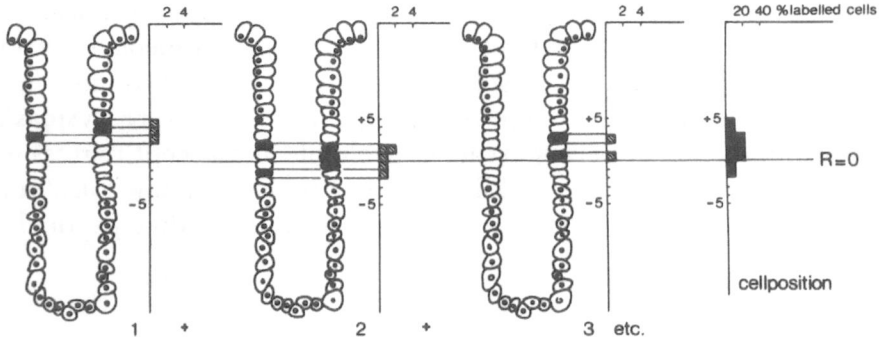

Figure 1. Principle of cell position analysis. The reference point (R) is the transition between the neckzone and the glandular area.

Table VI. Cell proliferation kinetics in the gastric remnant. Thymidine incorporation rate (TIR) in normal controls and asymptomatic post-gastrectomy patients.

	n	No of labelled cells	No of gastric pits	TIR mean	SD
Normal controls	5	421	564	0.74	0.50
Gastritis	23	5363	1201	4.63	3.24
Hyperplasia/metaplasia	26	12332	1519	8.12	5.46
Severe dysplasia	2	1664	127	13.12	4.91
Early stump cancer	2	4217	364*	11.59	

* Cell counts only made in pits without malignant change.

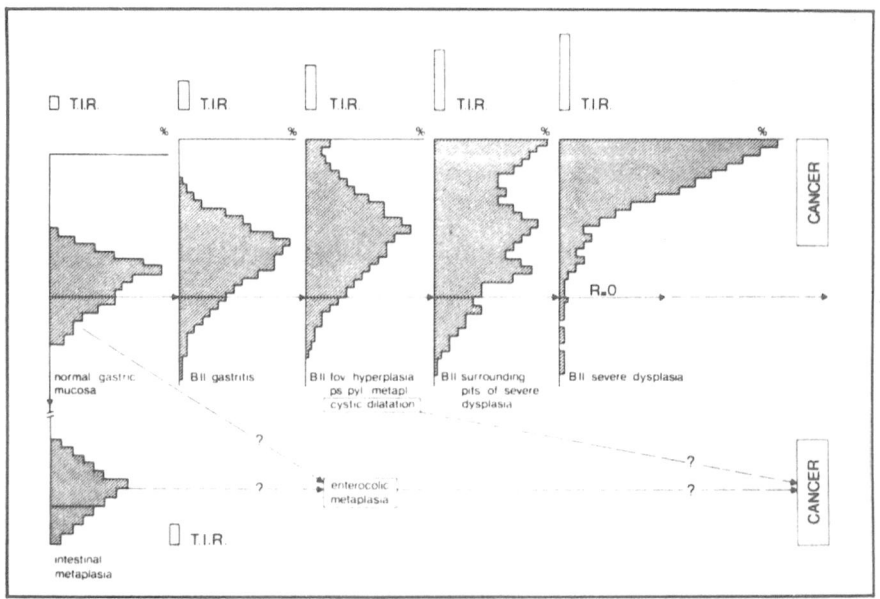

Figure 2. Schematic representation of proliferative activity defined as thymidine incorporation rate (TIR) and location of the proliferative compartment (shaded area) with respect to a reference point (R), in function of the degree of histological abnormality.

histogram is the parameter for the part of the gastric pit where the cell proliferation takes place.

The results of the study are given in Table VI and figure 2 and demonstrate that the number of labelled cells in the stomal area of the gastric remnant is higher than in the corresponding mid-corpus region of the normal gastric mucosa. With increasing evidence of a disordered growth pattern as seen histologically there was a parallel progressive increase in the thymidine incorporation rate, expressing the proliferative activity, and a parallel expansion and gradual upward shift of the proliferative compartment towards the luminal surface. These factors are indicative of a disordered growth pattern with enhanced proliferative activity rendering the mucosa more vulnerable to carcinogenic influences. Nitrosamines, reflux, achlorhydria, a disturbed mucosal barrier, an abnormal bacterial flora, disturbed motility and a resected antrum, probably all play an important role in this carcinogenic process.

The sequence of events suggests that early cancer formation takes place in the superficial gastric mucosa and should therefore be easily detectable at endoscopic biopsy. Presumably DNA-derepression starts in the progenitor cell region and extends from there to the luminal surface.

Practical recommendations – critical comments

As patients with previous gastric surgery are at increased risk for malignancy after 15 years, and especially after 20 years, some physicians recommend routine screening for visual inspection and multiple biopsies, especially of the stomal area, starting some 10 to 15 years after initial surgery.[30] Usually such endoscopic screening should be done at intervals of 2 or 3 to 5 years. If, however, severe dysplasia, or total atrophy with or without intestinal metaplasia is present in the biopsies, then a much closer follow-up is advisable, with intervals of 6 to 12 months. Indeed severe dysplasia may already be associated with early malignancy in the remnant in perhaps more than half the patients. If a malignancy is detected at an early stage, the surgical cure rate should be high: above 70%, in contrast to the cure rate of less than 10% when the lesion is discovered at the symptomatic stage.

A major problem occurs when severe dysplasia is detected in one, or in several of the biopsies. Because severe dysplasia is probably a true premalignant marker and because severe dysplasia may be associated with malignancy elsewhere in the remnant, some (especially American) authors feel that this abnormality is sufficient to recommend gastrectomy. This attitude seems logical, provided gastrectomy is a simple procedure with a low morbidity and mortality, which it is not. More conservative physicians feel at the present time that surgery is only indicated after a definite diagnosis of invasive malignancy is made. Indeed the difference between dysplasia grade I and III is not always sharply demarkated. Moreover, it is unknown how rapidly grade III dysplasia will develop into frank malignancy. It may be that such a transition takes many years. Instead of recommending immediate surgery, we too prefer a close surveillance of such patients with an interval of approximately 6 to 12 months between endoscopies. It is particularly important then to carefully map the biopsy sites in the stomal area, in order to be able to make proper comparisons.

Physicians should realize that bleeding is a potential complication after multiple endoscopic biopsies of a gastric remnant. The frequency of bleeding has been estimated at 0.8%.[31] Some of these bleeding episodes may be severe. When planning follow-up examination of such patients, the risk of bleeding should be taken into account and the patient should be appropriately informed and supervised. According to Domellöf et al,[31] all gastrectomized patients have an approximately 20-fold increased risk of bleeding after biopsy. It is perhaps advisable to use a small calibre biopsy forceps to sample tissue from the usually atrophic mucosa, to reduce the risk of bleeding. A disadvantage of such biopsies is that they are easily traumatized and crushed and more difficult for the pathologist to interpret.

Before physicians embark on screening programmes in post-gastrectomy patients, they should first answer three basic questions:

a) What is the magnitude of the risk in their geographical area?
b) Is the screening method acceptable?
c) What are the consequences of detecting an early lesion?

Many authors believe that the incidence of gastric cancer after gastric operation is not greater than in control population,[11,32] perhaps in part because patients die from diseases related to smoking.[33] Others feel that the increased risk is real, albeit small, but does not warrant screening.[34] Scandinavian and Mid-European authors[35,36] feel that the increased risk is such as to need repeated monitoring. Why there is so much diversity at present, is unknown. The risk will presumably be determined not only by the severity of the proliferative changes, but also by the environmental carcinogenetic factors. The latter almost certainly vary in different geographic areas. It may be relevant to mention that incidence of gastric cancer in Europe is between two and five times higher than in North America.[37] If gastric surgery predisposes to only one type of gastric cancer, such as the 'intestinal type', then a particular decline of this type of cancer may explain the differences in relative risk between North America and Europe. Another major problem in all the studies published is, that there is no proper cohort of ulcer patients not treated with gastric resection and followed-up for a similar time to calculate relative risks. The risk in the 'control' general population is usually taken as the denominator. In patients with duodenal ulcer the incidence of gastritis is lower[38] and it may be that incidence of gastric cancer in such patients is smaller.[39] This is in contrast with the incidence of gastritis and malignancy in the general population, which increases with age.[40] A comparison between the incidence of cancer after gastrectomy with malignancy in a true control group of longstanding unoperated duodenal ulcer disease patients has not yet been made. It is interesting to note that the risk of developing gastric cancer after operation is greatest in young patients.[41] That is, the comparative risk is greater when young post-operative patients are compared with young 'normal' controls, who have not yet developed atrophic gastritis.

Because it is very difficult to test clinically the efficacy of an endoscopic screening programme, Sonnenberg[42] approached this problem in a different way by applying known clinical observations on partial gastrectomy patients to a hypothetical cohort of 100,000 German or American partial gastrectomy patients. The possible benefits of regular endoscopic screening in such a population could be predicted. Markoff type of decision analysis was used on the hypothetical cohort to see if yearly endoscopy significantly improved outcome, compared with no endoscopic screening. Under the very liberal, but arbitrary, assumption that endoscopic screening could prevent death from gastric stump cancer in 80% of those diagnosed as having gastric stump cancer, 8.5% and 5.4% of German male and female gastrectomy patients respectively, and 2.2% and 1.3% of American male and female gastrectomy patients respectively would benefit from screening. Lives would be prolonged 10 and 13 years respectively for German men and women and 11 and 15 years for American men and women. Life expectancy of the total male and female cohort would increase by 9 and 8 months respectively for German and 2 and 2 months for American men and women respectively. Per 100 endoscopies, 6.4 and 4.3 versus 1.8 and 1.2 life years would be gained for German male and female and American male and female patients respectively. A sensitivity analysis shows the outcome of the calculations to depend most on the rate of 5 year survival gained by endoscopy and surgery: as the post-operative 5 year survival of gastric stump cancer patients falls below 80%, the benefit achieved by endoscopic screening becomes even less apparent. For American postgastrectomy subjects, the benefit of endoscopic screening would probably be too low to justify screening. Endoscopic screening could be beneficial only in populations with high incidence of gastric cancer.[42]

It would seem from all these data that the policy of routine screening is only applicable to areas where the risk is excessively high.

Many of the arguments against routine screening have recently been discussed by Logan and Langman.[34] These authors point out that the size of the increased risk is only one of several arguments against screening after gastric surgery. Equally, if not more persuasive arguments are the hazards of revisional gastrectomy in elderly patients and the relative unsuitability of endoscopy as a population screening procedure. Only a greatly increased risk, perhaps as high as 10-fold, would outweigh these other considerations. One should realize that patients with a stump cancer are usually elderly and that total gastrectomy carries a considerable morbidity and mortality. It seems unlikely that the mortality can fall much below $10-20\%$.[43] Screening can be justified ethically only when the risk of a serious adverse outcome is negligible compared with any benefit to the screened population as a whole. Moreover, it is not unlikely that many elderly patients if faced with a $10-20\%$ risk of immediate death traded for an uncertain longer term benefit, would decline surgery. Screening of the younger age group of the at risk population is likely to offer the best prospect for success, as operative risks are lowest and the years of life gained greatest.

Because of all these arguments, we feel that the risk of stump cancer, at least for The Netherlands, and the yield of endoscopic screening is too low, and the screening method too invasive to justify routine screening of all post-gastrectomy patients, especially those older than 55 years. However, now that endoscopy is increasingly used as primary screening technique for dyspepsia or epigastric discomfort, physicians should take advantage of endoscopic approach by taking multiple biopsies especially from the stomal area, whether or not endoscopic abnormalities are visible. For the others we have to await less invasive screening methods. Overall, the best prophylaxis is to avoid gastric resection whenever possible.

Acknowledgement

Figure 1 was reproduced by permission of the authors and the Editor of the European Journal of Cancer & Clinical Oncoloy from: Offerhaus GJA, van de Stadt J, Samson G et al. Cell proliferation kinetics in the gastric remnant. Europ J Can Clin Oncol 1984;21:73 – 79.

254

References

1. Farrands PA, Blake JRS, Ansell ID et al. Endoscopic review of patients who have had gastric surgery. Br Med J 1983;286:755–758.
2. Van de Stadt J. Premaligne en maligne verandering in de restmaag. Disseratie Universiteit van Amsterdam, 1984.
3. Van de Stadt J, Offerhaus J, Huibregtse K et al. Carcinoom en premaligne veranderingen in biopten uit de maag van patiënten die meer dan 15 jaar geleden een maagoperatie ondergingen. Ned T Geneesk 1984;128:606–611.
4. Morson BC, Sobin LH, Grundmann E et al. Precancerous conditions and epithelial dysplasia in the stomach. J Clin Pathol 1980;33:711–721.
5. Domellöf L, Erikson S, Janunger K-G. Carcinoma and possible precancerous changes of the gastric stump after Billroth II resection. Gastroenterology 1977;73:462–468.
6. Offerhaus GJA, Huibregtse K, de Boer J et al. The operated stomach: A premalignant condition. A prospective endoscopic follow-up study. Scand J Gastroenterol 1984;19:521–524.
7. Offerhaus GJA, van de Stadt J, Huibregtse K et al. Endoscopic screening for malignancy in the gastric remnant: The clinical significance of dysplasia in gastric mucosa. J Clin Pathol 1984;37:748–754.
8. Nicholls JC. Stump cancer following gastric surgery. World J Surg 1979;3:731–736.
9. Peitsch W, Becker HD. Was ist gesichert in der Pathogenese und Häufigkeit des primären Carzinoms im operierten Magen? Chirurg 1979;50:33–38.
10. Peitsch W, Becker HD. Frequency and prognosis of gastric stump cancer. Front Gastrointest Res 1979;5:170–177.
11. Fisher AB, Graem N, Jensen OM. Risk of gastric cancer after Billroth II resection for duodenal ulcer. Br J Surg 1983;70:552–554.
12. Pickford IR, Craven JL, Hall R et al. Endoscopic examination of the gastric remnant 31–39 years after subtotal gastrectomy for peptic ulcer. Gut 1984;25:393–397.
13. Lowenfels AB. Does bile promote extra-colonic cancer? Lancet 1978;2:667–670.
14. Langhans P, Heger RA, Hogenstein J et al. Gastric stump carcinoma – New aspects deduced from experimental results. Scand J Gastroenterol 1981;16 (Suppl 67):161–164.
15. Domellöf L, Eriksson S, Janunger K-G. Late precancerous changes and carcinoma of the gastric stump after Billroth I resection. Am J Surg 1976;132:26–31.
16. Meister H, Schlag P, Weber E et al. Frequency of cancerous and precancerous epithelial lesions in the stomach in different models for enterogastric reflux. Scand J Gastroenterol 1981;16(Suppl 67):165–168.
17. Offerhaus GJA. van de Stadt J, Huibregtse K et al. Is de geopereerde maag een premaligne toestand? N Tijdschr Geneesk 1983;127:2127–2132.
18. Scott RE, Whille JJ, Wier ML. Mechanisms for the invitation and promotion of carcinogenesis. A review and a new concept. Mayo Clin Proc 1984;59:107–117.
19. Correa P. Precursors of gastric and esophageal cancer. Cancer 1982;50:2554–2565.
20. Editorial. Bacteria in the stomach. Lancet 1981;2:906–907.
21. Tannenbaum SR. N-nitroso compounds: A perspective on human exposure. Lancet 1983;1:629–632.

22. Challis BC, Kyrkafoulos SA. The chemistry of nitroso-compounds. Part II. Nitrosation of amines by the two-phase interaction of amines in solution with gaseous oxides of nitrogen. J chem Soc 1979;I:299–304.
23. Glass GBJ, Pitchumoni CS. Atrophic gastritis. Human Path 1975;6:219–250.
24. Hansen OA, Larsen JK, Svendsen LB. Changes in gastric mucosal cell proliferation after antrectomy or vagotomy in man. Scand J Gastroenterol 1978; 13:947–952.
25. Assad RT, Eastwood GL. Epithelial proliferation in human fundic mucosa after antrectomy and vagotomy. Gastroenterology 1980;79:807–811.
26. Offerhaus GJA, van de Stadt J, Samson G et al. Cell proliferation kinetics in the gastric remnant. Europ J Can Clin Oncol 1984;21:73–79.
27. Miderer SE, Müller R, Kutz K et al. Multicentric early gastric carcinoma mimicking type I. Endoscopy 1977;9:50–53.
28. Osnes M, Lótveit T, Myren J et al. Early gastric carcinoma in patients with a Billroth II partial gastrectomy. Endoscopy 1977;9:45–49.
29. Oehlert W, Keller P, Henke M et al. Gastric mucosal dysplasia: What is its clinical significance? Front Gastroint Res 1979;4:173–182.
30. Schrumpf E, Serck-Hanssen A, Stadaas J et al. Mucosal changes in the gastric stump 20–25 years after partial gastrectomy. Lancet 1977;2:467–469.
31. Domellöf L, Enander L-K, Wilsson F. Bleeding as a complication to endoscopic biopsies from the gastric remnant after ulcer surgery. Scand J Gastroenterol 1983;18:951–954.
32. Schafer LW, Larson DE, Melton LJ et al. the risk of gastric carcinoma after surgical treatment for benign ulcer disease. N Engl J Med 1983;309: 1210–1213.
33. McLean Ross AH, Smith MA, Anderson JR et al. Late mortality after surgery for peptic ulcer. New Engl J Med 1982;307:519–522.
34. Logan RFA, Langman MJS. Screening for gastric cancer after gastric surgery. Lance 1983;2:667–670.
35. Dick W, Rösch W. Rezidivulkus und -karzinom im operierten Magen. Med Welt 1981;32:611–612.
36. Myren J. Markers of cancer risk and surveillance of the gastric stump. In: Sherlock P, Morson BC, Barbara L, Veronesi U (Eds). Precancerous lesions of the gastrointestinal tract. New York, Raven Press, 1983.
37. Correa P, Haenszel W. The epidemiology of gastric cancer. In: Correa P, Haenszel W (Eds). The epidemiology of cancer of the digestive tract. The Hague, Martinus Nijhoff 1982:59–84.
38. Kekki M, Saukkonen M, Sipponen P et al. Dynamics of chronic gastritis in the remnant after partial gastrectomy for duodenal ulcer. Scand J Gastroenterol 1980;15:509–512.
39. Lewis JH, Woods M. Gastric carcinoma in patients with unoperated duodenal ulcer disease. Am J Gastroenterol 1982;77:368–373.
40. Kekki M, Ihamäki T, Saukkonen M et al. Progression of gastritis at a population level. Scand J Gastroenterol 1980;15:651–655.
41. Giarelli L, Melato M, Stanta G et al. Gastric resection: A cause of high frequency of gastric carcinoma. Cancer 1983;52:1113–1116.
42. Sonnenberg A. Endoscopic screening for gastric stump cancer. Would it be beneficial? Gastroenterology 1984;87:489–495.
43. Pichelmayr R, Meyer HJ. Value of the gastrectomy 'de Principe'. In: Herfarth Ch, Schlag P (Eds). Gastric cancer. Berlin, Springer-Verlag 1979: 196–204.

44. Domellöf L, Janunger K-G. The risk for gastric carcinoma after partial gastrectomy. Am J Surg 1977;134:581–584.
45. Ewerth S, Bergstrand D, Hellers G et al. The incidence of carcinoma in the gastric remnant after resection for benign ulcer disease. Acta Chir Scand 1978; 482(Suppl):2–5.
46. Savage A, Jones S. Histological appearance of the gastric mucosa 15–27 years after partial gastrectomy. J Clin Path 1979;32:179–186.
47. Geboes K, Rutgeerts P, Broechaert L et al. Histological appearance of endoscopic mucosal biopsies 10–20 years after partial gastrectomy. Ann Surg 1980;192(2):179–182.
48. Helsingen N, Hillestad L. Cancer development in the gastric stump after partial gastrectomy for ulcer. Ann Surg 1956;143:173–179.
49. Krause U. Late prognosis after partial gastrectomy for ulcer. Acta Chir Scand 1957;114:341–354.
50. Liavåg K. Cancer development in gastric stump after partial gastrectomy for peptic ulcer. Ann Surg 1962;155:103–106.
51. Griesser G, Schmidt A. Statistische Erhebungen über die Häufigkeit des Karzinoms nach Magenoperation wegen eines Geschwürsleidens. Med Welt 1964;35:1836–1840.
52. Hilbe G, Salzer GM, Hussl H et al. Die Karzinomgefährdung des Resektionsmagens. Lengenbecks Arch Chir 1968;323:142–153.
53. Stalsberg H, Taksdal S. Stomach cancer following gastric surgery for benign conditions. Lancet 1971;2:1175–1177.
54. Peitsch W, Burkhardt K. Zur Pathogenese und Klinik des Magenstumpfscarzinoms. Langenbecks Arch Chir 1976;341:195–203.
55. Hakkiluoto A. Long-term follow-up study of patients operated on for benign peptic ulcer. Ann Chir Gynaecol 1976;65:361–368.
56. Clemençon G, Baumgartner R, Leuthold E et al. Das Karzinom des operierten Magens. Dtsch Med Wochensch 1977;9:169–172.
57. Schmid E, Vollmer R, Adlung J et al. Zur endoskopische Diagnostik des Karzinoms in operierten Magen. Z Gastroenterol 1976;5:521.
58. Cheli R, Molinari F, Santi L. Gastric stump cancer: statistical evaluation. Rendiconti Gastroenterol 1977;9:169–72.
59. Welvaart K, Warnsinck HH. Hoe vaak komt maagstomp-carcinoom voor? Ned T Geneesk 1982;126:2374–2376.
60. Rehner M, Soehendra N, Eichfusz HP et al. Frühkarzinome im (Billroth II-) Resektionsmagen. Dtsch Med Wochensch 1974;99:533–534.
61. Stokkeland M, Schrumpf R, Serck-Hanssen A et al. Incidence of malignancies of the Billroth II operated stomach: A prospective follow-up. Scand J Gastroenterol 1981;67(Suppl 16):169–171.
62. Graem N, Fischer AB, Hastrup N. Mucosal changes of the Billroth II resected stomach. A follow-up study of patients resected for duodenal ulcer with special reference to gastritis, atypia and cancer. Acta Path Microbiol Scand 1981; 89:227–234.
63. Hiltz SW, Schuman BM. The occurrence of gastric stump cancer in a US population. Gastrointest Endosc 1982;28:113A.
64. Pop P. Het carcinoom in de resectiemaag. Dissertatie Rijksuniversiteit Limburg, Maastricht, 1983.

20. Post gastrectomy syndromes and their management

T. KENNEDY, M.D. (hon.), M.S., M.R.C.S.

Department of Surgery, Royal Victoria Hospital, Belfast, N. Ireland

As vagotomy with or without drainage, but without gastric resection has been used in most patients, at least in the United Kingdom, during the past 15 – 20 years, I shall not limit my remarks to patients who have had gastrectomy. Dragstedt's advocacy of vagotomy was the start of an irreversible tide favouring conservative surgery. One of his best known remarks is: 'Any guy can cure a duodenal ulcer by gastrectomy, but when you are going out to dinner with an intact stomach, it is a mighty fine thing to take with you.'

Symptoms following gastric surgery

Following gastric surgery there may be three undesirable side effects of great importance: dumping, diarrhoea and bile reflux. These may be so severe that the patient becomes a 'gastric cripple', bringing disrepute to the operation. These patients tragically haunt the surgeon, leading to the concept of the Albatross Syndrome (Samuel Taylor Coleridges' Ancient Mariner) and most surgeons are afraid to reoperate. It is my purpose to explore this fear and consider whether we surgeons having produced severe side effects, can do anything to help these unfortunates.

Why do these symptoms occur? There is now overwhelming evidence that it is the removal, destruction, or bypassing of the pylorus that is the root cause. The pylorus is a beautiful mechanism that not only controls the rate of emptying of fluids and solids into the small bowel, but also prevents the unwanted reflux of duodenal content and bile into the stomach. Simply put, without pyloric function the stomach is 'incontinent'.

Dumping

Perhaps the commonest and most important symptom, particularly after partial gastrectomy, is dumping – the clinical features of which

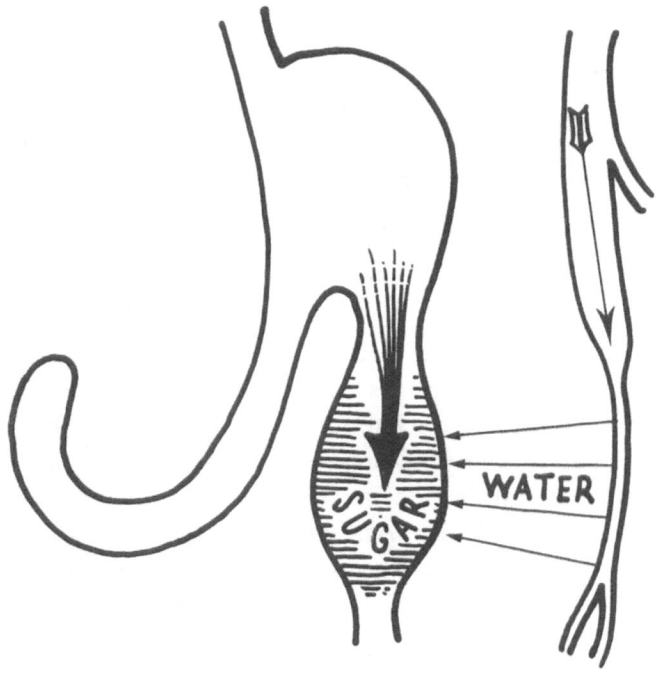

Figure 1. Mechanism of dumping.

are well known. Many workers have shown that when food, particularly carbohydrate, is rapidly emptied into the small bowel it has a profound osmotic effect. Large quantities of fluid, up to a quarter of the circulating blood volume, may be rapidly transferred to the small bowel lumen. (figure 1)This results in hypovolaemic shock causing tachycardia, palpitations, sweating and the need to lie down after even a small meal.

The rapid transfer of up to 3 or 4 litres of fluid into the gut causes a feeling of distension and very rapid transit, the head of the column reaching the ileo-caecal valve within five minutes, or less. This fluid load overwhelms the colon and causes the second cardinal symptom – *diarrhoea*.

Diarrhoea

This is urgent, watery and often post prandial – particularly after breackfast, where there may be a high sugar intake with coffee, cereal etc.

Bile reflux

Bile reflux into the stomach may also be caused by overflow from the distended small gut. Hogsley has stressed that all three of the unholy trinity have the same basic origin.

Medical management of dumping

Medical management of dumping is not very statisfactory. The standard advice is to eat dry meals and take drinks in between meals, or to take frequent, small meals. In my experience, much the most important advice is to avoid sugar in tea of coffee, or sugary biscuits, cake etc. This will also decrease the risk of the so-called 'late dumping'. This reactive hypoglycaemia due to insulin excess is actually quite rare. Certain drugs aimed at reducing the blood sugar have been tried with little success.

It is important to realize that the severity of dumping symptoms tends to decrease, with the passage of time, as patients learn to adjust their diet and eating habits. It is a cardinal rule that at least one year must elapse before a reconstructive operation is even considered.

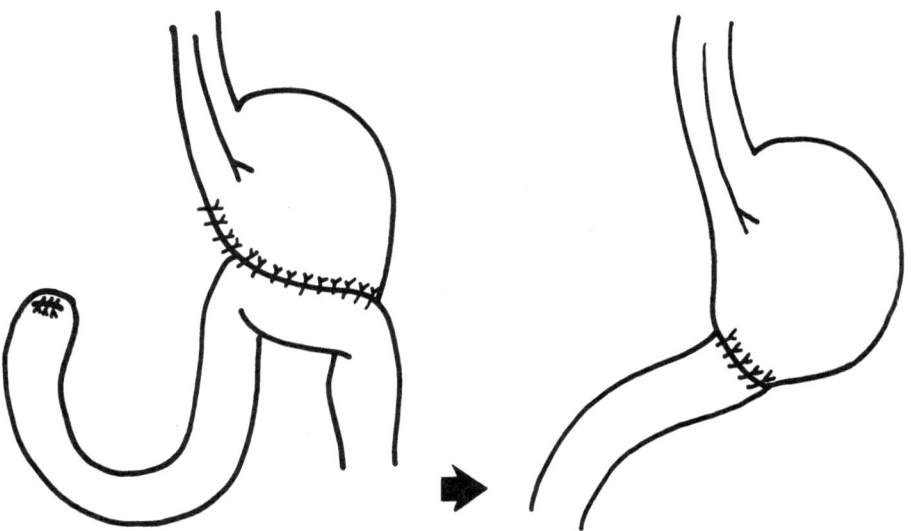

Figure 2. Conversion from Billroth II to Billroth I anastomosis

I have seen one patient who had multiple reconstructions, 6 within a 2 year period, all failed. She had in fact Münchhausen's Syndrome.

Surgical management of dumping

Billroth conversion (figure 2)

One of the earliest procedures used for dumping was conversion from Billroth II to Billroth I. This was attractive, because we knew that there was less dumping with the latter, more physiological anastomosis. In the long term, the results have been disappointing; I found a good result in only 4 of 10 patients.

Interposition (figure 3)

Many surgeons have interposed jejunal loops between stomach and duodenum. To slow gastric emptying further, the loop may be

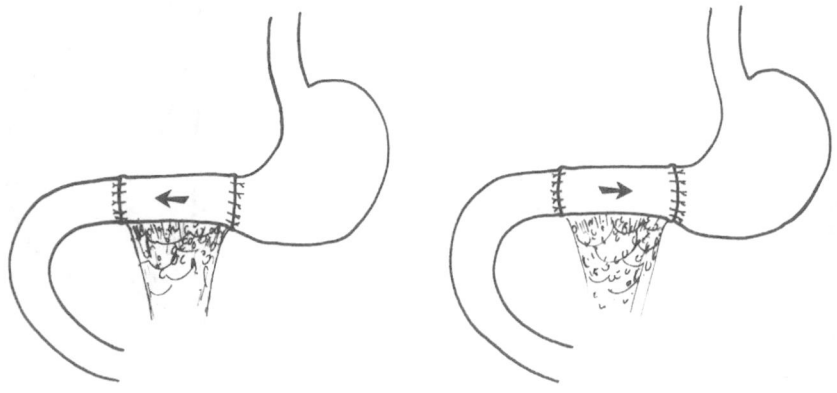

Figure 3. Jejunal loop interposition.

reversed, or an intussuscepting valve may as described by Svenson be used.

With reversed loops it is important to include a vagotomy and the length of the loop should not exceed 10 – 12 cm, otherwise intestinal obstruction may result. In my small experience a good result was obtained in only 43%.

Management of bile reflux gastritis

Dr W. Silen from Boston coined the phrase 'malevolent gall'. Bile in the stomach and oesophagus is highly irritant and plays an important part in the aetiology of benign gastric ulcer, and perhaps also carcinoma. In the colon it has a cathartic effect causing diarrhoea and again possibly colo-rectal cancer.

Duodenogastric reflux with bile reflux gastritis is characterized by constant burning epigastric pain, relieved by nothing, made worse by food and associated with weight loss. Not all patients actually vomit bile, but when they do the diagnosis is obvious. A curious feature of the pain and weight loss is that there may be a delay of several years before these symptoms manifest themselves, yet the reflux of bile into the stomach presumably starts from the time of operation. There is no obvious explanation for this delay.

The medical treatment of reflux is essentially the use of bile salt binders, of which the most effective is cholestyramine. This drug is not easy to take and many patients prefer either aluminium hydroxide or almasilate (Malinal). These drugs may give worthwhile relief to about half of the patients, but ultimately their efficacy tends to disappear.

The drugs are useful to try, because when they give a temporary relief you know that the bile reflux is causing the problem and that an operation may be helpful.

Roux-en-Y (figure 4)

Roux-en-Y diversion of bile is applicable after gastrectomy. Tanner's Roux 19 variant has, in my opinion, no advantage. The loop must be at least 45 cm in length and always covered by a vagotomy, because the diversion is inherently ulcerogenic.

Table I. Roux-en-Y diversions, overall results.

Number of patients operated: n = 62
Number of patients followed: n = 55
Mean duration of follow-up: 6 years (range 1 – 15)

Visick I	19	} 71%
Visick II	20	
Visick III	9	} 29%
Visick IV	7	

Table II. Roux-en-Y loop failures, Visick IV.

Visick IV	
death	1 (after Roux and reversal)
jejunal ulcer	4
gastric ulcer	1
reflux – loop too short	1
Total	7

Table III. Roux-en-Y loop failures, Visick III.

Visick III	
unexplained pain	4
nausea/vomiting	3
diarrhoea	3
dumping	2
malnutrition	1
depression	2
Total	9

Table IV. Long-term consequences of Roux-en-Y (5 – 10 yr, n = 12). (From Cuschieri A. Brit J Surg 1983)

Weight loss	mean 35 kg
Steatorrhoea	12/12
Anaemia ($<$ 10 g)	12/12
Bone disease	2/12

Table V. Roux-en-Y, personal results (average follow-up 5 years).

	Weight change
46 patients	34 gained
	12 lost
Average gain	2.58 kg

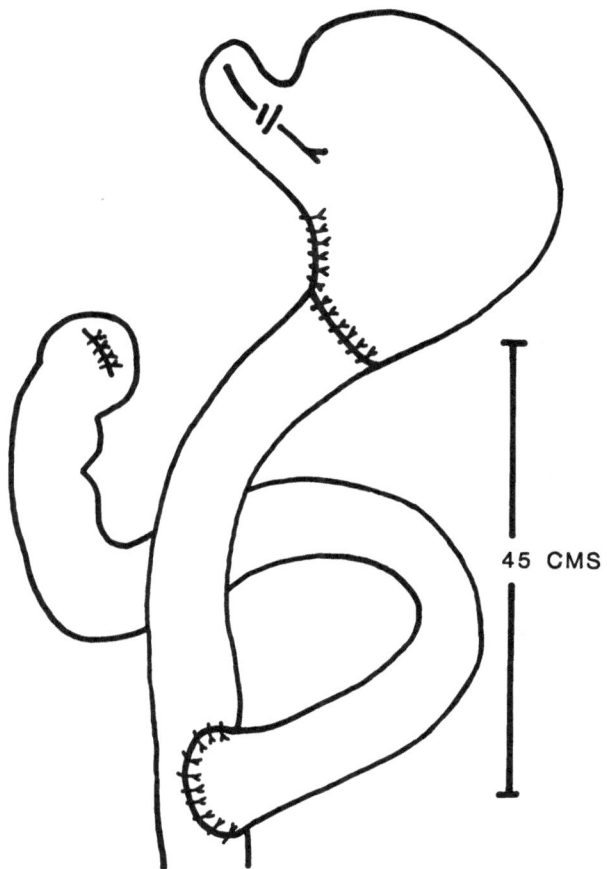

45 CMS

Figure 4. Roux-en-Y diversion.

In my series of 62 patients a good result has been obtained in 71%. There was one death – the only death in 139 patients having one or another of these reconstructions. (Table II)

Four of the failures were due to jejunal ulcerations in patients who had no vagotomy. Some of these patients after Roux-en-Y have quite severe delay in gastric emptying and this may in turn be associated with improvement in dumping.

In contrast, Cushieri recorded the long-term results after Roux-en-Y loop diversion summarized in Table IV, which included weight loss, steatorrhoea, anaemia and bone disease.

Patients I followed more than five years showed considerable weight gains with normal levels of haemoglobin, calcium and albumin.

Table VI. Roux-en-Y, metabolic consequences (follow-up 5 – 11 years).

	n	Mean	
Haemoglobin, g/100ml	18	13.7	<12.5: n = 4
			<11.0: n = 0
Albumin, g/l	12	40	<35 : n = 1
Calcium, mmol/l	13	2.3	< 2.2: n = 0

Roux-en-Y and reversal

Bile reflux is often associated with diarrhoea and with dumping. It is logical in these cases to reverse the proximal 10 cm of the loop. I have done this 6 times with considerable success in 4 patients, but one died. He suffered the calamity that is always threatened in these reversal operations – disruption of the anastomosis. It seems that peristalsis in opposite directions may literally pull an anastomosis apart. It is a difficult operation requiring a meticulous technique.

Table VII. Roux-en-Y and reversal (follow-up 3–7 years, n = 6).

Visick	I	II	III	IV
	3	1	1	1 (death)

Surgical management of post vagotomy diarrhoea

Post vagotomy diarrhoea can be a most distressing symptom and may prevent an otherwise healthy individual from going to work. Treatment is difficult, but some benefit from the use of bile salt binders. Metoclopramide and other drugs which accelerate gastric emptying must obviously be avoided. Reversal of a 10 – 15 cm loop of jejunum about 1 m below the ligament of Treitz has been advocated by Herrington. I have tried this 3 times with little success.

Closure of gastrojejunostomy (figure 5)

When any of the problems that we have discussed is associated with vagotomy and gastrojejunostomy, there is an attractive option. Provided that at least one year has elapsed *vide supra*), the stomach will empty satisfactorily after closure of the draininage even after a truncal

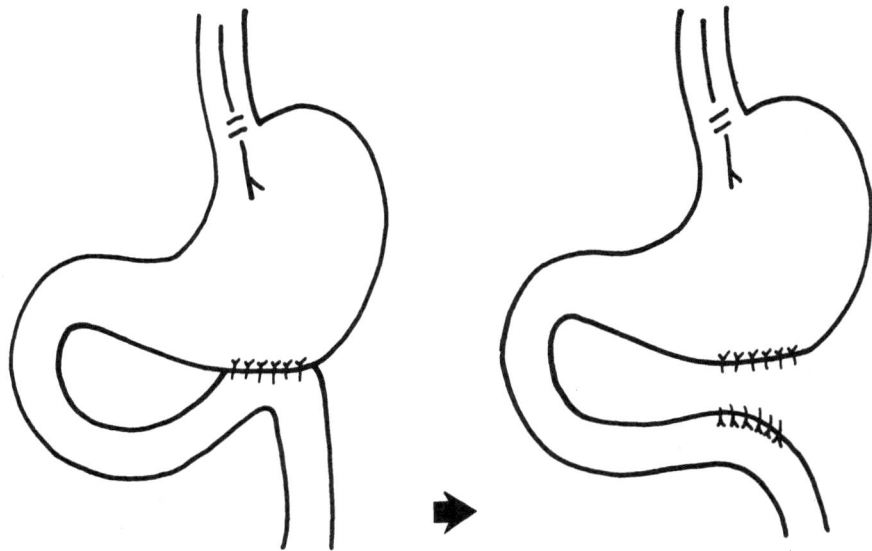

Figure 5. Closure of gastroe-jejunostomy.

vagotomy, because after one year adequate gastric muscle tone has been re-established.

In our experience of 45 closures the success rate has been 83%, all three symptoms being eliminated, or improved in nearly every case.

Table VIII. Closure of gastro-jejunostomy, overall results.

Number of patients operated: n = 62
Number of patients followed: n = 42
Mean duration of follow-up: 6 years (range 1 – 15)

Visick I	14	} 83%
Visick II	21	
Visick III	6	} 17%
Visick IV	1	

There have seven failures: it should be noted that only one has been due to food rentention and vomiting.

In no case in this series has it been necessary to re-institute drainage. In many of these patients the elimination of reflux has been demonstrated by pre- and post-operative HIDA scan.

266

Table IX. Gastrojejunostomy closure failures (n = 7).

Recurrent ulcer	1
Diarrhoea	2
Unexplained pain	3
Food vomiting	1

Reconstruction of pylorus (figure 6)

Most drainage procedures in recent years have been pyloroplasty of one sort or another. Here the problem is less simple, but it is possible to make a tolerably attractive reconstruction of the pyloric muscle ring, although it remains denervated. We have now done this in 15 patients with a 60% success rate. Two of the failures were due to recurrent ulceration close to the pylorus. (Table X)

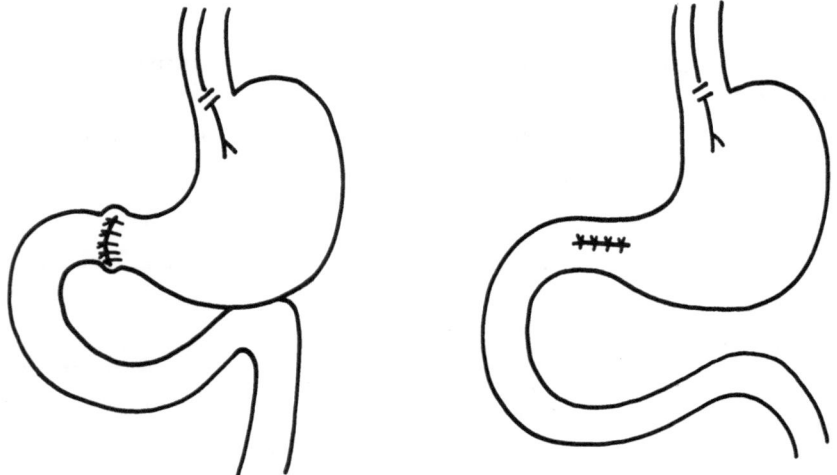

Figure 6. Reconstruction of the pylorus.

Table X. Reconstruction of pylorus (mean follow-up 4.1 yr).

Patients	Success		Recurrent ulcers
15	9	(60%)	2

Why this should be is not clear, but it does reinforce the message that none of these procedures should be done in the presence of a positive insulin test. Where reconstruction or closure of gastrojejunostomy is contemplated and the insulin test is found to be positive, the surgeon has a dilemma. Completion of vagotomy could lead to gastric retention; I have taken this risk in a few patients without cause for regret. In the past 15 years I have used one or other of these procedures in 139 patients with one dealth (0.7%). The overall success rate has been 59%.

Closure of gastrojejunostomy (83%) and Roux loop (71%) are the best operations. I do not think that jejunal interposition or reversal, or conversion of Billroth II to Billroth I should normally be used today. (Table XI) The results reported from the Mayo Clinic by Keith Kelly are remarkably similar to mine.

Table XI. Results of re-intervention.

Operation	n	Percentage success (Vis I + II)
Gastrojejunostomy closure	45	85
Roux loop	62	71
Reconstruction of pylorus	15	60
Jejunal interposition	7	43
Billroth II to Billroth I	10	40
Total	139	59

Other consequences of gastric resection

Anaemia

Anaemia which is nearly always microcytic is common after gastrectomy, less common after vagotomy and gastrojejunostomy and no problem after PGV without drainage. Old gastrectomy patients will require iron from time to time and after extensive gastrectomy it would be wise to keep a close look out for the occasional patient who develops a megaloblastic anaemia.

Calcium metabolism

Osteomalacia is rare after gastrectomy. I have never seen, nor heard of, osteomalacia after vagotomy without resection. Indeed calcium levels remain normal after vagotomy though alkaline phosphatase levels are raised after all forms of vagotomy.

Oesophageal reflux

Oesophageal reflux is a not uncommon problem after all forms of gastric surgery, particularly vagotomy, when there has been extensive mobilization of the cardia. After PGV it is simple to do a fundoplication, but unfortunately in our experience this may lead to lesser curve necrosis. Others, notably Jordan of Houston, has not had this experience.

Stump cancer

Stump cancer following gastrectomy is well recognized. Less well recognized is the incidence of cancer for the stomach following vagotomy and drainage. This was noted many years ago by Capper and Johnston and we too have seen this. We have analysed 735 patients treated by vagotomy and drainage more than 15 years previously and the follow-up was remarkably close to completeness. In this study the overall mortality was considerably in excess of the expected mortality and this increase up to a $1-1.79$ ratio was mainly in the later years. The commonest causes of the excess deaths were cardio pulmonary and various diseases related to smoking, but cancer of the stomach occurred in excess in a ratio of $3.30-1$. There was also an increase in colorectal cancer. One might speculate that the speed of the intestinal transit and the entry of bile into the colon had a possible carcinogenic effect. There were 16 patients with cancer of the stomach in this study. This lead us to look at mucosal changes after vagotomy and gastrojejunostomy and we compared the history of patients 15 years after operation with age and sex-matched patients with chronic duodenal ulcer who had had no operation. We found a highly significant excess of moderate and severe dysplasia in the post-operative group.

It is a fair assumption that dysplasia had at least something to do with the operation. So we then asked whether this dysplasia was reversible if bile and duodenal content had been diverted from the stomach. We studied a group of 33 patients who had had diversion either by a Roux-en-Y loop, or by closure of gastrojejunostomy, with biopsy before and at least one year after re-operation. We found a highly significant improvement in the dysplastic state after surgery. Other mucosal changes such as chronic superficial gastritis, mucosal atrophy and intestinal metaplasia, were not influenced by the diversion of bile. It seems therefore that it may be possible at least in part, to reverse a pre-malignant change.

My message is that it is worthwhile treating the gastric cripples – even if they are not all cured, at least most are improved.

In the words of William Edward Hickson: 'If at first you don't succeed, try, try again.'

21. The role of mucosal blood flow in the pathogenesis and healing of peptic ulcer

P.H. GUTH, M.D.

Medical and Research Services, Wadsworth V.A. Medical Center CURE and UCLA School of Medicine, Los Angeles, California USA

Introduction

In recent years there has been a considerable increase in our knowledge of the role of mucosal blood flow in the pathogenesis of experimental acute gastroduodenal mucosal injury and in the healing of human gastric ulcer. Improved techniques to measure mucosal blood flow in man and in animals have played a major role in this advance. A relationship between acid back diffusion and mucosal blood flow has been demonstrated by these techniques.

In the stomach a barrier to acid back diffusion comprises the mucus-bicarbonate layer and the actual cell layer. These can be overwhelmed by high concentrations of acid; the addition of barrier breakers such as indomethacin and acetylsalicylic acid facilitates this process. A recently developed concept is that increased acid back diffusion is accompanied by an increase in blood flow to the gastric mucosa. If the increase in gastric mucosal blood flow is sufficient to neutralize, dilute and carry away the back diffusing acid, lesions at the mucosal surface do not occur. But if the quantity of acid back diffusion is too great, or if blood supply is inadequate, then lesions do occur.

Mucosal blood flow in the pathogenesis of experimental gastroduodenal injury

Mersereau and Hinchey used an *ex vivo* gastric chamber technique to study acute gastric mucosal lesions induced by haemorrhagic shock in the rat.[1] This permitted direct observation of development of the lesion. Immediately after induction of haemorrhage, the glandular mucosa blanched uniformly. As the blood pressure stabilized at 20 mm Hg, some colour returned to the mucosa and, under stereomicroscopic observation, sluggish flow was observed in mucosal collecting veins. Small white superficial areas were then seen and these slowly enlarged. With retransfusion of blood, bleeding began in the base of these lesions. In the normotensive rat superfusion with 150 mM HCl caused no gastric damage, while in the hypotensive rat as little as 50 mM HCl produced lesions in all animals. In the totally ischemic stomach (clamping of the blood supply for 10 minutes), as little as 25 mM HCl produced mucosal lesions. These studies led to the hypothesis that 'at adequate hydrogen ion concentration, ulceration occurs at pre-existing focal breaks in the mucosa when the mucosal blood flow is so reduced that it cannot prevent the build up of toxic concentration of hydrogen ions'.

Using a lucite gastric chamber technique in dogs, Ritchie studied the effect of topical 100 mM HCl alone, HCl + 5 mM sodium taurocholate, and HCl + sodium taurocholate topically + close intra-arterial vasopressin infusion.[2] Mucosal blood flow was measured by the aminopyrine clearance technique. No lesions were observed in the mucosae exposed to HCl or HCl + taurocholate. However, mucosal blood flow was almost doubled by the combination of HCl + sodium taurocholate. Vasopressin infusion markedly reduced blood flow, but lesion formation in the presence of HCl was minimal. However, when taurocholate in acid was applied to the mucosa and vasopressin infused, there was a marked reduction in blood flow and marked gross mucosal damage occurred. Ritchie also measured hydrogen ion back diffusion and found a similar H^+ loss whether taurocholate was applied with, or without the vasopressin infusion. He postulated that the increased blood flow during HCl + taurocholate application might be a compensatory mechanism to protect against the increased back-diffusion of H^+, and that under ischemic condition lesion formation was the result of the inability to effectively clear or neutralize H^+, which entered the mucosa as a consequence of permeability changes induced by the bile salts.

The thesis that the pathogenesis of acute mucosal lesions was the result of bile salt-induced H^+ back-diffusion plus gastric mucosal ischemia was further tested by Ritchie and Shearburn.[3] They repeated the previously-described studies by Ritchie,[2] with addition of the close intra-arterial infusion of the beta-adrenergic agonist isoprenaline.

Animals subjected to HCl + taurocholate + shock but receiving iso-prenaline still demonstrated an increased H^+ loss, but mucosal blood flow returned to near normal levels and there was a significant decrease in lesions.

Whittle[4] studied acid back diffusion and mucosal blood flow in the rat. Perfusion with $100-150$ mmol hydrochloric acid did not produce mucosal lesions. If sodium taurocholate was added to the perfusate the barrier to acid back diffusion was broken, resulting in an increase in acid back diffusion. Simultaneously there was an increase in mucosal blood flow and few lesions developed. After pre-treatment with indomethacin acid back diffusion was unaffected, but mucosal blood flow significantly decreased and severe lesions developed. This reduction in mucosal blood flow and the development of lesions could be prevented by the administration of exogenous prostaglandins in the same experimental design.

Moody[2] studied the ratio of acid back diffusion and blood flow in an acetylsalicylic acid-injury model and demonstrated a significant relationship between the severity of mucosal lesions and this ratio. (Table I)

Table I. The relation between mucosal lesions, acid back diffusion and mucosal blood flow following acetylsalicylic acid injury in the rat.[5] (mean ± SD)

Severity of lesion	H^+-loss μ Eq/min	Blood flow ml/min	Ratio
None	-17.3 ± 2.2	36.3 ± 3.4	0.51 ± 0.1
Mild	-21.7 ± 1.3	26.5 ± 3.1	0.98 ± 0.1
Severe	-22.3 ± 1.7	8.8 ± 0.8	3.44 ± 0.5

These findings suggest that increased blood flow protects against lesion formation under these experimental conditions. In these cir-cumstances the intramural pH will fall and possibly it is ultimately the low intramucosal pH which causes the cell damage. This hypothe-sis has been tested by Kivilaakso, Fromm and Silen who studied the pH of the lamina propria of the fundus and the antrum in rabbits and dogs during haemorrhagic shock.[6] A small area of the gastric wall was denuded of its seromuscular coat and, using a micromanipulator, an antimony microelectrode was advanced vertically into the mucosa so that its tip was in the mid-portion of the mucosa. The millivoltage was recorded continuously by a high-input impedance pH/electro-meter. In the rabbit fundic mucosa, a relatively permeable membrane, pH rapidly and profoundly decreased (from 7.35 to 6.62), and this was associated with severe lesion formation. In canine fundic mucosa, a less permeable membrane, intramural pH decreased much more slowly.

However, when the mucosal barrier was disrupted by the addition of 5 mM taurocholate to the acidic mucosal solution, a more rapid and profound decrease in intramural pH to 6.50 occurred, with severe and extensive mucosal lesion formation. These findings suggest that the critical determinant of lesion development during shock is an impaired capacity of the mucosa to remove, or buffer the influx of acid.

Relationship between the extent of decreased mucosal blood flow and increased susceptibility to gastroduodenal injury

Leung et al[7] studied the question of whether decreases in mucosal blood flow produce a similar pattern of increased susceptibility to mucosal injury by exogenously administered acid in the stomach and duodenum. In the anaesthetized rat, antral and corpus mucosal blood flows were measured by the hydrogen gas clearance technique using platinum contact electrodes and 3% hydrogen in air.[8] Three percent hydrogen is non-explosive and does not produce hypoxia during inhalation. One platinum contact electrode was positioned gently against the antral mucosa and one against the corpus mucosa. Reference electrodes were placed inside the abdominal cavity. This technique takes advantage of the dissociation of molecular hydrogen into hydrogen ions and electrons at the surface of the platinum electrode. With a completed circuit, a current can be registered. The magnitude of this current is proportional to the concentration of molecular hydrogen in the tissue, in this case, the antral and corpus mucosae. As the animal breathes the 3% hydrogen, the current tracing gradually rises and finally reaches a plateau in about 10 – 15 minutes, indicating tissue saturation with hydrogen. At this point the external source of hydrogen is removed. The current tracing gradually falls. Since the hydrogen in the mucosa can only be removed by blood perfusing it, the rate at which the current tracing falls provides an estimate of blood flow in the mucosa. (fig. 1)

Points along the desaturation curve are graphed on semilogarithmic paper. The half-time, t-½, can be determined from this.

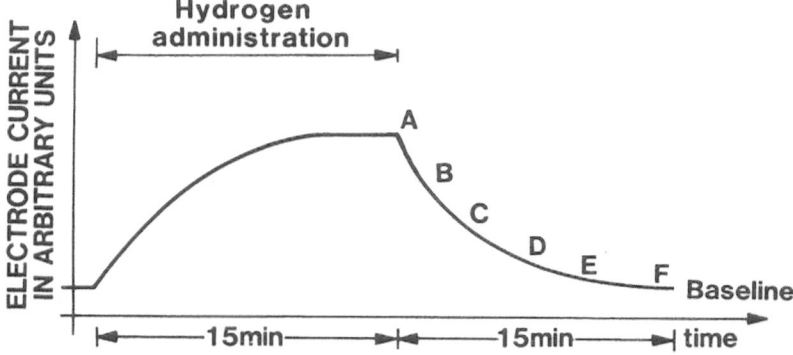

Figure 1. Idealized tracing of the current recorded during a hydrogen gas clearance determination.

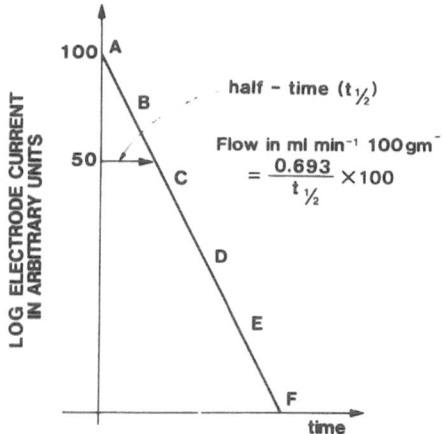

Figure 2. Semilog plot of the data presented in figure 1. The letter points correspond to the letter points in figure 1. Flow can be determined from the half-time obtained from the plot.

Mucosal blood flow in ml.min^{-1}.100 gm^{-1} is calculated from the equation $\frac{0.693}{t_{1/2}}$ × 100. (fig. 2) Readers who desire a more detailed discussion of the theoretical basis of this technique should consulte reference 8. Antral and corpus mucosal blood flows were obtained before and during graded hypotension (produced by removing blood

276

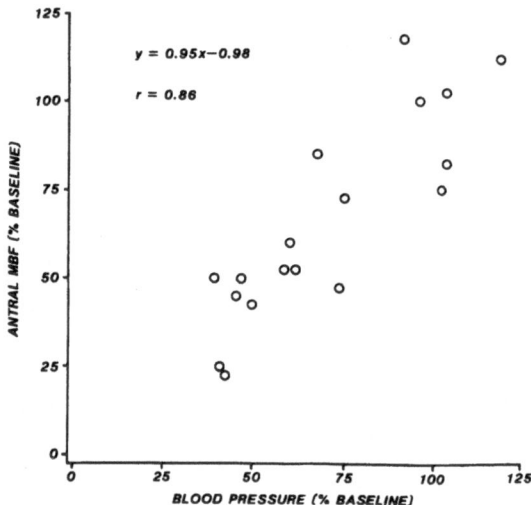

Figure 3. Correlation between corpus mucosal blood flow and systemic blood pressure (both expressed as percent of initial baseline values).

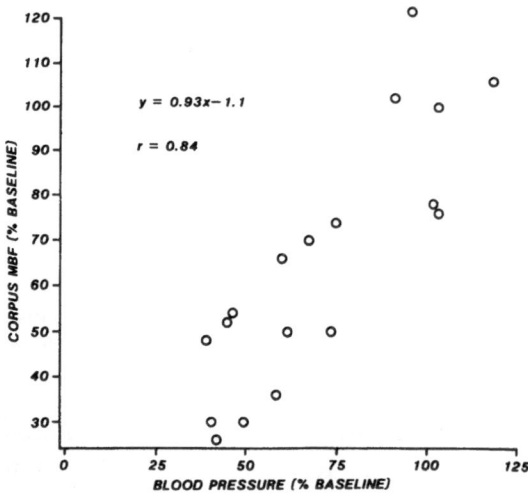

Figure 4. Correlation between antral mucosal blood flow and systemic blood pressure (both expressed as percent of initial baseline values.

via a carotid artery cannula) to a mean systemic blood pressure of either 80 or 50 mm Hg. An attempt to measure mucosal blood flows at a mean systemic blood pressure of 25 mm Hg was unsuccessful as flows were so slow that they were beyond the sensitivity of the method. For the measurement of duodenal mucosal blood flow, before and during graded hypotension, the platinum contact electrode was positioned gently against the duodenal mucosa within 0.5 to 1 cm of the pylorus. For studying the effect of reduced blood flow on susceptibility to acid-induced gastric mucosal injury, one ml 0.1 N HCl/100 gm was instilled into the pylorus-ligated stomachs of anesthetized rats.

For studying the effect of reduced blood flow in susceptibility to acid-induced duodenal mucosal injury, the duodenum was perfused with 0.1 N HCl via a catheter passed through the stomach to just beyond the pylorus. Experimental animals were individually bled and blood pressure was maintained at a graded level of hypotension for 20 minutes. The drawn blood was then retransfused and 20 minutes later the stomach or duodenum was removed, opened and gently rinsed free of debris. The percent area of the corpus antrum or duodenum occupied by lesions was then determined.

Results

Effect of graded hypotension on gastric and duodenal mucosal blood flow

As blood pressure was reduced to 64% and 46% of initial baseline values, antral mucosal blood flow was reduced to 61% and 40% of baseline. Corresponding corpus mucosal blood flows were reduced to 61% of baseline and 37% of baseline. When the blood pressure was reduced to between 20–30 mm Hg, blood flow was too slow to measure in either the antrum or corpus. Regression analysis of all the data revealed a significant correlation between mucosal blood flow and blood pressure during hypotension.

In the duodenum, when blood pressure was reduced to 87%, 68%, 52% and 39% of initial baseline values, mucosal blood flow was reduced to 81%, 57%, 51% and 39% of initial baseline values. Regression analysis of all the data revealed a significant correlation between duodenal mucosal blood flow and blood pressure during hypotension. (figs 3–5)

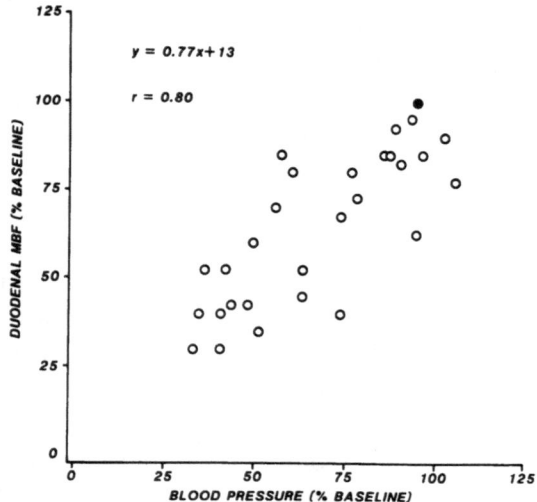

DUODENAL MUCOSAL BLOOD FLOW VS BLOOD PRESSURE

$y = 0.77x + 13$

$r = 0.80$

Figure 5. Correlation between duodenal mucosal blood flow and systemic blood pressure (both expressed as percent of initial baseline values.

Effect of graded hypotension on susceptibility to acid-induced gastric and duodenal mucosal injury

In rats subjected to haemorrhagic shock (25 mm Hg blood pressure or 20% of baseline) plus intragastric 0.1 N HCl fairly large erosions developed primarily in the corpus.

In the stomach, lesions did not appear when blood pressure was reduced to 64% of baseline. Antral and corpus mucosal lesions began to appear as blood pressure was reduced to 33% of baseline. The area of lesion involvement in the corpus and the antrum were 6.4 ± 2.3% and 3 ± 1.3%, respectively. As blood pressure was reduced to 26 ± 1 mm Hg (20% of baseline), corpus and antral mucosal lesions markedly increased to 26.8 ± 4.5% and 5.3 ± 1.4% respectively. Both were significantly greater (p < 0.05) than in control animals. Regression analysis of all the data revealed poor correlation between antral and corpus lesions and blood pressure expressed as percent of baseline. The mucosa of both the corpus and antrum remained resistant to injury, no lesions developing, until the blood pressure fell to well below 40% of baseline.

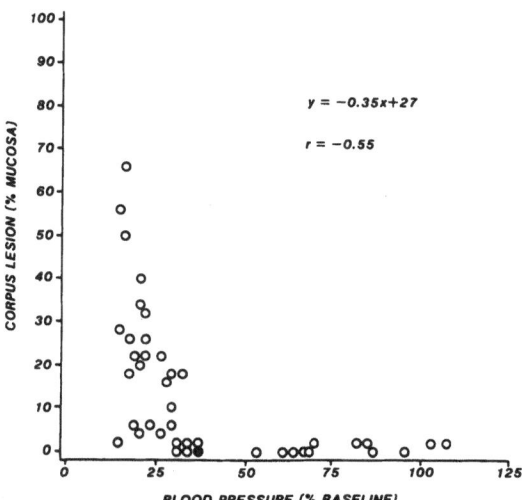

Figure 6. Surface area of mucosal lesions in the gastric body (expressed as percent of corpus area) vs changes in systemic blood pressure (expressed as percent of baseline value).

In the duodenum, as blood pressure was reduced to 84 ± 1, 65 ± 1, and 41 ± 2 mm Hg or 71, 52 and 32% of baseline, respectively; there was a progressive increase in the area of mucosal lesions to 25 ± 10, 3 ± 11 and 77 ± 12%. Regression analysis of all the data revealed a significant negative correlation between mucosal lesions and blood pressure, both expressed as percent of baseline. (figs 6–8)

In the blood flow studies of Leung et al,[7] a significant correlation was found between blood pressure during hypotension, and antral, corpus and duodenal mucosal blood flows. In their gastric mucosal injury study, there was a poor correlation between step-wise reductions in systemic blood pressure and lesion formation in the antrum and the corpus. A threshold appeared to exist for the formation of antral and corpus mucosal lesions. Systemic blood pressure had to be reduced to 40% of baseline value before mucosal lesions began to appear and to 25% of baseline for fairly severe lesion formation. On the other hand, in the duodenal mucosal injury study, a significant correlation was found between duodenal mucosal lesion formation and reductions in systemic blood pressure.

280

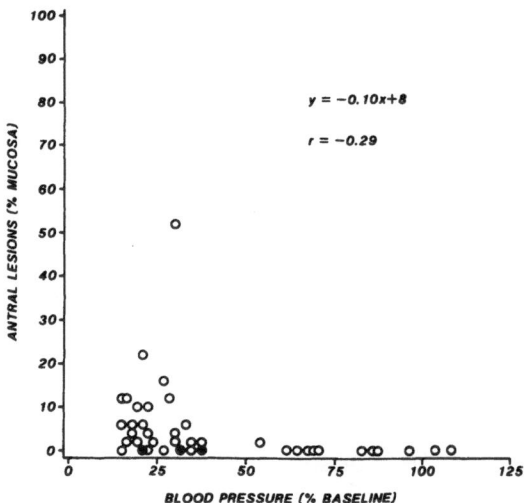

ANTRAL LESION VS BLOOD PRESSURE

$y = -0.10x + 8$

$r = -0.29$

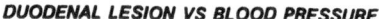

Figure 7. Surface area of mucosal lesions in the gastric antrum (expressed as percent of antral area) vs changes in systemic blood pressure (expressed as percent of baseline value).

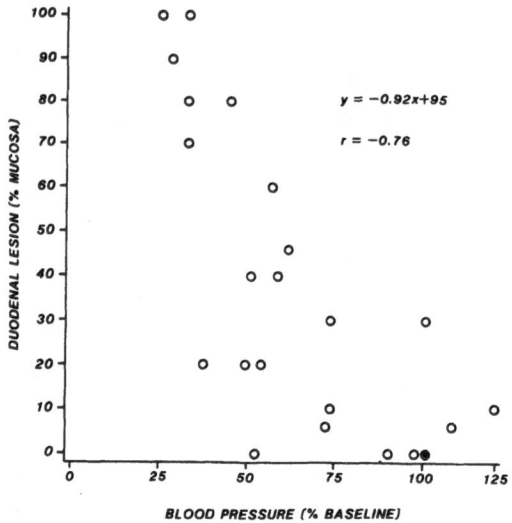

DUODENAL LESION VS BLOOD PRESSURE

$y = -0.92x + 95$

$r = -0.76$

Figure 8. Surface area of mucosal lesions in the duodenum (expressed as percent of duodenal area) vs changes in systemic blood pressure (expressed as percent of baseline value).

It can be inferred from these findings that mucosal blood flow is a less important factor in resisting acid induced injury in the stomach than in the duodenum. In the stomach the resistance to mucosal injury did not break down until mucosal blood flow was reduced to less than 40% of baseline, but in the duodenum, the mucosal injury progressively increased with fall in mucosal blood flow. Other defensive mechanisms must be stronger in the stomach than the duodenum. Since the stomach continually faces a much higher concentration of acid than does the duodenum, this is not surprising. Nevertheless, this study, as did previous ones, demonstrated that a marked reduction in mucosal blood flow renders both the gastric and duodenal mucosae susceptible to acid-induced injury.

Mucosal blood flow in the healing of peptic ulcer

Nearly all studies of blood flow in experimental ulcer disease have involved acute mucosal injury. This is largely due to the lack of a good animal model that closely mimics human chronic peptic ulcer. Until recently there has also been a dearth of mucosal blood flow studies in human peptic ulcer disease. This was because of the lack of methods to measure local mucosal blood flow in man. In the past few years, however, the new techniques have been successfully used in man.

The hydrogen gas clearance technique has been used to measure gastric mucosal blood flow in man by passing the platinum electrode through the biopsy channel of an upper gastrointestinal endoscope. Two types of electrodes have been used: a needle electrode that is inserted no more than 3 mm into the gastric mucosa and a contact electrode. The reference electrode is applied to the skin of an extremity.

Fukutomi et al[9] used the needle electrode to study blood flow in 35 patients with gastric ulcer and 27 normal controls. Blood flow was similar in the corpus and antrum in both ulcer patients and controls, and blood flow was slightly higher in the corpus than in the antrum (about 60 vs 50 ml/min/100 g) in both groups. Blood flow in an acctive gastric ulcer was lowest at the center (31 ± 12 ml/min/100 g – mean $\pm$ SD, and rose at the ulcer margin (41 ± 10 ml/min/100 g). With healing blood flow in the ulcer margin increased, being 62 ± 14 during healing and 70 ± 9 ml/min/100 g with complete healing. When blood flow in the ulcer margin was compared with that in the surrounding normal mucosa, it was lower during the active stage, higher during healing and the same with complete healing. While this was true of ulcers that healed readily, in intractable or recurring ulcers blood flow at the ulcer margin remained significantly below that of the surrounding normal mucosa(39 ± 2 vs 59 ± 2 ml/min/100 g, mean $\pm$ SE).

Using a contact platinum electrode through an endoscope, Murakami et al[10] described a similar low blood flow at the margin of an active ulcer in one patient, with a progressive rise to normal levels as the ulcer healed.

Kamada, Sato and their colleagues have developed a reflectance spectrophotometric method to measure gastric mucosal haemoglobin concentration.[11] A coaxial optical fiber bundle is gently touched to the gastric mucosal surface. Light from an external source passes down the outer bundle to the mucosa. Light reflected from the mucosa passes back up the center bundle to an external spectrophotometer and the resultant spectral data stored in a computer. In animal studies, they demonstrated a good correlation between the difference in absorption between 569 and 650 nm with the concentration of haemoblogin in the gastric mucosa.[11] They have successfully used this method in man by passing the coaxial optical fiber bundle through the biopsy channel of an upper gastrointestinal endoscope.

The main advantage of this method is the possibility to perform multiple measurements very quickly, the hydrogen gas clearance technique being more time consuming as an equilibration phase and a washout phase is necessary with each measurement. The disadvantage of the reflectance spectrophotometric method is that it is essentially a volume measurement. A rise in the haemoglobin concentration does not necessarily reflect an increase in mucosal blood flow, but can also be due to stasis.

This technique was used to study human gastric ulcer disease.[12] The mucosal blood volume in patients with active gastric ulcer was significantly lower than that of controls in almost all portions of the stomach. With healing of the ulcer, it returned to the same level as the control group. During healing, mucosal blood flow at the ulcer margin increased to a greater extent (33%) than the more distant surrounding mucosa. With complete healing it fell to the same normal level as the latter. In 9 patients whose ulcer failed to heal in 3 months, however, mucosal flow at the ulcer margin failed to increase

(2 ± 14% increase in the non-healing group vs 33 ± 20% in the healing group). The difference between these values was significant, $p < .05$.

Comment

The experimental animal studies clearly demonstrate the role of mucosal blood flow in defense of the gastric and duodenal mucosa against acute injury. A decrease in blood flow renders the mucosa more susceptible to injury, and raising blood flow protects against injury.

The studies of gastric ulcer in man demonstrate the importance of mucosal blood flow in the healing of peptic ulcers. During active ulceration, blood flow and blood volume in the margin of the ulcer is low. With healing, both measurements rise even above normal. With complete healing, both return to normal levels.

In recalcitrant or recurring gastric ulcers, blood flow and blood volume at the ulcer margin remain low. Although only limited numbers of patients have been studied, the similarity of results using two different techniques suggests that mucosal blood flow at the ulcer margin is an important factor in ulcer healing, and its increase predicts healing. Conversely, it appears that an impaired blood supply is a factor in persisting or recurring gastric ulcer disease in man.

References

1. Mersereau WA, Hinchey EJ. Effect of gastric acidity on gastric ulceration induced by hemorrhage in the rat, utilizing a gastric chamber technique. Gastroenterology 1973;64:1130–5.
2. Ritchie WP Jr. Acute gastric mucosal damage induced by bile salts, acid, and ischemia. Gastroenterology 1975;68:699–707.
3. Ritchie WP Jr, Shearburn EW III. Influence of isoproterenol and choleystyramine on gastric mucosal ulcerogenesis. Gastroenterology 1977;73:62–5.
4. Wittle BJR. Mechanism underlying gastric mucosal damage induced by indomethacin and bile salts, and the actions of prostaglandins. Br J Pharmacol 1977;60:455.
5. Moody FG, McGreavy J, Salewsky C et al. The cytoprotective effect of mucosal blood flow in experimental erosive gastritis. Acta Physiol Scand 1977;Special Suppl 35.
6. Kivilaakso E, Fromm D, Silen W. Relationship between ulceration and intramural pH of gastric mucosa during haemorrhagic shock. Surgery 1978;84:70–8.

7. Leung FW, Itoh M, Hirabayashi K, Guth PH. Role of blood flow in gastric and duodenal mucosal injury in the rat. Gastroenterology 1985;88:281–9.
8. Leung FW, Guth PH, Scremin OU et al. Regional gastric mucosal blood flow measurements by hydrogen gas clearance in the anesthetized rat and rabbit. Gastroenterology 1984;87:28–36.
9. Fukutomi H, Miyamoto J, Sakita T. Endoscopical measurement of gastric blood flow of patients suffering from gastric ulcer. In: Tsuchiya M, Asano M, Oda M (Eds). Basic Aspects of Microcirculation. Exerpta Medica, Amsterdam 1982:251–258.
10. Murakami M, Morriga M, Miyake T et al. Contact electrode method in hydrogen gas clearance technique: A new method for determination of regional gastric mucosal blood flow in animals and humans. Gastroenterology 1982;82:457–467.
11. Sato N, Kamada T, Shichiri M et al. Measurement of hemoperfusion and oxygen sufficiency in gastric mucosa in vivo. Gastroenterology 1979;79:814–9.
12. Kamada T, Kawano S, Sato N et al. Gastric mucosal blood distribution and its changes in the healing process of gastric ulcer. Gastroenterology 1983;84:1541–6.

22. Duodenal ulcers produced in rats by indomethacin plus bile duct ligation

A. ROBERT, J.E. NEZAMIS, and C. LANCASTER

Diabetes and GI Diseases Research, The Upjohn Company, Kalamazoo, MI 49001, USA

Abstract

Duodenal ulcers were produced in rats by ligating the common bile and giving indomethacin immediately after. Neither indomethacin alone nor bile duct ligation alone was ulcerogenic. When the two conditions were combined, the ulcers developed within 24 hours and began to perforate after 48 hours. No gastric ulcers were performed. The incidence of duodenal ulcers and perforations increased with the dose of indomethacin. The optimal conditions were: fed animals given a single administration of 10 – 20 mg/kg of indomethacin orally or subcutaneously, given after bile duct ligation, and killed two days later. The ulcers were prevented by antisecretory agents (methscopolamine bromide, 16,16-dimethyl PGE_2 at a subcutaneous antisecretory dose) and an antacid, as well as by 16,16-dimethyl PGE_2 given orally at a non-antisecretory dose (cytoprotection). The mechanism by which indomethacin plus bile duct ligation is duodeno-ulcerogenic appears to involve reduction of bicarbonate in duodenal contents due to lack of alkaline bile (from bile duct ligation) and to inhibition of bicarbonate secretion by the duodenal mucosa (an effect of indomethacin). Reduction of prostaglandin content of the duodenal mucosa, by indomethacin administration, may sensitize the mucosa to the damaging effect of unbuffered gastric acid.

Introduction

Most non-steroidal anti-inflammatory compounds (NOSAC) can damage the gastrointestinal mucosa in animals[1-3] as well as in humans.[4-10] In humans, the lesions consist of petechiae, erosions and ulcers, usually accompanied with bleeding. They occur in the stomach and the duodenum. In experimental animals most NOSAC (*e.g.*, aspirin, indomethacin) produce gastric lesions, but only a few cause duodenal lesions.[11-14] Mepirizole[12,13] and dulcerozine, an analog of mepirizole,[14] are particularly potent in producing duodenal ulcers in rats. Indomethacin, on the other hand, produces gastric ulcers and intestinal lesions, but very rarely duodenal ulcers.

We report here the production of duodenal ulcers in rats by indomethacin when administered after ligation of the common bile duct. Part of the results were published in abstract form before.[15]

Methods

Female Upjohn rats, derived from the Sprague-Dawley strain, of an average body weight of 210 g were used. They were fed Purina laboratory chow throughout the duration of each experiment. Indomethacin was administered either orally or subcutaneously at various dose levels in a volume of 1 ml of water or saline containing Tween 80 as a suspending agent (1 drop/20 ml). Indomethacin was administered immediately after bile duct ligation or a sham operation, which were performed under ether anesthesia. The common bile duct was identified and sectioned between two ligatures. In sham-operated animals, forceps were inserted under the common bile duct.

The following experiments were performed:

a. In a dose-response study, the animals were killed three days after a single administration of indomethacin at doses ranging from 2 to 20 mg/kg, given either orally or subcutaneously immediately after bile duct ligation or sham operation.
b. In a time course study, the animals were killed from one to five days after oral administration of 10 mg/kg of indomethacin, given immediately after bile duct ligation.
c. The effect of fasting was studied. Indomethacin, 10 mg/kg, was given orally immediately after bile duct ligation. Half of the animals were then fasted for three days whereas the other half were fed ad libitum.

d. The following agents were studied for their effect on duodenal ulcers produced by indomethacin (10 mg/kg) given orally immediately after bile duct ligation: methscopolaminebromide (an anticholinergic agent) given subcutaneously at 0.1, 1 and 2.5 mg/kg in 1 ml of saline, twice a day, the first dose being given 30 minutes before indomethacin and bile ligation; 2 ml of an antacid (Malcogel®) containing 133 mg of magnesium trisilicate and 66 mg of aliminum hydroxide per ml, given orally twice a day for three days, starting immediately after indomethacin and bile duct ligation; 16,16-dimethyl PGE_2 given orally at 50 μg/kg, or subcutaneously at 50 μg/kg or 100 μg/kg, twice a day, starting 30 minutes before indomethacin and bile duct ligation. The animals were killed three days after surgery.

e. The effect of indomethacin and bile duct ligation on gastric secretion was also studied. The bile duct was first ligated, or a sham operation was performed. Then, indomethacin (20 mg/kg) or its vehicle was administered orally. Two hours later, all the animals were reanesthetized and their pylorus was ligated. They were killed four hours after pylorus ligation. The stomachs were dissected out, their contents emptied into a graduated test tube and the volume measured to the nearest 0.1 ml. Gastric acidity was determined by titration with 0.1 M NaOH to pH 7, and the results were expressed in μEq of acid per 4 hour.

Results

Dose-response of indomethacin (Table I)

Indomethacin, given either orally or subcutaneously at doses up to 20 mg/kg to sham-operated animals produced no ulcers (gastric or duodenal). When given to bile duct ligated animals, a dose of 4 mg/kg produced duodenal ulcers in 18% of animals, but no gastric ulcers. The incidence of duodenal ulcers and of perforations increased dose dependently up to 15 mg/kg. The duodeno-ulcerogenic effect of indomethacin was similar after oral and subcutaneous administration. Bile duct ligation by itself did not produce any lesions. The duodenal ulcers are illustrated in Figure 1.

As reported earlier,[16-18] indomethacin produced multiple ulcerations throughout the small intestine. These ulcers perforate, produce

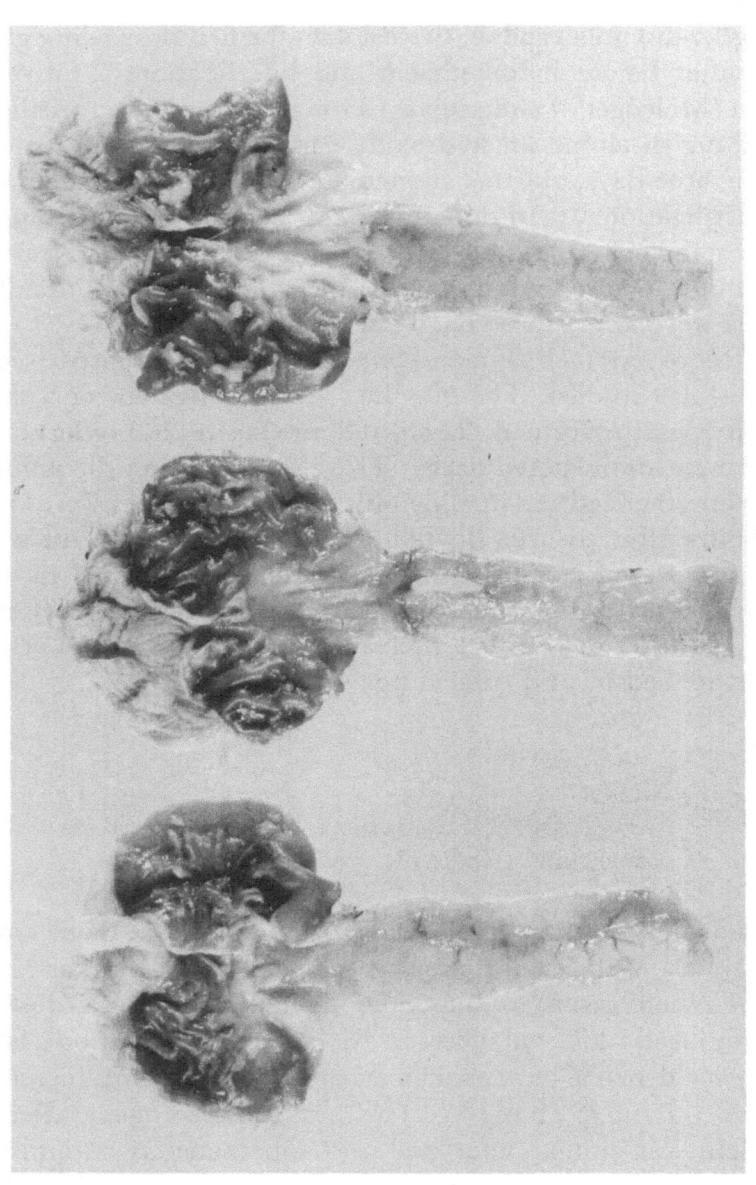

Figure 1. Duodenal ulcers produced by indomethacin plus bile duct ligation. Stomachs and duodenums after opening along the greater curvature of the stomach and the mesenteric attachment of the duodenum. Left: Sham-operated control. No ulcer. Middle: indomethacin 10 mg/kg given orally only once, after bile duct ligation, animals killed 3 days later. Perforated duodenal ulcer. Right: indomethacin plus bile duct ligation, and treatment with 16,16-dimethyl PGE$_2$, 25 μg/kg orally twice a day. No ulcer.

Table I. Duodenal ulcers produced by indomethacin in bile duct ligated rates.

Indomethacin	Mortality (%)		Duodenal ulcer (%)		Duodenal perforation (%)	Intestinal lesions (%)	
	sham	bdl	sham	bdl	bdl	sham	bdl
Oral (mg/kg)							
0	0(18)	0(46)	0	0	0	0	0
2	0(10)	0(10)	0	0	0	0	0
4	0(10)	0(10)	0	18	3	0	0
6	0(10)	0(10)	0	52	13	10	0
8	0(10)	3(28)	0	66	21	86	0
10	0(82)	8(108)	0	77	31	80	0
12	0(53)	8(78)	0	86	63	100	0
14	0(10)	10(10)	0	70	60	100	0
Subcutaneous							
0	0(12)	0	0	0	0	0	0
4	0(8)	0	0	0	0	0	0
6	0(24)	0	0	0		25	0
10	0(21)	0		89	22	73	0
20	10(12)	10		80	50	100	0

Indomethacin given only once, immediately after bile duct ligation or sham-operation. The animals were killed after 3 days. (%): Percent of animals. bdl: bilde duct ligation. (): Number of animals.

an exudative peritonitis and adhesions of intestinal loops. This syndrome was observed in sham-operated animals, the threshold dose being 6 mg/kg, but was completely prevented by bile duct ligation. (Table I) This confirms previous reports.[18,19]

Time course (Table II)

The animals were killed from one to five days after a single oral administration of indomethacin, 10 mg/kg, given after bile duct ligation. After one day, half of the animals already had duodenal ulcers but none were perforated. The incidence of animals with duodenal ulcers nearly doubled after five days, whereas the incidence of duodenal perforations remained constant from the second to the fifth day. No duodenal ulcers developed in sham-operated animals given indomethacin, nor in bile duct ligation animals given only the vehicle.

Fed vs fasted state

Indomethacin given at an oral dose of 10 mg/kg was slightly more duodeno-ulcerogenic in fed animals than in animals fasted for three

Table II. Time course of duodenal ulcers produced by indomethacin and bile duct ligation.

Days post-operation	Number of animals	Operation	Treatment	Duodenal ulcers incidence (%)	Duodenal perforations incidence (%)
1	12	sham	ind	0	0
2	12	sham	ind	0	0
3	13	sham	ind	0	0
4	12	sham	ind	0	0
5	12	sham	ind	0	0
1	12	bdl	ind	50	0
2	12	bdl	ind	67	42
3	11	bdl	ind	63	27
4	9	bdl	ind	56	33
5	10	bdl	ind	90	40
5	5	bdl	vehicle	0	0

Ind: Indomethacin, 10 mg/kg given orally, only once, after bile ligation or sham operation.
Bdl: Bile duct ligation. Animals killed 3 days later.

days from the time of indomethacin administration and bile duct ligation (an incidence of 69% in fed animals vs 45% in fasted animals). However, the incidence of duodenal perforations was comparable (23% in fed animals and 20% in fasted animals). On the other hand, the incidence of intestinal lesions due to indomethacin was markedly reduced by fasting (80% of intestinal lesions in fed animals vs 10% in fasted animals). The preventive effect of intestinal lesions by fasting confirms published results.[18]

Effect of various agents (Table III)

Methscopolamine bromide, an anticholinergic agent, inhibited formation of duodenal ulcers dose dependently. The ED_{50} was around 0.5 mg/kg subcutaneously twice a day. An antacid, given at 2 ml twice a day, completely prevented formation of duodenal ulcers. 16,16-dimethyl PGE_2 given orally at 25 µg/kg (a non-antisecretory dose)[20] reduced the incidence of duodenal ulcers from 66% to 17%, and completely prevented duodenal perforations. When given subcutaneously at the same dose, it did not reduce the incidence of duodenal ulcers but prevented the perforations. At 100 µg/kg subcutaneously (an antisecretory dose),[20] it significantly reduced the incidence of duodenal ulcers.

Table III. Effect of an anticholinergic agent, a prostaglandin and an antacid on duodenal ulcers produced in rats by indomethacin plus bile duct ligation.

	Number of animals	Duodenal ulcers incidence (%)	Duodenal perforations incidence (%)
Sham operation			
Vehicle	5	0	0
Ind	10	0	0
Bile duct ligation			
Vehicle	10	0	0
Ind			
+ vehicle	12	75	25
+ methscopolamine bromide:			
0.1 mg/kg	10	40	20
1.0 mg/kg	10	20	20
2.5 mg/kg	10	0	0
+ dmPGE$_2$: 25 μg/kg oral	6	17	0
50 μg/kg oral	6	67	0
100 μg/kg oral	6	17	0
Ind			
+ vehicle	10	90	30
+ antacid: 2 ml	10	0	0

Ind: Indomethacin given immediately after pylorus ligation. Methscopolamine bromide, 16,16-dimethyl PGE$_2$ (dmPGE$_2$) and an antacid given twice a day, the first injection being 30 minutes before indomethacin. Antacid: Malcogel® .

Gastric acid secretion (Table IV)

Indomethacin given at 20 mg/kg, orally, with or without bile duct ligation reduced gastric acid secretion by approximately the same degree (35 – 45%) in pylorus ligated rats. Bile duct ligation alone reduced acid secretion by 38%, although the difference did not reach statistical significance.

Table IV. Effect of indomethacin and bile duct ligation on gastric acid secretion

	Sham operation		Bile duct ligation	
	vehicle	ind	vehicle	ind
Number of animals	9	7	8	8
Acid output: μEq/4hr	861.6 ± 99.7	562.0 ± 68.7*	535.6 ± 119.5	464.0 ± 52.1*

Ind: Indomethacin, 20 mg/kg, given orally immediately after bile duct ligation or sham-operation. Two hours later, the pylorus was ligated, and the animals were killed 4 hours after pylorus ligation. *: p < 0.05 vs sham vehicle group.

Discussion

These results show that bile duct ligation sensitizes the duodenum to ulcer formation by indomethacin. The optimal conditions are: fed rats of approximately 200 g, indomethacin given only once either orally or subcutaneously at a dose of 10 to 20 mg/kg immediately after bile duct ligation, and animals killed two days later. For statistical evaluation, groups of ten rats are adequate. The absence of gastric ulcers after indomethacin administration is probably due to the fact that the animals were fed throughout the experiments. In the only study where the animals were fasted prior to indomethacin (for collection of gastric juice after pylorus ligation), indomethacin did produce multiple gastric ulcers.

The mechanism by which such duodenal ulcers are produced is unknown, but the following hypotheses can be considered.

a) The duodenal ulcers are not due to hypersecretion of gastric acid. In fact, indomethacin, bile duct ligation, or both, instead of stimulating gastric secretion reduced such secretion by 35% to 45%. Therefore, duodenal ulcers develop in indomethacin-treated bile duct ligated rats in spite of a reduced acid load in the duodenum.

Bile duct ligation was reported earlier to inhibit gastric acid secretion in rats.[21,22] Our results confirm such inhibition of acid output by bile duct ligation. Indomethacin also reduced acid secretion, but the combined procedure of indomethacin administration and bile duct ligation was not more antisecretory than either condition applied separately. The reason for the reduction in acid secretion by indomethacin may be that portions of the gastric mucosa were damaged by the drug: the dose used (20 mg/kg), given to animals that had been fasted for 24 hours, produced numerous gastric ulcers. It is likely that the extensive necrosis at the ulcer sites reduced the parietal cell mass; this may account for the reduction in acid secretion.

Conflicting results have been reported on the effect of mepirizole, a duodeno-ulcerogenic drug, on gastric acid secretion. Okabe et al[12] reported inhibition in the pylorus ligated rat, whereas Tabata et al[13] found no effect on acid secretion from gastric fistula rats. On the other hand, dulcerozine, another drug causing duodenal ulcers, was shown to stimulate gastric acid secretion in the pylorus ligated rat.[14]

b) Although the ulcers produced by indomethacin plus bile duct ligation are not associated with gastric hyperacidity, the presence of some acid in the duodenum appears to be necessary since methscopolamine bromide, at a dose shown earlier to reduce gastric acid secretion,[23] as well as an antacid, did inhibit the ulcers. As in the case of several other models for duodenal ulcer, gastric acid must be present, although not necessarily in excessive quantities, to allow the ulcers to develop.

c) Bile ducht ligation may have promoted duodenal ulcer formation by preventing biliary bicarbonate from being delivered to the duodenal mucosa. such a reduction in luminal bicarbonate would result in less neutralization of acid coming from the stomach, and therefore would produce relative duodenal hyperacidity. Since the duodenum is particularly sensitive to injury by acid, reduced neutralization might be sufficient to damage the mucosa.

The sensitization to duodenal ulcer by bile duct ligation shown in the present studies is similar to that reported earlier for cysteamine. Cysteamine produces duodenal ulcers in rats,[24] and the incidence is increased about three-fold when it is administered after bile duct ligation.[25] The ulcer promoting effect of bile duct ligation in such animals was also ascribed to the absence of neutralization of duodenal contents by biliary bicarbonate. This results in gastric acid flowing unbuffered over the duodenum.

d) The duodenal ulcers may be due to inhibition by indomethacin of bicarbonate secretion by the duodenum itself. Such inhibition was demonstrated *in vitro* in amphibians[26,27] and *in vivo* in cats.[28] The reduced bicarbonate secretion by the duodenum, combined with the lack of biliary bicarbonate, may have prevented adequate neutralization of gastric acid and thus favoured ulcer formation. Mepirizole, a duodeno-ulcerogenic agent, also reduces the secretion of bicarbonate by the duodenum.[13]

e) Since indomethacin is a potent inhibitor of prostaglandin synthesis,[29] the duodenal ulcerations seen after indomethacin plus bile duct ligation could be due to a duodenal depletion of prostaglandins. The lack of prostaglandin in the duodenal mucosa may have reduced its resistance and led to ulceration. However, indomethacin given without bile duct ligation was not duodeno-ulcerogenic. One can postulate that either the inhibition of prostaglandin synthesis by indomethacin is more marked in bile duct ligated animals than in sham-operated animals, or that the reduction in prostaglandin levels by indomethacin sensitizes the duodenal mucosa to the reduced luminal bicarbonate. The reduction in duodenal bicarbonate by itself is not ulcerogenic nor is the reduction in prostaglandin content; however, when both conditions are present, an ulcerogenic situation may be created.

16,16-dimethyul PGE_2 prevented formation of the duodenal ulcers in part by inhibiting gastric acid secretion, when given at a subcutaneous dose of 100 μg/kg. However, an oral dose of 25 μg/kg, which is not antisecretory,[19] still prevented the ulcers, presumably through duodenal cytoprotection.

In conclusion, the combination of indomethacin plus bile duct ligation produces duodenal ulcers within 24 hours in rats. These ulcers are not due to hyperacidity, although some acid in the duodenum is necessary, since antisecretory agents and antacids prevent their formation. The mechanism by which these ulcers develop appears to involve a reduction of acid neutralization in the duodenal lumen due to the lack of biliary bicarbonate (caused by the bile duct ligation) and to inhibition of duodenal secretion of bicarbonate (caused by indomethacin). The depletion of prostaglandin content of the duodenum, induced by indomethacin, may lower the resistance of the duodenal mucosa to acid.

References

1. Robert A. Antisecretory, antiulcer, cytoprotective and diarrheogenic properties of prostaglandins. In: Samuelsson B, Paoletti R (Eds). Advances in Prostaglandin and Thromboxane Research, Vol. 2. New York, Raven Press, 1976:507–520.
2. Whittle BJR. Mechanisms underlying gastric mucosal damage induced by indomethacin and bile salts, and the actions of prostaglandin. Br J Pharmacol 1977;60:455–460.
3. Rainsford KD, Fox SA, Osborne DJ. Comparative effects of some nonsteroidal anti-inflammatory drugs on the ultrastructural integrity and prostaglandin levels in the rat gastric mucosa: Relationship to drug uptake. Sand J Gastroenterol 1984;19(Suppl 101):55–69.
4. Silvoso GR, Ivey KJ, Butt JH, Lockard OO, Holt SD, Sisk C, Baskin WN, Mackercher PA and Hewett. Incidence of gastric lesions in patients with rheumatic disease on chronic aspirin therapy. Ann Int Med 1979;91:517–520.
5. Lanza FL, Royer GL Jr, Nelson RS. Endoscopic evaluation of the effects of aspirin, buffered aspirin, and enteric-coated aspirin on gastric and duodenal mucosa. New Engl J Med 1980;303:136–138.
6. Morris AD, Holt SD, Silvoso GR, Hewitt J, Tatum W, Grandione J, Butt JH, Ivey KJ. Effect of anti-inflammatory drug administration in patients with rheumatoid arthritis. An Endoscopic assessment. Scand J Gastroenterol 1981;16(Suppl 67):131–135.

7. O'Loughlin JC, Hoftiezer JW, Ivey KJ. Effect of aspirin on the human stomach in normals: Endoscopic comparison of damage produced one hour, 24 hours, and 2 weeks after administration. Scand J Gastroenterol 1981;16(Suppl 67): 211–214.
8. Piper DW, McIntosh JH, Ariotti DE, Fenton BH, MacLennan R. Analgestic ingestion and chronic peptic ulcer. Gastroenterology 1981;80:427–432.
9. Cohen MM, MacDonald WC. Mechanism of aspirin injury to human gastroduodenal mucosa. Prostgl Leukotr Med 1982;9:241–255.
10. Konturek SJ, Obtulowicz W, Kwiecien, Oleksy J. Generation of prostaglandins in gastric mucosa of patients with peptic ulcer disease: Effect of non-steroidal anti-inflammatory compounds. Scand J Gastroenterol 1984;19(Suppl 101):75–77.
11. Robert A, Nezamis JE, Lancaster C. Duodenal ulcers produced in rats by non-steroidal anti-inflammatory compounds. VIth International Congress on Pharmacology. Helsinki, July 1975:117.
12. Okabe S, Ishihara Y, Inoo H, Tanaka H. Mepirizole-induced duodenal ulcers in rats and their pathogenesis. Dig Dis Sc 1982;27:242–249.
13. Tabata K, Jacobson ED, Chen M-H, Murphy RF, Joff SN. Decrease in alkaline secretion during duodenal ulceration induced by mepirizole in rats. Gastroenterology 1984;87:396–401.
14. Kurebayashi Y, Asano M, Hashizume T, Akashi A. Dulcerozine-induced duodenal ulcers in rats: A simple, highly-reliable model for evaluating anti-ulcer agents. Arch Int Pharmacodyn 1984;271:155–168.
15. Robert A, Nezamis JE, Lancaster C. Duodenal ulcers produced by nonsteroidal antiinflammatory compounds plus bile duct ligation. Fed Proc 1975;34:442.
16. Somogyi A, Kovács K, Selye H. Jejunal ulcers produced by indomethacin. J Pharm Pharmacol 1969;21:122–123.
17. Kent TH, Cardelli RM, Stamler FW. Small intestinal ulcers and intestinal flora in rats given indomethacin. Am J Pathol 1969;54:237–249.
18. Brodie DA, Cook PG, Bauer BJ. Indomethacin-induced intestinal lesions in the rat. Toxicol Appl Pharmacol 1970;17:615–624.
19. Wax J, Cling WA, Vamer P, Bass P, Winder CF. Relationship of the entero-hepatic cycle to ulcerogenisis in the rat small bowel with flufenamic acid. Gastroenterology 1970;58:772–780.
20. Robert A, Schultz JR, Nezamis JE, Lancaster C. Gastric antisecretory and antiulcer properties of PGE_2, 15-methyl PGE_2, and 16,16-dimethyl PGE_2. Intravenous, oral and intrajejunal administration. Gastroenterology 1976;70: 359–370.
21. Menguy R, Koger E. Mechanism of inhibition of gastric secretion in the rat following bile duct ligation. Proc Soc Exp Biol Med 1959;101:666–668.
22. Guth PH, Paulsen G, Lynn D, Aures D. Mechanism of prevention of aspirin-induced gastric lesions in bile duct ligation in the rat. Gastroenterology 1976; 71:750–753.
23. Robert A, Nezamis JE. Effect of an anti-acetylcholine drug, methscopolamine bromide, on ulcer formation and gastric mucus. J Pharm Pharmacol 1964;16: 690–695.
24. Selye H, Szabo S. Experimental model for production of perforating duodenal ulcers by cysteamine in the rat. London, Nature 1973;244:458–459.
25. Robert A, Nezamis JE, Lancaster C. Aggravation of cysteamine-induced duodenal ulcers by bile duct ligation. Gastroenterology 1977;72:1121.
26. Flemström G. Stimulation of HCO_3 transport in isolated proximal bullfrog duodenum by prostaglandins. Am J Physiol 1980;239:G198–G203.

27. Simson JNL, Silen W. Bicarbonate secretion by amphibian duodenum *in vitro*. In: Case RM et al (Eds). Electrolyte and Water Transport across gastrointestinal epithelia. New York, Raven Press 1982:95–106.
28. Smeaton LA, Hirst BH, Allen A, Garner A. Gastric and duodenal HCO_3 transport *in vivo*: Influence of prostaglandins. Am J Physiol 1983;245: G751–G759.
29. Vane JR. Inhibition of prostaglandin synthesis as a mechanism of action of aspirin-like drugs. Nature (New Biol) 1971;231:232–235.

23. Cytoprotection and adapted cytoprotection

A. ROBERT, M.D., PH.D.

Experimental Biology Research, The Upjohn Company, Kalamazoo, USA

Cytoprotection in the stomach can be defined as the phenomenon that damage to the gastric mucosa by irritating agents can be prevented. Data will be outlined below to show that two different forms of cytoprotection exist:
1. direct cytoprotection
2. adapted cytoprotection
As prostaglandins play an important role in the concept of cytoprotection, a short outline is given of the structure of prostaglandins.

Structure of prostaglandins

Prostaglandins are a group of oxidized long chain fatty acids. The natural prostaglandins are present in practically every body cell. The nomenclature of prostaglandins makes use of letters and numbers. The letters refer to the structure of the C_5-carbon ring and the numbers refer to the number of double bonds present in the side chains. (fig. 1)

Prostaglandins are synthesized from essential fatty acids with arachidonic acid as the main precursor of all natural prostaglandins. Endoperoxides are formed from arachidonic acid by the enzyme cyclooxygenase. The endoperoxides are very rapidly converted into prostaglandins by specific prostaglandin synthetases. Indomethacin and other nonsteroidal anti-inflammatory drugs interfere with cyclooxygenase and thereby inhibit prostaglandin formation.

In the stomach prostaglandins are synthesized in the subepithelial tissues while degradation takes place in the superficial epithelium.[1] After oral administration of natural prostaglandins rapid degradation by 15-hydroxyprostaglandin dehydrogenase, which is present in gastric juice, takes place.

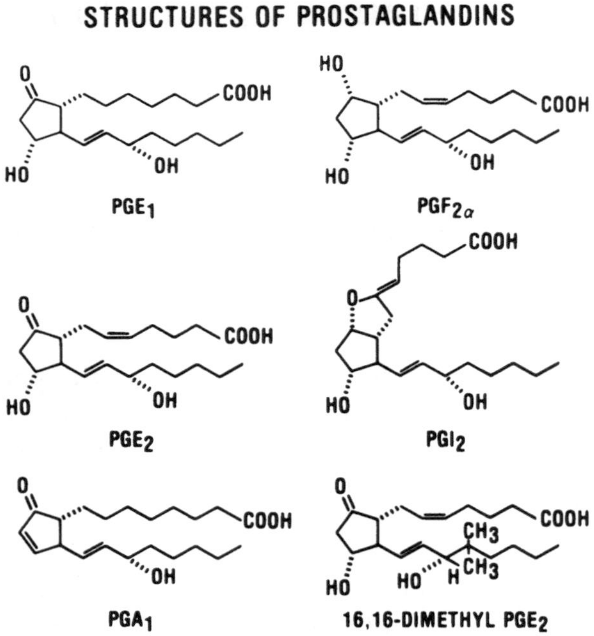

STRUCTURES OF PROSTAGLANDINS

Figure 1. The structure of prostaglandins.

Synthetic analogues produced by methylation at the 15 or 16 position, such as for example 16,16-dimethyl prostaglandins E_2 have been developed to prolong the half life of the natural prostaglandins. The methyl group protects against oxidation at the 15-position, hence preserving the biological activity of the molecule. The methylation at the 16-position also renders the prostaglandin analogues to be active after oral adminsitration. Prostaglandins inhibit gastric acid secretion.[2,3] The dose-response curve in figure 2 demonstrates a linear inhibition of gastric acid secretion with increasing doses of 15(R)-15-methyl prostaglandin E_2, with anacidity at high doses. The cytoprotection by prostaglandins is, however, unrelated to the inhibition of gastric acid secretion.[4]

Direct cytoprotection

Direct cytoprotection is achieved by the administration of exogenous prostaglandins. The first demonstration of cytoprotection was in rat

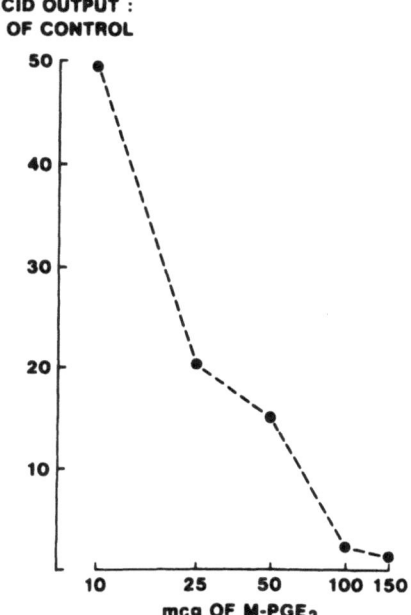

15(R)-15-METHYL PGE$_2$ INHIBITS MEAL-INDUCED ACID SECRETION IN HUMANS

ACID OUTPUT :
% OF CONTROL

mcg OF M-PGE$_2$

15(R)-15-METHYL PGE$_2$: GIVEN ORALLY.

10% PEPTONE MEAL.

FIVE SUBJECTS PER POINT.

(Robert, Kane, Reele : GUT. 22 : 728-731. 1981.)

Figure 2. Dose-response curve of the inhibition of meal-stimulated gastric acid secretion by 15(R)-15-methyl prostaglandin E$_2$.

stomachs, in which ulcers were produced by the administration of indomethacin. Within four hours after oral indomethacin bleeding ulcers can be observed in the gastric corpus mucosa. If the animals were pre-treated with prostaglandins, these lesions did not develop. (fig. 3) This preventive action of exogenous prostaglandins was observed with 16,16-dimethyl prostaglandins E$_2$ in very low doses, not inhibiting acid secretion. The same results could be obtained with the administration of prostaglandin F$_{2\beta}$ which does not inhibit acid secretion at any dose. Obviously in this model the cytoprotective action of prostaglandins was unrelated to their influence on gastric acid secretion.

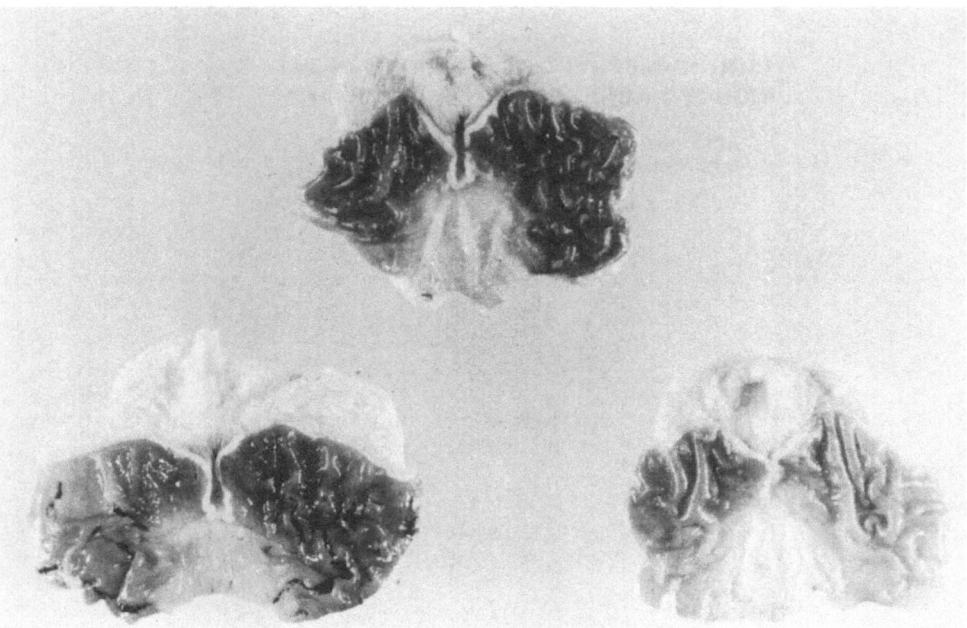

Figure 3. Protection from indomethacin-induced ulcers in the rat stomach by pre-treatment with prostaglandins. *Below, left:* ulcers induced by the administration of indomethacin; *below, richt:* protection obtained by pre-treatment with 16,16-dimethyl prostaglandin E$_2$ at doses which do not affect gastric acid secretion; *top:* control stomach.

To investigate gastric cytoprotection an experimental design in which ulcers are not prevented by the inhibition of gastric acid secretion was preferred. Such experimental conditions are the intra-gastric instillation of absolute ethanol (100%, 1 ml), a strong acid (HCl 0.6 M), a strong base (NaOH 0.2 M), hypertonic solutions (NaCl 25%) or boiling water. After the instillation of one of these agents severe necrotic lesions invariably develop, sometimes involving whole thickness of the mucosa. Using this model of damage, prostaglandins were administered to investigate whether those lesions could be prevented. Figure 4 shows the data obtained with 16,16-dimethyl prostaglandins E$_2$ at various dose levels, administered 30 minutes before various necrotizing agents. The number of lesions in animals given only the necrotizing agent ranged from 12 – 15, while a decrease in the number of lesions to zero was observed with increasing doses of the prostaglandin in a linear relationship. The doses given were very small. These cytoprotective doses are far below the threshold anti-secretory dose: – it would have needed at least a 100-fold higher

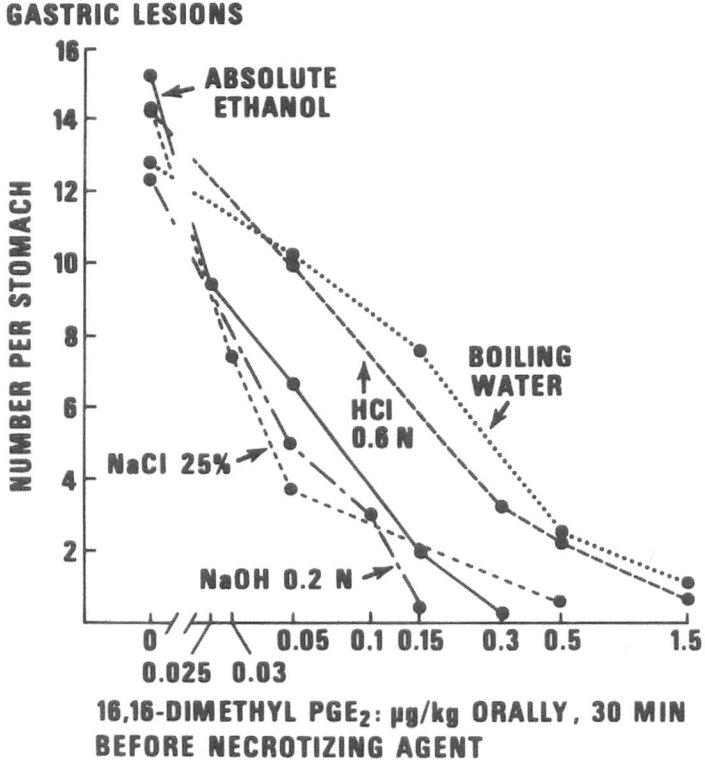

GASTRIC LESIONS

Figure 4. Protection from gastric lesions induced by various necrotizing agents by increasing doses of 16,16-dimethyl prostaglandin E_2; rat stomach.

dose of prostaglandins to obtain the slightest inhibition of gastric acid secretion.

Cohen,[5] Johansson et al.[6,7] and Kachel et al.[8] demonstrated the presence of cytoprotection in humans. After labelling erythrocytes with ^{51}Cr, volunteers were given acetylsalicylic acid or indomethacin in doses used clinically. The amount of blood lost in the faeces was determined by counting the ^{51}Cr radioactivity. With acetylsalicylic acid and indomethacin a certain amount of blood, approximately 6 ml per day, is invariably lost. If various doses of natural prostaglandin E_2 were given together with the damaging agent there was nearly complete prevention of gastric bleeding. (fig. 5, Table I) These doses of prostaglandin were very low and well below any anti-secretory activity.

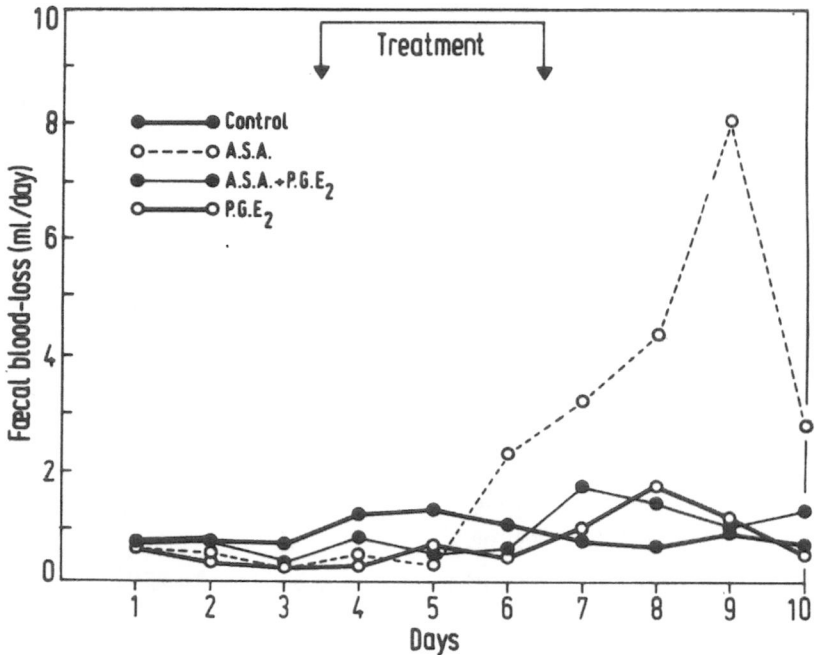

Figure 5. Prostaglandins prevent gastric blood loss produced by acetylsalicylic acid.

Table I. Faecal blood-loss during treatment with indomethacin 50 mg t.i.d. (I) combined with placebo (P), or prostaglandin E_2 (PGE$_2$), or 15(R),15-dimethyl prostaglandin E_2 (15-PGE$_2$). Values are means $\pm$ S.E.M. Adapted from: Johansson et al.[7]

	n	Faecal blood loss ml/day	p
Controls	20	0.8 $\pm$ 0.2	
I + P	10	3.4 $\pm$ 0.8	
I + PGE$_2$, 1 mg t.i.d.	10	1.0 $\pm$ 0.6	<0.01
I + P	5	3.7 $\pm$ 0.8	
I + PGE$_2$, 33 mcg t.i.d.	5	1.5 $\pm$ 0.2	<0.05
I + P	5	2.3 $\pm$ 0.7	
I + 15-PGE$_2$, 40 mcg t.i.d.	5	0.9 $\pm$ 0.5	<0.025

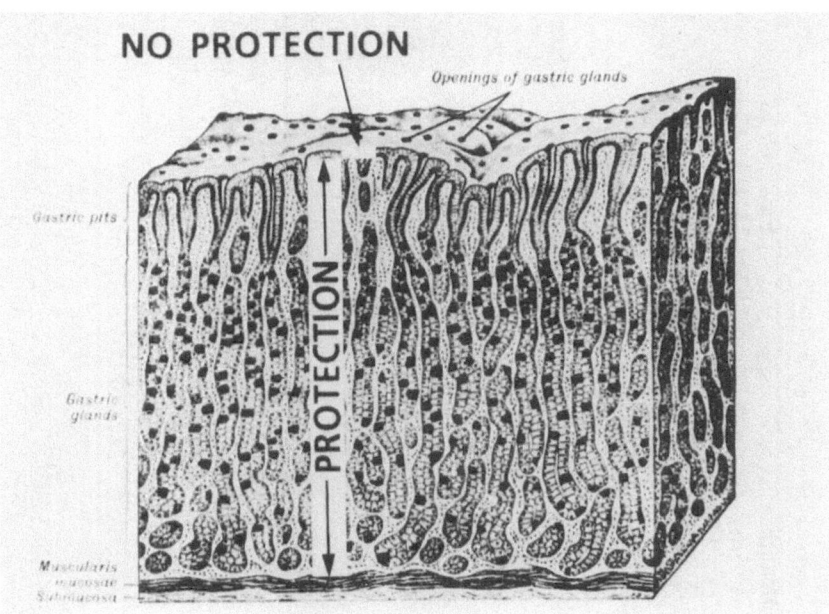

Figure 6. Diagram of the gastric mucosa showing the extent of cytoprotection by prostaglandins.

Instillation of ethanol 100% causes a massive necrosis of the mucosa and submucosal oedema. Lacy and Ito[9] demonstrated that the superficial layer of the surface epithelium desquamated despite pretreatment with prostaglandins, but the underlying parts of the mucosa remained intact. (fig. 6) The term cytoprotection' has been challenged, because the superficial epithelial layer is not adequately protected by prostaglandins from necrosis. As over 95% of the cells are protected from damage, the term 'cytoprotection' seems adequate and a definition could be: *Cytoprotection is the property of many prostaglandins to protect the mucosal tissue located under the surface epithelium and the submucosa from becoming inflamed and necrotic after exposure to noxious agents.*

This kind of cytoprotection can be called *direct cytoprotection* because it is obtained by the administration of exogenous prostaglandins.

Direct cytoprotection can be distinguished in two forms:

a. Cytoprotection by replacement.

With indomethacin-induced ulcers it is very likely that these lesions are the result of a blockade of prostaglandin synthesis by the drug and that replacement of this deficiency is the reason for cytoprotection.

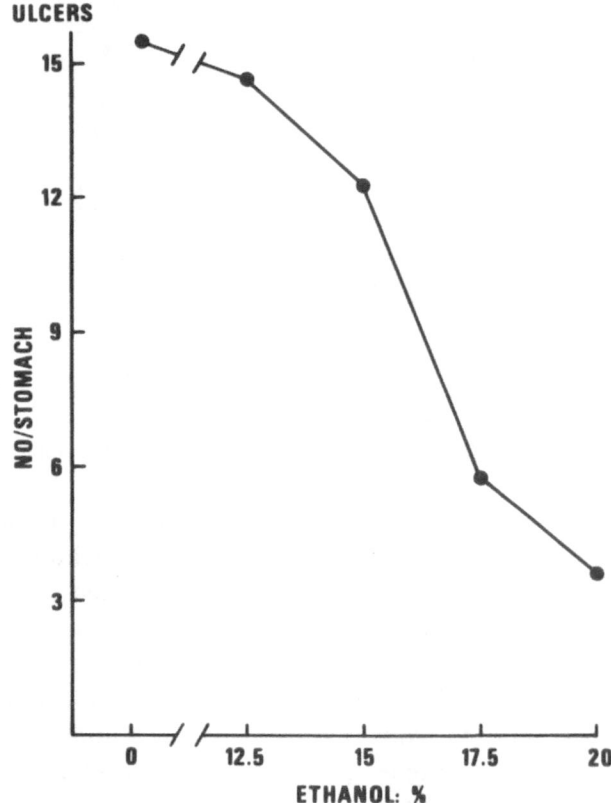

Figure 7. Number of gastric lesions produced by 100% ethanol and their prevention by prior administration of 12.5 – 20% ethanol.

b. Cytoprotection by supplemental amounts of prostaglandins.
    With ethanol-induced lesions prostaglandin concentration in the gastric mucosa remains normal (see below) and supplemental amounts of prostaglandins, greater than those normally present in the mucosa, are needed to obtain cytoprotection.

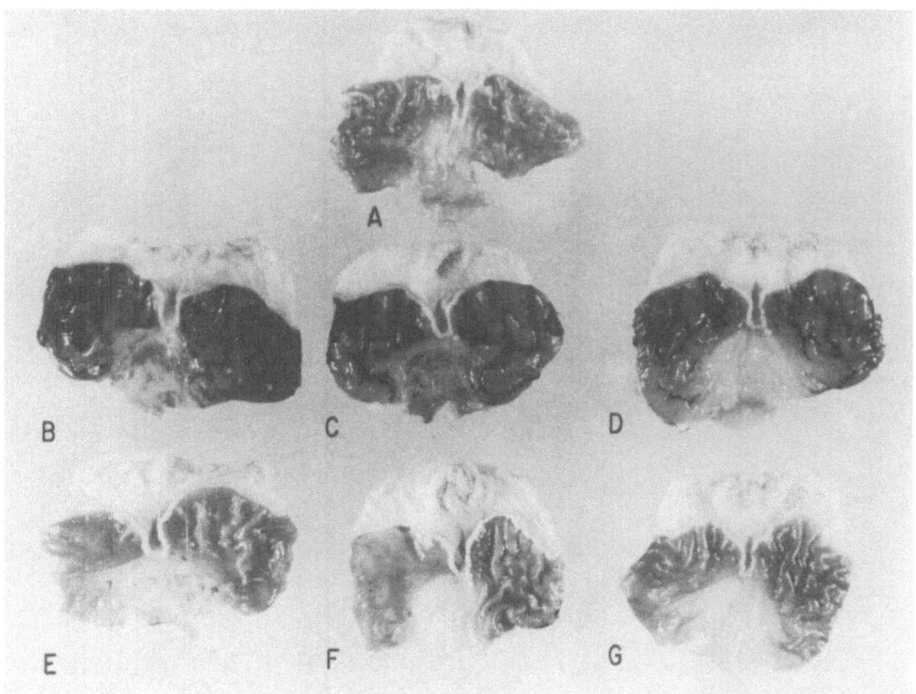

Figure 8. Induction of gastric lesions by strong irritants and their prevention by the prior administration of mild irritants. *Top row:* control stomach, untreated; *middle row:* prevention of lesions by pre-treatment with ethanol 20% (*left*), HCl 0.6 M (*middle*) and NaOH 0.2 M (*right*); *bottom row:* prevention of 100% ethanol-induced lesions by pre-treatment with 20% ethanol (*left*), prevention of 0.6 M HCl-induced lesions by pre-treatment with HCl 0.3 M (*middle*) and prevention of 0.2 M NaOH-induced lesions by pre-treatment with 20% ethanol.

Adapted cytoprotection

This form of cytoprotection is different from direct cytoprotection. As shown before, strong irritants such as ethanol 100% produce severe necrotic lesions in the rat stomach. If a rat is given 1 ml of ethanol in low concentrations (15 – 20%) and 15 minutes later 1 ml of ethanol 100%, the large number of lesions that absolute ethanol alone will produce is decreased and the ulcers are more superficial. (figs. 7 and 8).

Lesions resulting from a necrotizing agent were thus prevented by the prior administration of that agent in low concentrations. The results obtained by pre-treatment with low concentration of necrotizing agents are comparable to the cytoprotective effect of prostaglandins.

Not only could the effects of a strong irritant be prevented by prior

306

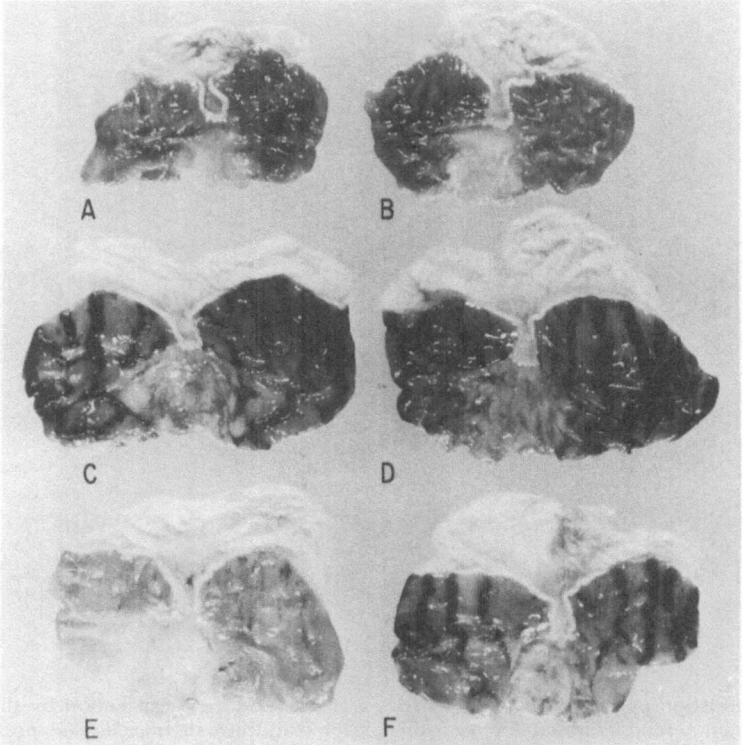

Figure 9. Prevention of adaptive cytoprotection by inhibition of prostaglandin synthesis with·
indomethacin administered orally. *Top row, left and right:* control stomachs; *middle row, left and
right:* lesions induced by 100% ethanol; *bottom row, left:* 100% ethanol-induced lesions prevented by pre-treatment with 20% ethanol; *bottom row, right:* indomethacin blocks the protection by 20% ethanol of gastric ulcers induced by 100% ethanol.

administration of a mild irritant of the same nature, but also by mild
irritants of unrelated chemical structure. As shown in figure 8, ethanol
20% protects against lesions induced by ethanol 100% as well as
against lesions produced by NaOH 0.2 M. In further experiments it
was shown that mild irritants of any nature can protect the stomach
against the damaging effect of any necrotizing agent regardless its
nature. This is called: *adapted cytoprotection*

Mechanism of adapted cytoprotection

The phenomenon of adapted cytoprotection is similar to the cytoprotection achieved by the administration of exogenous prostaglandins.
It was therefore hypothesized that when a mild irritant was placed in

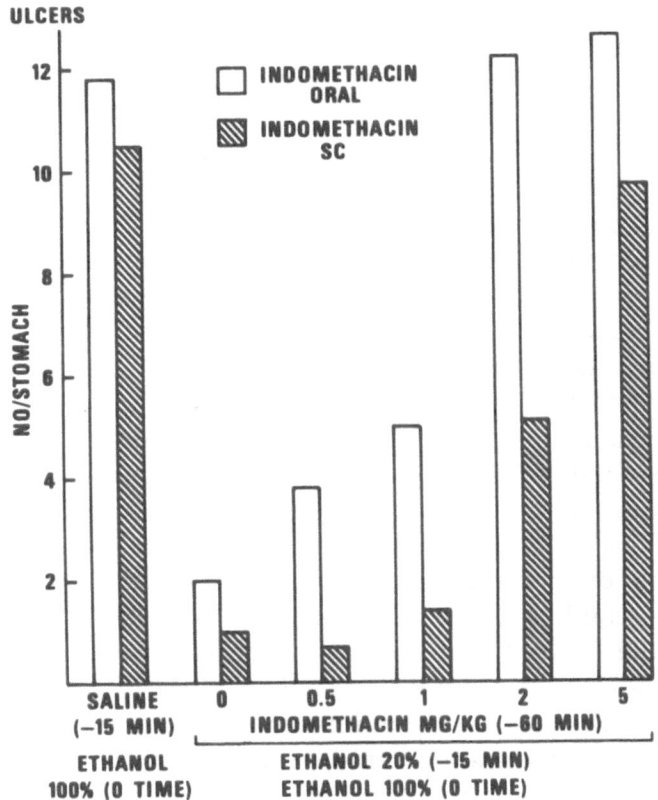

Figure 10. Dose-response curve of the blocking action of indomethacin orally and subcutaneously on the protection by 20% ethanol of gastric ulcers induced by 100% ethanol.

the stomach, the mucosa would start synthesizing and releasing prostaglandins locally, which then would protect the cells. To test this hypothesis indomethacin was used as a blocker of prostaglandin synthesis.

Figure 9 shows the initial results. It was demonstrated that indomethacin prevented the protective effect of ethanol 20% on gastric necrosis induced by ethanol 100%.

Figure 10 shows a dose-response curve of the effect of indomethacin on adapted cytoprotection. In the control animals 11 – 12 lesions/ stomach were present after exposure to ethanol 100%, which can be decreased to $1 - 2$ lesions/stomach by pre-treatment with ethanol 20%. When indomethacin is administered in various doses, there is a return to the number of lesions observed in the control animals which occurs in a dose-dependent way. After oral indomethacin the effect is more pronounced than after subcutaneous administration, probably because oral indomethacin causes local inhibition in the target organ, while it takes time for the drug to reach the stomach when given subcutaneously.

It was provisionally concluded that by blocking the synthesis of prostaglandins by administration of an inhibitor of the cyclooxygenase enzyme, the stomach could not synthesize prostaglandins. The lack of cytoprotection was probably due to the absence of prostaglandin synthesis in the stomach. This was an tentative conclusion based on circumstantial evidence, but direct evidence would only be obtained if, by determining the prostaglandin concentration in the gastric mucosa, it could be shown that the formation of prostaglandins was increased by administering a mild irritant. Mucosal concentration of prostaglandin E_2 and F_2 were measured in the gastric body and antrum 15 min after oral administration of three mild irritants: HCl 0.35 M, NaOH 0.075 M and NaCl 4%. None of these agents produced visible damage to the mucosa. By and large there was a marked increase in the formation of prostaglandins by the gastric mucosa in the body and antrum. The only mild irritant that did not produce an increase was HCl 0.35 M. Only prostaglandin E_2 increased by 40% in the antrum, but in the other tissues the prostaglandins did not increase. A possible explanation for this observation could be that these acid-labile natural prostaglandins were destroyed when preparing the mucosa shortly after the instillation of acid. The other mild irritants, NaOH 0.075 M and NaCl 40%, resulted in a $20 - 60\%$ increase in prostaglandin formation by the gastric mucosa. (fig. 11) One study used various concentrations of NaOH to investigate whether there was a stepwise response in the formation of prostaglandins. Using NaOH in various concentrations from 0.005 to 0.1 molar, it was demonstrated that the mucosal content of prostaglandin E_2, $F_{2\alpha}$ and tromboxane B_2 increased linearly with the increase in the concentration of NaOH.

It was concluded that adapted cytoprotection is the protection of the gastric mucosa against a strong irritant by prior administration of mild irritants. This protection is mediated by formation of cytoprotective prostaglandins in the gastric mucosa, induced by these mild irritants.

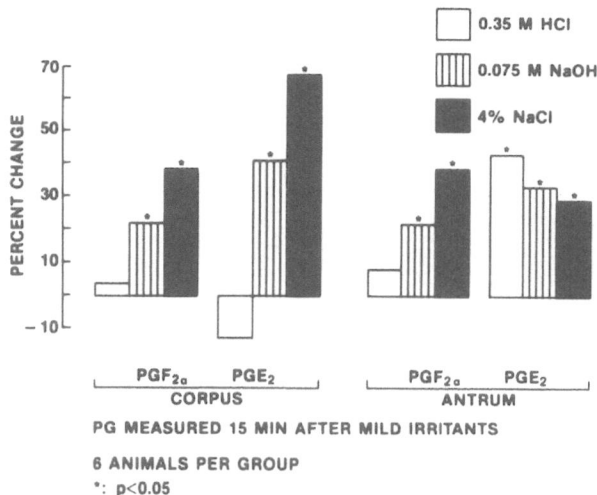

MILD IRRITANTS STIMULATE
PROSTAGLANDIN SYNTHESIS

Figure 11. Prostaglandin synthesis in the gastric corpus and antrum mucosa of rats by oral administration of mild irritants.

Adapted cytoprotection as a physiological phenomenen

Based on the experimental facts that:
a. indomethacin blocks adapted cytoprotection by mild irritants
b. these mild irritants stimulate the formation of prostaglandins in the gastric mucosa

adapted cytoprotection can be considered to be a physiological phenomenon. The normal stomach contains a variety of substances at various pH, various temperatures and various consistency. In the stomach micro-organisms, bile acids, enteric juice, enzymes etc. are regularly present. If such contents were introduced into any other body cavity, they would produce inflammation, necrosis and probably the host would die. Yet the stomach and the intestine have contact with these substances while maintaining their cellular integrity. One possible reason could be that defense substances are constantly formed in response to exposure to mild irritants. The family of prostaglandins would be a good candidate for such a defensive substance. Given their short half-life and their constant presence in the gastric mucosa at each measurement, they are probably formed continuously. One of the hypotheses is that prostaglandins are formed

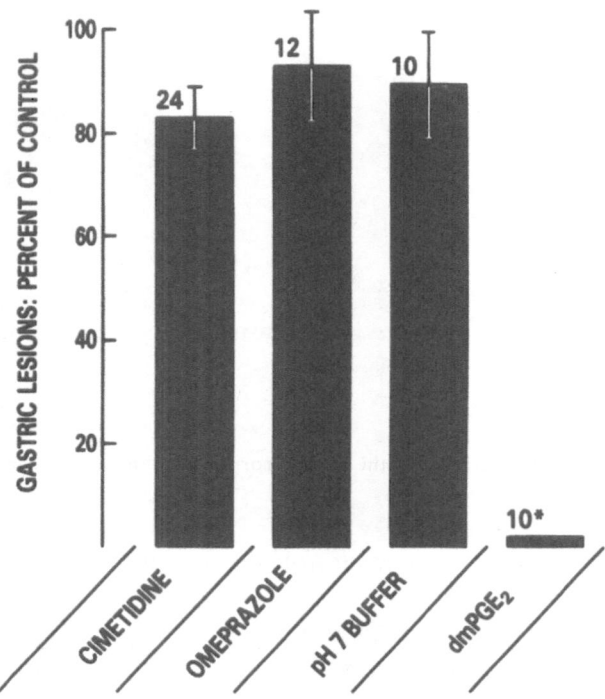

Figure 12. The influence of antisecretory agents, antacids and 16,16-dimethyl prostaglandin E$_2$ on ethanol-induced gastric lesions.

in the mucosa on demand, in response to the presence of mild irritants, in order to maintain cellular integrity.

How do prostaglandins protect the gastric mucosa?

It is not known how prostaglandins protect the gastric mucosa, but several hypotheses have been postulated:
a. inhibition of acid secretion
b. stimulation of gastric bicarbonate and mucus secretion
c. changes in mucosal blood flow

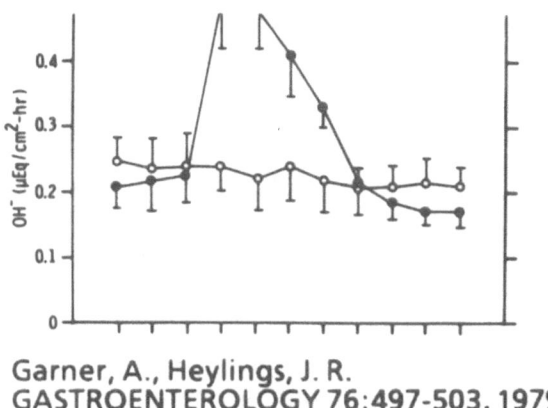

Garner, A., Heylings, J. R.
GASTROENTEROLOGY 76:497-503, 1979

Figure 13. The influence of 16,16-dimethyl prostaglandin E₂ on gastric bicarbonate secretion.

d. prevention of the penetration of necrotizing agents into the gastric mucosa
e. cellular resistance.

Cytoprotection by inhibition of acid secretion?

One possible reason for the cytoprotective action of prostaglandins is the anti-secretory action, but prostaglandins are effective in doses that are too low to inhibit acid secretion. Moreover, cimetidine and omeprazole at doses that cause nearly total antacidity are not protective against ethanol-induced lesions. Neither does constant neutralization of the gastric lumen with a pH 7 buffer protect against those lesions. (fig. 12) This excludes inhibition of gastric acid secretion as the mechanism of cytoprotection.

Cytoprotection by stimulation of gastric bicarbonate and mucus secretion

It has been shown that prostaglandins enhance gastric bicarbonate secretion in amphibians[10] (fig. 13) and this could possibly play an important role in some forms of protection, for example in aspirin-induced lesions. The stimulatory effect of prostaglandins on bicarbonate secretion has been confirmed in humans and *in vivo*.[11,12] Uncertainty remains whether this is a physiological or a pharmacological effect of prostaglandins.[13] An increase in the gastric mucus layer and an alteration in its composition by prostaglandins has been described.[14-16] This may be a favorable factor in cytoprotection.

Cytoprotection by changes in mucosal blood flow?

If prostaglandins were to increase gastric mucosal blood flow, one might expect that the mucosa would be better nourished and that it could remove toxic substances better, resulting in cytoprotection. Using the hydrogen gas clearance technique to measure gastric mucosal blood flow, it was shown that 16,16-dimethyl prostaglandin E_2 in cytoprotective doses decreased mucosal blood flow by 15%, instead of increasing blood flow.[17] Based on the demonstration that mucosal perfusion rates decreased by haemorrhage, or infusion of vasopressin considerably damage the gastric mucosa, it becomes highly unlikely that the suppressing effect of prostaglandins on gastric mucosal blood flow is the basis for cytoprotection.

Cytoprotection by prevention of the penetration of necrotizing agents into the gastric mucosa?

Are prostaglandins cytoprotective by preventing necrotizing agents such as absolute ethanol from penetrating the gastric mucosa? To test this hypothesis, ^{14}C-labelled ethanol was administered intragastrically to rats and the ^{14}C-content of the mucosa was measured after pretreatment with 16,16-dimethyl prostaglandin E_2, or placebo. Figure 14 shows that in this experiment the number of lesions was reduced from 12/stomach in the animals receiving the vehicle only, to 2/stomach in the animals receiving the active treatment. However, the ^{14}C-ethanol content of the mucosa was comparable in both groups.

It was concluded from these studies that cytoprotection is not dependent on the prevention of the penetration of necrotizing agents into the gastric mucosa.

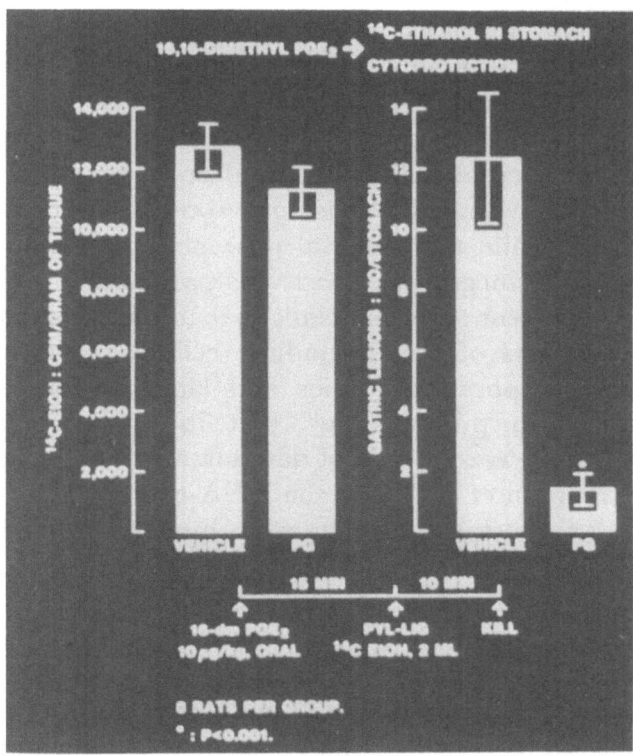

Figure 14. 16,16-dimethyl prostaglandin E$_2$ protects the gastric mucosa against lesions induced by ethanol, but does not prevent ethanol accumulation in the mucosa.

Table II. Gastric epithelial cell desquamation estimated from washout of DNA-P (ng atoms/min). Values given as mean ± S.D. Adapted from Ruppin et al.[20]

	Mean	S.D.
Saline, controls	10.5	2.4
PGE$_2$ 1 mg in 50 ml	9.2	2.6
Ethanol 40%, 50 ml	25.7*	3.7
Ethanol 40%, 50 ml + PGE$_2$ 1 mg	12.9**	4.8

* p < 0.05 versus controls.

** p < 0.05 versus ethanol alone and p > 0.05 versus PGE$_2$ alone.

Cytoprotection by cellular resistance?

The electrical potential difference between the blood and the gastric lumen is a good indicator of mucosal integrity. Mueller et al.[18] demonstrated, that in humans a drop in the potential difference was induced by the administration of acetylsalicylic acid, suggestive of mucosal damage. If 16,16-dimethyl prostaglandin E_2 was given together with the acetylsalicylic acid, the drop in potential difference was prevented. This was achieved using low doses of the prostaglandin: 0.1 mcg/subject, while the minimal dose needed to inhibit gastric acid secretion is 25 mcg/subject with this particular prostaglandin.

This could represent a mechanism closer to the explanation of the cytoprotective effects of prostaglandins: cellular resistance. Using ^{3}H-thymidine incorporation studies and labelling indices, Tijtgat shows elsewhere in this volume[19] that in the normal stomach prostaglandins decrease the rate of desquamation of the surface epithelial layer. Ruppin et al.[20] used the DNA-content of gastric washings as an index of cellular exfoliation in humans. After instillation of ethanol 40% into the stomach there was a sharp increase in the DNA-content of the gastric washings, indicating an increased exfoliation of surface eptithelium. By pre-treatment with prostaglandin E_2 15 min before the instillation of ethanol 50%, this rise in DNA-content was completely abolished. This suggests that in the presence of a damaging agent (Table II) prostaglandins appear to be preventing the shedding of cells into the lumen.

Conclusion

Cytoprotection by prostaglandins can be either *direct*, brought about by exogenous administration of prostaglandins, or *adaptive* by formation of endogenous prostaglandins in the gastric mucosa in response to contact with mild irritants. Cytoprotection by prostaglandins is not mediated by inhibition of gastric acid secretion, changes in mucosal blood flow or prevention of penetration of necrotizing agents into the mucosa. It is more likely that the cytoprotective effect is due to stimulation of bicarbonate and mucus secretion and, above all, by maintaining cellular integrity after exposure to necrotizing agetns. How cytoprotection works at the level of the cell membranes or in terms of molecular biology, is still unknown.

It remains to be established in which clinical situations this mechanism is profitable to the individual.

Acknowledgements

Figure 2 has been reproduced with permission of the authors and the Editor of Gut from: Robert A, Kane G, Reele SB. Dose response inhibition in man of meal-stimulated gastric acid secretion by 15(R)-15-methyl prostaglandin E_2, given orally. Gut 1981;22: 728 – 31.

Figure 5 has been reproduced with permission of the author and the Editor of The Lancet from: Cohen MM. Mucosal cytoprotection by prostaglandin E_2. Lancet 1978;2:1253 – 4.

Figure 13 has been reproduced with permission of the authors and the Editor of Gastroenterology from: Garner A, Heylings JR. Stimulation of alkaline secretion in amphibian isolated gastric mucosa by 16,16-dimethyl PGE_2 and $PGF_{2\alpha}$. A proposed explanation for some of the cytoprotective actions of prostaglandins. Gastroenterology 1979;76:497 – 503.

References

1. Smith GS, Warhurst G, Turnberg LA. Synthesis and degradation of prostaglandin E_2 in the epithelial and sub-epithelial layers of the rat intestine. Biochim Biphys Acat 1982;713:684 – 7.
2. Robert A, Nezamis JE, Phillips JP. Effect of prostaglandin E on gastric secretion and ulcer formation in the rat. Gastroenterology 1968;55:481.
3. Robert A, Kande G, Reele SB. Dose response inhibition in man of meal-stimulated gastric acid secretion by 15(R)-15-methyl prostaglandin E_2, given orally. Gut 1981;22:728 – 31.
4. Robert A. Antisecretory, antiulcer, cytoprotective and diarrhoegenic properties of prostaglandins. In: Samuelsson B, Paoletti R (Eds). New York, Raven Press 1957:507 – 20.
5. Cohen MM. Mucosal cytoprotection by prostaglandinm E_2 Lancet 1978;2: 1253 – 4.
6. Johansson C, Kollberg B, Nordemar R, Bergström S. Protection of gastrointestinal mucosa by E_2 prostaglandins. Lancet 1979;1:317.
7. Johansson C, Kollberg B, Nordemar et al. Protective effect of prostaglandin E_2 in the gastrointestinal tract during indomethacin treatment of rheumatic diseases. Gastroenterology 1980;78:479.
8. Kachel G, Ruppin H, Hagel J et al. Gastrale Mikroblutung und Acetylsalicylsäure. Dtsch Mediz Wochenschr 1983;108:1145 – 7.

316

9. Lact ER, Ito S. Microscopic analysis of ethanol damage to rat gastric mucosa after treatment with a prostaglandin. Gastroenterology 1982;83:613 – 25.
10. Garner A, Heylings JR. Stimulation of alkaline secretion in amphibian-isolated gastric mucosa by 16,16-dimethyl PGE_2 and $PGF_{2\alpha}$. A proposed explanation for some of the cytoprotective actions of prostaglandins. Gastroenterology 1979;76:497 – 503.
11. Johansson C, Aly A, Nilsson E, Flemström G. Stimulation of bicarbonate secretion by E_2 prostaglandins in man. In: Samuelsson B, Paoletti R, Ramwell P (Eds). Advances in prostaglandin, Thromboxane, and Leukotriene Research. New York, Raven Press 1983:395 – 401.
12. Feldman M, Barnett CC. Gastric bicarbonate secretion in humans. Effects of pentagastrin, betanechol and 11,16,16-trimethyl prostaglandin E_2. J Clin Invest 1983;72:295 – 303.
13. Rees WDW, Gibbons LC, Warhurst G, Turnberg LA. Studies of bicarbonate secretion by the normal human stomach *in vivo* effect of aspirin, sodium taurocholate and prostaglandin E_2. In: Allan A, Flemström G, Garner A (Eds). Mechanism of mucosal protection in the upper gastrointestinal tract. New York, Raven Press 1983:119 – 23.
14. Bickel M, Kauffman GL. Gastric mucus gel thickness: effect of distension, 16,16-dimethyl prostaglandin E_2 and carbonoxolon. Gastroenterology 1981;80:770 – 5.
15. Johansson C, Kollberg B. Stimulation by intragastrically administered E_2 prostaglandin on humans mucus output. Eur J Clin Invest 1979;9:229 – 32.
16. Domschke W, Domschke S, Hornig D, Demmling L. Prostaglandin stimulated gastric mucus secretion in man. Acata hepatogastroenterol 1978;25:292 – 4.
17. Guth PH. The role in mucosal blood flow in the pathogenesis and healing of peptic ulcer. In: Nelis GF, Boevé J, Misiewicz JJ (Eds). Peptic ulcer disease: basic and clinical aspects. Dordrecht, Martinus Nijhoff 1985:271 – 84.
18. Mueller P, Fischer N, Kather H, Simon B. Prevention of aspirin-induced drop in gastric potential difference with 16,16-dimethyl prostaglandin E_2. Lancet 1981;1:333 – 4.
19. Tijtgat GNJ. Medical treatment of peptic ulcer with prostaglandins. In: Nelis GF, Boevé J, Misiewicz JJ (Eds). Peptic ulcer disease: basic and clinical aspects. Dordrecht, Martinus Nijhoff 1975:143 – 53.
20. Ruppin H, Person B, Robert A, Domschke W. Gastric cytoprotection in man by prostaglandin E_2. Scand J Gastroenterol 1981;16:647 – 52.

24. Discussion V

Westerveld:
Mr Kennedy, on what criteria do you establish the diagnosis of biliary reflux gastritis, or alkaline gastritis and how do you select the patients which are suitable for successful surgery?

Kennedy:
I suppose the most obvious case is the patient who actually vomits bile, either daily or every few days. The presence of bile in the stomach on endoscopy doesn't prove biliary reflux gastritis and histologically the relationship is not really very obvious. The criteria for choosing the patient for operation are: crippling persistent burning epigastric pain with anaemia, weight loss and general misery. These are the patients one selects for operation.

Westerveld:
Do you consider weight loss to be important?

Kennedy:
No, actually this whole question of weight gain and loss in the assessment of gastric surgery is very deceptive. I looked at this in patients having regular annual follow-up. I examined the relationship between yearly weight change and changes in the Visick grading. We had expected patients who did well to gain weight, but not a bit of it, it works the other way round. Very often the patient who develops recurrent ulcer, gains weight because he has to take a lot of milk to control the symptoms and once one has treated his recurrent ulcer, he looses weight as he stops taking an excess of milk. So, weight loss and gain, unless it is excessive, is not a very important criterium.

Johnston:
I was very impressed with the demonstration of the high incidence of cancer, not only after Billroth II resection, but as mr Kennedy

said, also after vagotomy with drainage. I think some studies may have underestimated the problem, because as dr Tijtgat emphasized, we have to make a great number of precise biopsies before one may diagnose it. But the pattern which is coming through is of about a 3 times expected risk, though in some high risk areas it more looks like 6 times. If you pick up the cases at such an early stage as dr Tijtgat does, I presume that the surgical results will be pretty good. We have 18 cases of stump cancers in our review of gastric cancer I mentioned yesterday and a third of them are still alive after radical surgery at varying periods of follow-up. So it is not a hopeless stage. We have also to ask ourselves how long the rather early mucosal lesion takes to involve into invasive cancer, because in some old decripit patients maybe radical surgery is not indicated.

Tijtgat:

I think you are very right. There is some evidence that stump cancers take a long time to grow and they can stay at a stage of early superficial malignancy for many years, even 5 – 10 years. And this is one of the problems with screening too, because these patients are quite elderly when one detects these lesions. One may wonder whether it is worthwhile to do a total gastrectomy, because their life expectancy is rather limited anyhow and these cancers may take a long time to grow. So if you believe in screening you should concentrate on the younger patients, who have another 20 – 30 years to go.

Can I say something on the biliary reflux gastritis. To my knowledge there is not one single drug which has been shown to be effective in controlling these symptoms: neither cholestyramine, nor the combination of cholestyramine and alginate, which was called Gaviscamine in our study. We have just finished a study with prostaglandin and to our surprise we could not improve either symptoms, nor histology. Dr Robert, ar you not surprised that prostaglandins are ineffective in biliary reflux gastritis?

Robert:

Yes, I am surprised at that. We have been able to demonstrate in animals prevention of gastric damage. There is very little done in the reversal of such damage, produced by either necrotizing agents, or bile salts. So it could be that in the patients you and others have treated with biliary reflux gastritis it may be much more difficult to reverse the process back to a normal mucosa, than it might be if the treatment was started immediately after surgery.

Kennedy:

Our experience is that symptoms of bile reflux gastritis appear only many years after the operation. It appears as if these patients are initially protected (*e.g.* by prostaglandins). Do you have this experience of the delay in symptoms coming on?

Tijtgat:

Your question about definition is something we all struggle with. There is no good definition of biliary reflux gastritis. To be honest, when we are sick and tired of listening to the complaints of burning pain, then we refer the patients to the surgeon.

I was surprised to see your 75% of excellent results: it is certainly less in our hands. At least 50% keep complaining of different symptoms which are difficult to interpret. They don't vomit bile anymore, but have got something else instead. I wish somebody could come up with a definition that we could all agree on and then make the proper selection of the patients who will truly benefit from revisional surgery.

Rees:

Could I ask two questions. One is for dr Tijtgat about the very interesting radio-labelled thymidine studies. Have such studies been performed in other subjects who have not had surgery, such as in patients with pernicious anaemia who also have malignant potential and perhaps also in patients with other forms of gastritis, which do not share such a malignant potential, for example patients on non-steroidal anti-inflammatory drugs for long periods of time. I would like to know whether this is a peculiar finding confined to the postgastrectomy state or whether it extends to other circumstances.

The second question is directed to dr Robert on adaptive cytoprotection: Do you know how long this phenomenon lasts when the stomach is exposed to an irritant compound. One may apply the more damaging compound very soon after the initial exposure to the mild irritant and show adaptive cytoprotection. But what happens if the time lag between the applications increases? As the turnover of prostaglandins is rather fast, one would imagine then a long lasting effect must be synthesis, or degradation of prostaglandins. Could conditions such as bile reflux gastritis, gastritis in patients taking non-steroidal anti-inflammatory drugs for long periods of time, or indeed chronic peptic ulcer, represent a failure of adaptive cytoprotection.

Robert:

To answer your question on the duration of the effects of adaptive cytoprotection: If we give a mild irritant, cytoprotection is demonstrated within 1 minute and lasts for about 3 hours. If after 3 hours we again apply the mild irritant, we then have another 3 hours of adaptive cytoprotection. We repeated this experiment for 16 hours in one study to find out if there would be exhaustion. The capacity of adaption by production of prostaglandins could not be exhausted.

Your second question whether gastritis, or peptic ulcer might be an example of lack of adaptive cytoprotection is a very nice suggestion, but I don't think there is any evidence at the moment.

Johnson:

May I come bakc to the first question about the definition of biliary reflux gastritis. There are two diagnostic procedures available: One is the alkaline provocation test, comparable to the Bernstein test for the oesophagus, where the reproduction of symptoms after instillation of an alkaline bile salt solution into the stomach as opposed to saline is analyzed.

Secondly there is an interesting study from England, where patients before operation were interviewed by a psychiatrist who recorded in a sealed envelope what he predicted the results of the surgery would be and he was nearly always right. In other words, if one has a patient who has a lot of other symptoms, who has a great deal of anxiety, consultation with a psychiatrist might be useful.

Tijtgat:

You raise a very important problem. To me as a physician the majority of the problems that I see post-operatively are usually as a result of ill-advised operations. And it is usually that type of patient that keeps coming back.

Van Blankenstein:

We have used the provocation test, but we don't find it very useful. What we do is this; We admit the patient and we flush the stomach with about 6–8 liters of water per 24 hours continuously and if the complaints disappear during infusion and reappear when you stop the infusion, we consider that a reasonable evidence of biliary reflux gastritis and go on to operation.

Guth:

I agree completely with mr Johnson's and dr Tijtgat's remarks. A few years ago dr Ippoliti at the centre for Ulcer Research and Education looked at this question and tried to devise a diagnostic test. He investigated a group of post-gastrectomy patients, some with symptoms that could be called bile reflux symptoms and some without, with endoscopy, biopsy and bile acid concentration in the gastric content and he could not find any significant differences between those complaining of symptoms and those who were relatively asymptomatic.

Soll:

I must admit there are so many things to talk about that I hardly know where to start. First of all on the question dr Robert raised. I believe there is evidence that, at least in treating duodenal ulcer patients, the effects of the prostaglandins correlate with their anti-secretory effect and not with their cytoprotective effect at all. I'm still concerned with the term 'cytoprotection' and would argue with your conclusion at this point: Do you have evidence that the cells themselves are directly protected, or could blood flow be the point where prostaglandins act in the process of 'cytoprotection'?

Robert:

Concerning the term 'cytoprotection', dr Soll, the main reason why I think it is still a good term is the histological appearance of these cells. We know something about the function of these cells, whether they have been damaged by ethanol or whether the damage has been prevented by prostaglandins. If we measure acid secretion from the stomach after ligation of the pylorus, comparing two groups: ethanol and ethanol + prostaglandins, we find that in the ethanol-alone-group there is anacidity, the barrier is broken, there is pH 7.5, for hours, for days. Only after about a week there is a beginning of return of acid secretion. The protected stomach begins to secrete acid again within the same day. Knowing that this cannot be done by new cells (the turnover is much slower than that), is strongly suggestive that these cells have been protected not only histologically, but also functionally. So this is a second line of evidence to show that these cells are really protected, therefore cytoprotected.

Guth:

Blood flow studies in the alcohol-treated animal show that blood flow is totally absent in the area of the damaged mucosa, but it is normal in the adjacent, normal-appearing mucosa. In the animals pretreated with prostaglandins, even although total blood flow is not increased, blood flow was normal throughout the mucosa. So prostaglandins somehow do maintain blood flow, even although they don't increase total flow. We have an *in vivo* microscopy technique where we can directly observe blood cells flowing in the capillaries of the surface mucosa, and a fluorescein-labelled albumin technique to measure permeability. Almost immediately after alcohol was applied to the mucosa, a marked plasma leak from the small blood vessels and at the same time a marked slowing of blood flow was observed. So I suspect the alcohol lesion involves plasma exsudation with marked increase in viscosity and stasis. Prostaglandins completely prevent this permeability change. I think that is why they maintain blood flow and I would postulate that by maintaining blood flow, prostaglandins enable the cells to withstand better the onslaught of alcohol.

Robert:

It is indeed possible that what we are showing in our experiments is more vasoprotection, than epithelial protection.

Tijtgat:

Dr Guth, do you think we can use mucosal perfusion studies in the future to subdivide peptic ulcer patients into those that are going to heal and those that are not going to heal? Because if we see reactive hyperaemia around an ulcer, this is a sign that an ulcer is on its way to healing. If we do not see reactive hyperaemia endoscopically, then we are less certain. The point is: endoscopy informs us only about one moment in time. If a patient has an iatrogenic ulcer after indomethacin immediately after stopping the medication, there is usually no reactive hyperaemia at endoscopy, but if one looks again after 10 days, then these ulcers have definite reactive hyperaemia. My question is: Will we use these studies in the future to separate ulcers that are going to heal from those that are not?

Guth:

The Japanese studies of mucosal blood flow and ulcer healing have not been particularly well described. I suspect they studied different groups of patients at different stages of healing, rather than take one patient through all the stages of healing. Until we have a large number of patients who have been so followed and so studied, I don't think we can really answer your question.

Festen:

Dr Robert, there are a lot of drugs for which it is claimed in the literature that they act as a cytoprotective agent: several come from Konturek in Poland. Some of these data are conflicting; I would like your view on that. On the other hand, I could imagine a drug such as cimetidine could act as an adaptive cytoprotective agent, being a mild irritant to the stomach. I have found some data in the literature on omeprazole acting only as a cytoprotective given orally but not when given intravenously, or intra-peritoneally, which would support this hypthesis.

Robert:

Dr Guth and dr Konturek have reported that cimetidine in doses which don't inhibit acid secretion can decrease gastric lesions produced by aspirin. I cannot explain that; but I can say that in my hands when I use a model that has nothing to do with gastric secretion such as ethanol, cimetidine does not work at all. There is something special about the aspirin model that is so responsive to agents that will lower acid secretion; even if it is not detectable in the lumen, there may still be some inhibition of acid production near the parietal cells and that may explain the protection.

Omeprazole: I agree with you. When we give it orally there is a dose-response cytoprotection agains ethanol. This is partially reversible by pretreatment with indomethacin. There are so many agents which, if given directly into the stomach will exert some protection, that I am inclined to think that many more drugs are irritating than we think. It may be true that that mild irritation protects. If I find an agent that is cytoprotective orally, I immediately give it parenterally to be sure: if it is a specific effect of the compound it will be effective regardless of the route of administration. If it is a local effect, that could be in many cases related to mild irritation.

Soll:

How do you establish the causal relationship of changes in blood flow to ulcer formation? You suggested an ulcer is being described with these techniques by having a lower blood flow or is the lower blood flow a causal factor in the failure of the ulcer to heal?

Guth:

This has not been established with certainty.

Tijtgat:

Mr Kennedy, in what kind of patients do you reconstruct a pyloroplasty?

Kennedy:

In the patients who have one, or more of these problems: dumping of sufficient severity to interfere with their way of life, diarrhoea of sufficient severity, or severe bile reflux gastritis. It is a small operation and a no-risk operation with no guarantee of success.

Tijtgat:

But do you have any evidence, you really restore pyloric function.

Kennedy:

No, I haven't any evidence that we can restore pyloric function, but one is slowing down the rate of emptying. If the patient is getting symptomatic improvement, it will not matter whether his stomach is emptying more, or less rapidly.

Tijtgat:

What was the exact localization of the cancers that you have seen after vagotomy and drainage?

Kennedy:

I cannot give exact data as that series was taken many years ago and many of the cancer patients had died. The one I showed you after pyloroplasty was adjacent to the pyloroplasty ring.

Johnston:

I would like to comment about stoma's, gastroenterostomies and pyloroplaties. This is not to disagree with what mr Kennedy has said. These are difficult patients and the alternatives such as Roux-en-Y procedures are usually more dangerous. However, we should be quite clear that this is an anatomical approach to a physiological problem.

It was noticeable from mr Kennedy's figures that the success rate was around 60% for the reversal of pyloroplasty, against 80% for the closure of gastroenterostomy. In mr Kelly's paper that you quoted, the success rate was lower: 45 – 50%. With increasing experience, we have been increasingly disillusioned with our results: We have about one third success, one third no worse and one third worse.

Going back to physiology, we used to say that the stomach gets its tone back in the long term after a truncal vagotomy, but we do not really know what tone is. It has been shown that the disruption in myoelectrical activity in the antrum does not return to normal after truncal vagotomy, even on long term testing.

Tijtgat:

Do you add a Roux-en-Y anastomosis and truncal vagotomy routinely to a Billroth II gastrectomy? Is the increase in morbity and mortality related to that procedure sufficiently low to warrant that addition?

Kennedy:

First of all let us get mortality out of this. The concept that gastric surgery is dangerous is surely out of date. Any competent gastric surgeon can do any of these operations we have discussed with a mortality of less than 1%. Billroth II gastrectomy is a terrible operation, because there is so much trouble with bile reflux. So I believe the right operation is an antrectomy and (re)vagotomy. If one is going to do an antrectomy and if one is going to hitch it up as a Billroth II, then one should always do a Roux-loop to prevent bile reflux.

Johnson:

Mortality does matter; these operations can be extremely difficult. I am sure we cannot restore the physiology of the pylorus by sewing it together again. The problem is not the pylorus: probably the motility of the duodenum is at fault. Just by narrowing the pyloric ring will not restore antro-duodenal co-ordination and motility. I do not favour a primary Roux-en-Y procedure with a Billroth II resection routinely, because the operation carries a considerable morbidity, can give rise to distrubances of gastric emptying and one will have to perform a reliable vagotomy.

Johnston:

The necessity to add a vagotomy may be a distinct disadvantage in the sense that receptive relaxation is lost. This is a very valuable property of the fundus and corpus, which may contribute to the very good functional results that many patients have after an ordinary Billroth II gastrectomy without vagotomy.

Westerveld:

Dr Guth, in Intensive Care Unites many patients are treated with vasoactive drugs to stabilize their haemodynamics. Do you consider the changes in gastric mucosal blood flow induced by these agents a contribution to the aetiology of stress ulceration?

Secondly, once stress ulcer bleeding occurs, what is your opinion of treatment with vasopressin in this situation?

Guth:

Superselective angiography is mandatory for controlling active bleeding with vasoactive drugs in order to get the catheter as close to the bleeding site as possible. Intravenous administration of vasopressin is not effective in bleeding duodenal ulcer. In prophylaxis of stress ulcer, I have been impressed in the last 5 years with the rarity of severe stress ulcer bleeding. I think it is a disappearing disease, because patients are given optimal care in Intensive Care Units watching blood pH and nutrition. In studies reported in the literature claiming a beneficial effect of cimetidine, or antacids on stress ulcer bleeding, stress ulcer bleeding is usually defined as 3 successive guaiac-positive nasogastric aspirations. That may be statistically significant, but is clinically unimportant. So I don't think that at present prophylaxis is a problem. How to manage established stress bleeding is a real problem, because the few that bleed can do so excessively and I have no good thoughts about that.

Westerveld:

But would you suspect a deleterious effect by diminishing the blood flow to the gastric mucosa?

Guth:

Well, there are two problems really. I do emphasize that a decreased blood flow renders the mucosa more susceptible to injury. But once there is a bleeding lesion the first goal has to be stopping that bleed.

That will prevail over the concern over mucusal blood flow, which might theoretically aggravate the lesion.

Tijtgat:

An alternative could be somatostatin, or secretin in high doses, which work a bit differently.

Guth:

I am very sceptical about the efficacy of somatostatin and secretin in stress ulcer bleeding. In the majority of patients with major stress ulcer bleeding there is gross vascular damage which will only be controlled surgically.

Soll:

One last comment and question. I am a little disturbed when talking about gastric surgery as having a 1% mortality. Earlier I heard that the risk of carcinoma in patients who generally have a benign disease may get into an increase of several percent over time. It seems that is an incredible risk. We operate on patients with ulcerative colitis and take their colons out just to prevent that kind of risk and yet we induce it in these other patients. So I don't think we can take this lightly.

I have a few questions pertaining to that. It seems that duodenal ulcer patients which are unoperated have an extremely low risk of gastric carcinoma as if they are protected. Secondly it has been stated that there is a great deal of variation in the studies that report gastric carcinoma following surgery. Is this variation a regional variation and is there solid evidence for that?

Tijtgat:

There is certainly geographical variation. In Scandinavia and Hungary the incidence is high, whereas in the USA and in Japan it is low. The problem in Japan is that the natural incidence of gastric cancer is so high that it might obscure the extra risk that might follow Billroth II gastrectomy. There are two papers from the USA reporting roughly the same figures as in Europe. In England I would think it is around 2 – 3 times the expected incidence for the matched unoperated population. These figures are not terribly accurate, because no study has been following exactly the same way a cohort of population; that is impossible. But it is certainly a big regional difference.

Kennedy:

I am sure that this is right. In just the same way there is a considerable regional variation for duodenal ulcer. In the United Kingdom to the North and West from the more prosperous South-East corner the incidence of ulcers increases steadily and a maximum incidence of ulceration is in the rather deprived area of South-West Scotland around Glasgow. There is this tremendous difference across even one country.

Rees:

Could I ask dr Tijtgat whether the observations on the thymidine incorporation have been extrapolated to other patients?

Tijtgat:

As soon as you touch, or irritate, or damage the epithelium virtually immediately proliferation is speeded up. That is the reason why most of us do not develop ulcers constantly, there is a continuous battle of exfoliation and immediate repair of the mucosa. The number of labelled cells increase, but they stay in the right position, in the proliferative zone. The big difference between pre-malignancy is the upward shift of the proliferative zone towards the lumen which is also seen in other conditions associated with an increased cancer risk.

This has been documented in the Barrett oesophagus, in some cases of ulcerative colitis, but especially in all the polyposis-adenomatosis syndromes. It has been quite a uniform pattern in all the quoted premalignant conditions that we know of in the GI-tract at present. So one should not only measure the proliferative activity, but also locate exactly where these cells are situated.

25. The management of severe haemorrhage

W. RÖSCH, M.D.

Department of Medicine, Krankenhaus Nordwest der Stiftung Hospital zum Heiligen Geist, Frankfurt, Federal Republic of Germany

Gastrointestinal haemorrhage is the most common complication of peptic ulcer disease. Its frequency depends on anamnestic data[1] while mortality is governed by previous haemorrhagic epidsodes,[2] severity of bleeding[3] and the patient's age.[4-6] Despite the apparent decline in the prevalence of peptic ulcer, the annual incidence of this complication seems to be constant as measured by hospital admissions with 50 to 100 per 100,000 population and 3500 deaths per annum in the United Kingdom. The critical factors determining outcome are the patient's age, the site of bleeding, its severity and the presence or absence of other disease. The past history gives an indication of the risk of future haemorrhage. The patient who has bled once will bleed again within a ten year period in about 60% of the cases.

When a patient with acute upper alimentary bleeding is admitted to the hospital, the questions to be answered are:
1. Is he still bleeding?
2. Why is he bleeding?
3. Where is he bleeding from?
4. How much has he bled?
5. Is he likely to bleed again?
6. What needs to be done now?
7. What may need to be done in the near future?

Many of these questions can be answered by early endoscopic examination after restoration of the patient's vital functions, although the value of urgent endoscopy on the final outcome of the patient is debated.[7-9]

In Dronfield's series 1037 patients were randomly allocated to endoscopy or radiology. With early endoscopy an increase in diagnostic accuracy was obtained in up to 97% of the cases, but early surgery, frequency of operation, duration of stay in hospital and mortality were not different in the two groups.[9]

Both Pertson and Graham found no significant differences between patients in whom endoscopy results were available and in those in whom they were not, in the duration of hospital stay, recurrent bleeding and mortality. The total numbers of patients in these series was however, small.[7,8]

A survey of the literature describing 6922 patients showed an overall mortality rate of 12.2% and an operation rate of 24.1%. Spontaneous arrest of bleeding was recorded in 63% of patients with duodenal ulcer and 67% of patients with gastric ulcer.

There is no doubt that in some patients prognosis is dependent on the endoscopic findings when FORREST's criteria[10] are applied. (Table I) Griffiths, Foster and Storey have all stressed the importance of active haemorrhage and the presence of a visible blood

Table I. Classification of bleeding activity of peptic ulcer, modified from Forrest et al.[10]

Active bleeding	Forrest Ia	spurting
	Forrest Ib	oozing
Recent Bleeding	Forrest IIa	visible vessel
	Forrest IIb	adherent blood clot
	Forrest IIc	black base
No bleeding	Forrest III	lesion without above stigmata

vessel in deciding the management, so that all further therapeutic recommendations should be based on the classification given by Forrest et al in 1974[11-13] Griffiths observed an overall incidence of 9% Forrest IIa haemorrhages in 317 patients admitted with upper gastrointestinal haemorrhage. Of his 28 patients, 4 had primary uncontrolable bleeding and the other 24 patients all rebled. Of the remaining 289 patients with Forrest IIb, IIc or III bleeding, rebleeding occurred in 53 (18%) and surgery was necessary in 25 (9%). The incidence of Forrest IIa bleeding in ulcer patients was 28/152 (18%). In Storey's series a visible vessel was present in 56/292 (19%) for all patients and in 56/117 (48%) of the patients with peptic ulcers. Of the 34 patients managed initially by conservative means, 19 (56%) rebled and 17 (50%) underwent emergency surgery. From the Forrest IIb bleeds only 8% rebled and from the Forrest III series none. Foster observed a rebleeding rate of 56% patients with duodenal ulcer and 30% patients with gastric ulcer admitted with endoscopic stigmata of recent haemorrhage (Forrest IIa, IIb, IIc) and of 4.8% in duodenal ulcer patients and none of gastric ulcer patients in Forrest III category.

The mortality of Forrest IIa bleeding category was $14-17\%$ in this series. Although Hunt and colleagues from Melbourne have shown by an aggressive policy of endoscopy, early surgery and intensive care for all poor-risk and post-operative patients that mortality from bleeding ulcer can be reduced to 4%, there is still no standardization of how to manage the bleeding patient. A prospective randomized trial in Birmingham showed some favourable results for early surgery in patients over age 60 but the problem remains when to operate and when to try a more conservative approach.[14,15]

As about 60% of all bleeding episodes stop spontaneously, all therapeutic recommendations should start with a precise Forrest classification. This is especially true for all endoscopic attempts to arrest spurting, or oozing haemorrhage by electro- or photocoagulation using the Argon or Nd-YAG laser or injection therapy.[16-24]

The tables II – IV are based on figures published by Rutgeerts, Matek and Frühmorgen, Soehendra and Grimm, Swain et al, and Salmon, and compare the three different methods in relation to initial haemostasis, recurrence and mortality under the three conditions spurting haemorrhage, oozing and visible vessel.[20-24] There is increasing evidence that patients with stigmata of recent haemorrhage profit from laser photocoagulation[25] but this rather expensive method is available in only a few gastroenterological centers. We would therefore recommend to try injection therapy with noradrenaline 1 : 10,000 combined with aethoxysclerol, or electrocoagulation with the electro-hydro-thermo-probe, or the BICAP probe first. Then delayed surgery can be done in patients with a visible vessel, or spurting haemorrhage. In case of successful treatment or oozing haemorrhage, prophylaxis of recurrent bleeding is mandatory as mentioned later. It has, however, to be stressed that in about 10% of bleeding ulcers the lesion is inaccessible to all endoscopic maneuvers, especially when the bleeding point is situated on the posterior aspect of the duodenal bulb.

There are many reports on the use of levarterenol, cyclocaprone, antacids, histamine H_2-receptor antagonists, vasopressin etc., but most studies are uncontrolled and do not take into account the endoscopic findings. Trials with the antifibrynolytic agent tranexamic acid have produced a small but consistent benefit in mortality, but the drug had no beneficial effect on arrest of bleeding or on the rebleeding rate.[26] The mortality rate in this study on 676 patients was 11% with placebo, 8% with cimetidine and 4% with tranexamic acid. The

Table II. Forrest Ia haemorrhage: Results of endoscopic therapy. **Based on studies published** by Rutgeerts, Matek and Soehendra.

	Percentage		
	Initial haemostasis	Recurrent haemorrhage	Mortality
Laser	87	55	30
Coagulation	89	18	
Injection therapy	100	30	18

Table III. Forrest Ib haemorrhage: Results of endoscopic therapy. **Based on studies publis-**hed by Rutgeerts, Matek and Soehendra.

	Percentage		
	Initial haemostasis	Recurrent haemorrhage	Mortality
Laser	100	7	13
Coagulation	96	4	
Injection therapy	100	11	8

Table IV. Forrest IIa haemorrhage (visible vessel): Results of laser therapy. **Based on data** published by Swain and Salmon.

	n	Percentage		
		Recurrent haemorrhage	Urgent surgery	Mortality
Argon	17	24*	24*	0*
Controls	24	54	50	21
Nd-YAG	22	9*	8*	5*
Controls	24	50	32	29

* Significantly better results.

Table V. Drug therapy in Forrest Ib haemorrhage.

	Gastric ulcer	Duodenal ulcer	Stress lesion
Antacids	−	−	(+)
Terlipressin	−	−	(+)
Cimetidine	+ ?	0	0
Ranitidine	+ ?	0	0
Somatostatin	+	+	+
Secretin	+	+	+

−   Not tested.
0   No effects.
?   Positive in only few trials
+   Superior to other drugs.

rebleeding rate was 23%, 24% and 21% respectively and surgery had to be performed in 16%, 20% and 14% of the patients respectively.

Despite of the small number of patients treated, somatostatin and secretin seems to be the only agents which can be recommended, based with evidence in several published series.[27-30] These studies indicate that persistent Forrest Ib haemorrhage can be arrested in 80% by either somatostatin (250 μg/h) or secretin (0.25–0.5 μ/kg BW/h). Because of the high cost, this treatment should be restricted to patients not suitable for operative measures. In Table V the results of drug therapy in oozing peptic ulcers are summarized.

Finally we have to deal often with peptic ulcers which have bled and where we have to prevent recurrent haemorrhage. There are two studies indicating that combined therapy with histamine H_2-receptor antagonists and pirenzepine[31] and histamine H_2-blockers with antacide[32,33] are superior to treatment with one agent only. The value of treatment with one drug is questioned by Zuckerman et al.[34] In published data on prevention of bleeding relapse are summarized in Table VI.

Table VI. Drug therapy to prevent bleeding relapse.

Cimetidine	?
Ranitidine	? (+ duodenal ulcer)
Antcids	(+)
Somatostatin	(+)
Secretin	(+)
Cimetidine + pirenzepine	+
Cimetidine + antacids	+

Evidence available at present suggests that gastrointestinal bleeding from a peptic ulcer is best managed by a policy of early investigation by endoscopy and if the standard surgical care allows, early surgery for those patients with visible vessels. Endoscopic measures to arrest haemorrhage are primarily indicated to bring the patient to a better condition for elective surgery, although there is some recent evidence that laser coagulation may in many patients bring not only temporary, but permanent arrest of a spurting haemorrhage. In case of persistent oozing over more than 24 hours a trial with secretin or somatostatin can be done, if surgery is contraindicated. Successful staunching by endoscopy, or spontaneously should be followed by combined drug therapy for about one week leading finally to treatment with an histamine H_2-receptor antagonist.

Many of our treatments used at present are based on the experience of well-trained endoscopists, or on therapeutic trials which can be critized because of the small number of patients or imperfect design. However, if we stick to Forrest's criteria and analyze all data in accordance with this classification we should soon be able to determine what kind of patient benefits from our therapeutic efforts to decrease mortality from bleeding peptic ulcer.

References

1. Stolte JB. Gross bleeding from the digestive tract. 2. The frequency of manifest bleeding in peptic ulcer with respect to the duration of the disease and to the age of the diseased. Acta Med Scand 1944;16:584.
2. Wastell C. Chronic duodenal ulcer. London, Butterworth, 1972.
3. Jensen HE, Amdrup E, Christiansen P, Fenger C, Lindskov J, Nielsen J, Damgaard-Nielsen SA. Bleeding gastric ulcer. Surgical and non-surgical treatment of 225 patients. Scand J Gastroenterol 1972;7:535.
4. Kim U, Dreiling DA, Kark AE, Rudick J. Factors influencing mortality in surgical treatment of massive gastrointestinal haemorrhage. Am J Gastroenterol 1974;62:24.
5. Rumpf P, Hoffmann E, Jacobs G, Kremer K. Operationsindikation bei der massiven Gastrointestinalblutung mit besonderer Berücksichtigung der Magen-Duodenalblutung. Zbl Chir 1973;98:1531.
6. Wilkinson RH. Management of acute upper gastrointestinal haemorrhage. Can J Surg 1973;16:92.
7. Graham DY. Limited value of early endoscopy in the management of acute upper gastrointestinal bleeding. Amer J Surg 1980;140:284.
8. Peterson WL, Barnett CC, Smith HJ, Allen MH, Corbett DB. Routine early endoscopy in upper gastrointestinal tract bleeding, a randomized controlled trial. N Engl J Med 1981;403:925.
9. Dronfield MW, Langman MJS, Atkinson M, Balfour TW, Bell GD, Vellacott KD, Amar SS, Knapp DR. Outcome of endoscopy and barium radiography for acute upper gastrointestinal bleeding: a controlled trial in 1037 patients. Brit Med J 1982;284:545.
10. Forrest JAH, Finlayson NDC, Shearman DJC. Endoscopy in gastrointestinal bleeding. Lancet 1974;ii:394.
11. Griffiths WJ, Neuman DA, Welsh JD. The visible vessel as an indicator of uncontrolled or recurrent gastrointestinal haemorrhage. N Engl J Med 1981; 305:915.
12. Foster DN, Miloszewski KJA, Losowski MS. Stigmata of recent haemorrhage in diagnosis and prognosis of upper gastrointestinal bleeding. Br Med J 1978; 1:1173−7.
13. Storey DW, Bown SG, Swain CP, Salmon PR, Kirkham JS, Northfield TC. Endoscopic prediction of recurrent bleeding in peptic ulcers. N Engl J Med 1979;300:1411.

14. Hunt PS, Francis JK, Hansky J, Hillman H, Korman MG, McLeish J, Marshall R, Schmidt G. Reduction in mortality from upper gastrointestinal haemorrhage. Med J Austral 1983;70:552.
15. Morris DL, Hawker PC, Brearley S, Simms M, Dykes PW, Keighley MRB. Optimal timing of operation for bleeding peptic ulcer: A prospective randomized trial. Gut 1982;23:A888.
16. Domschke W. Nutzen der Notfallendoskopie bei oberer Gastrointestinalblutung. Dt Ärztebl 1983;80:23.
17. MacLeod IA, Mills PR, Mackenzie JF, Russel RI, Carter DC. Neodymium YAG laser photocoagulation for major acute upper gastrointestinal haemorrhage. Gut 1982;23:A905.
18. Soehendra N, Kempeneers I, de Heer K. Endoskopische Injektionsmethode zur Blutstillung im Verdauungstrakt. Dtsch Med Wschr 1982;107:1474.
19. Vallon AG, Cotton PB, Laurence BH, Armengol Miro JR, Salord Oses JC. Randomized trial of endoscopy argon laser photocoagulation in bleeding peptic ulcers. Gut 1981;22:228.
20. Matek W, Frühmorgen P. Elektro-Hydro-Thermo-Sonde. Klinische Erfahrungen und Einsatzmöglichkeiten der modifizierten Elektrokoagulation im Gastrointestinaltrakt. Dtsch Med Wschr 1983;108:816.
21. Rutgeerts P, Vantrappen G, Broeckaert L, Janssens J, Coremans G, Geboes K, Schurmans P. Controlled trial of YAG laser treatment of upper gastrointestinal haemorrhage. Gastroenterology 1983;83:410.
22. Salmon PR. Controlled trials of laser therapy in upper alimentary haemorrhage. Z Gastroenterol 1984;22, in press.
23. Soehendra N, Grimm H, Tietze B. Gastrointestinale Blutung-Therapeutische Sklerosierung. Z Gastroenterol 1984;22:102.
24. Swain CP, Bown SG, Salmon PR, Kirkham JS, Northfield TC. Controlled trial of Nd-YAG laser photocoagulation in bleeding peptic ulcers. Gut 1982; 23:A915.
25. Swain CP, Bown SG, Kirkham JS, Northfield TC. Controlled trial of ND-YAG laser photocoagulation in bleeding peptic ulcers. Abstract Book International Congresses of Gastroenterology, Lisbon 1984.
26. Baker D, Ogilvie A, Henry D, Dronfield M, Coggon D, French S, Ellis S, Atkinson M, Langman M. Cimetidine and tranexamic acid in the treatment of acute upper gastrointestinal tract bleeding. N Engl J Med 1983;308:1571.
27. Kayasseh L, Gyr K, Keller U, Stalder GA, Wall M. Somatostatin and cimetidine in peptic ulcer haemorrhage. Lancet 1980;i:844.
28. Berg P, Bär U, Hausamen TU, Lingenberg G, Pfleiderer TH, Raedsch R, Saeger HD, Sailer S, Schwigon CD, Seidel G, Stiehl A. Vergleichende Behandlung gastroduodenaler Blutungen mit Sekretin und Cimetidin. Dtsch Med Wschr 1982;107:1831.
29. Rothmund M, Wagner PK. Wirkung von Cimetidin und Sekretin bei akuten Blutungen aus gastroduodenalen Ulzera und Erosionen. Dtsch Med Wschr 1982;107:245.
30. Wagner PK, Rothmund M, Gröninger J. Sekretin versus Somatostatin bei akuter Blutung aus gastroduodenalen Ulcers and Erosionen, eine randomisierte Studie. Klin Wschr 1983;61:285.
31. Londong W, Hasford J, Sander R, Sommerlatte Th, Überla K, Ultsch B, Weinzierl M. Kombination von Cimetidin und Pirenzepin zur Rezidivprophylaxe der akuten gastroduodenalen Blutung – eine multizentrische Doppelblindstudie. Z Gastroenterol 1981;19:514.
32. Engelhardt D, Karl R, Possinger K. Cimetidin/Pirenzepin versus Antazida

zur Stressblutungsprophylaxe bei Intensivpatienten. Zwischenbericht einer randomisierten, kontrollierten klinischen Studie. Intensivmedizin 1983;20: 164.

33. Welch R, Douglas A, Cohen S. Effect of cimetidine on upper gastrointestinal haemorrhage. Gastroenterology 1981;80:1313.
34. Zuckerman G, Welch R, Douglas A, Troxell R, Cohen S, Lorber S, Melnyk C, Bliss C, Christiansen P, Kern F. Controlled trial of medical therapy for active upper gastrointestinal bleeding and prevention of rebleeding. Am J Med 1984;76:361.

26. Discussion VI

Johnston:

The great difficulty is that the elderly patient with ischemic heart disease and severe bleeding ulcer is not only a high surgical risk, but also does badly on conservative therapy. How do you weigh up the costs and benefits of medical versus surgical treatment in these high risk elderly people?

Rösch:

The best results in bleeding peptic ulcer are obtained in Australia, in dr Hunt's department. In his department physicians and surgeons together are looking after patients with bleeding ulcer, discussing the clinical situation hourly. They have very strict criteria when to operate. In my department I do an endoscopy and ask the surgeon to have a look at the ulcer and then we jointly decide, based on the patients condition, whether I shall try to stop the haemorrhage with endoscopic means, or whether the surgeon considers this patients for operation. We don't lose time, we decide in 10 – 20 minutes.

Johnston:

What criteria do you use?

Rösch:

If there is arterial haemorrhage, the patient goes straight to the surgeon, unless the patient's condition is too poor. If there is a visible vessel of 2 – 3 mm diameter, this patient goes directly to surgery, even if the bleeding has stopped, because he will rebleed in the next few hours. Coagulation, or injection therapy will only give a temporary solution of the problem. In all these endoscopic treatment studies certain ulcers or bleeding sites were excluded at the beginning: the posterior wall ulcer in the stomach and the duodenal bulb. This is the location which also causes problems to the surgeon. It is never mentioned, but it is the prerequisite for endoscopic therapy.

Van Rooyen:

When do you adivse surgery in cases of uncontrollable Forrest Ib bleeding?

Rösch:

In the oozing haemorrhage I would start with secretin or somatostatin only if the bleeding persists for longer than 24 hours. In some university hospitals obviously everybody who was admitted with tarry stools received as the first measure somatostatin, but that is very expensive.

27. Management of recurrent duodenal ulcer after highly selective vagotomy, as seen by the physician

M. VAN BLANKENSTEIN, B.Sc., M.B.

Department of International Medicine II, University Hospital Dijkzigt, Rotterdam, The Netherlands

A physician encoutering a patient with symptoms suggesting recurrent ulcer after highly selective vagotomy (HSV) will have to consider the diagnosis, the aetiology, the treatment and finally the prevention of this form of ulcer disease. The diagnosis is of particular importance as is illustrated by the study of Poppen et al,[1] who found that in 20 out of a group of 54 patients with symptoms suggestive of recurrent ulcer, no ulcer could be demonstrated.

Differential diagnosis should include: irritable bowel disease, non-ulcer dyspepsia, which seems to be particularly prevalent in this group of patients, pancreatic disease and biliary tract disease. These diagnoses should be particularly borne in mind in patients in whom the presence of an ulcer pre-operatively was not altogether certain. Endoscopic verification of recurrent ulcer is therefore mandatory in all suspected cases.

If a recurrent ulcer is found, it is necessary to analyse the cause of recurrence.

Potential mechanisms are:
a) technical failure of the vagotomy procedure;
b) true recurrence;
c) complications of the operation;
d) new disease; and
e) exogenous factor like medication and smoking.

A diagnosis of failed vagotomy can be made of peak acid output after pentagastrin or similar maximal acid stimulation is undiminished post-operatively in comparison to the pre-operative value. In cases where no pre-operative acid studies were performed, a positive insulin

test can confirm that the vagus is still functioning. In view of the wide
variety of interpretations of the insulin test and its potential dangers,
a modified sham-feeding test is preferred for testing vagal integrity.

True recurrent ulcer can be defined as an ulcer in the same anatomical region as before the operation in a patient in whom an un-
equivocal reduction in acid output was achieved by the operation. In
the event stimulated acid production at the time of diagnosis of a recurrent ulcer is comparable to pre-operative levels, it will not always
be possible to distinguish between true recurrence from a failed vagotomy, unless systematic post-operative testing has been done.

Aetiologically a large number of factors can be involved.

There is probably a tendency for the number of recurrences to increase with time. This was nicely shown in the study of Jensen et al[2]
who demonstrated a constant risk of recurrence. Other authors have
claimed that recurrences level off after a number of years,[3] but this
may be an artefact due to the small number of patients followed up
for a long time. A number of factors have been cited in the literature
which may be associated with ulcer recurrence. The experience, or
lack of it, of the surgeon, a relatively small post-operative decrease in
acid secretion and the development of a positive insulin stimulation
test are frequently mentioned. The length of ulcer history, the anatomical location of the ulcer and pre-operative hypersecretion are
more controversial, the last mentioned factor finds few adherents. A
number of mechanisms has to be considered.

The first is vagal reinnervation. Support for this mechanism has
been found in animal studies.[4] Another mechanism is based on the
fairly obvious assumption that the vagus should posses a feedback inhibition on acid output. A hypothesis has recently been advanced that
vagotomy may remove a vagus-dependent inhibiting mechanism in
the fundic mucosa.[5]

The inability to predict recurrent ulcer by pre-operative acid secretion studies indicates that defective epithelial resistance may also be
involved.

Another, somehwat vaguer, mechanism is suggested by an observation recently reported by Hansen and Knigge[6] who found a 44%
recurrence rate after HSV in a group of 'cimetidine resistant'
patients. This was followed by an observation in which a 28% recurrence rate was recorded in 104 patients, who underwent proximal
gastric vagotomy between 1970 and 1973 while, in spite of a shorter

follow-up, this percentage rose significantly to 44% in 80 patients operated between 1975 and 1980. The authors explained this paradoxal result by postulating a selection of patients with more aggressive ulcer disease for operation after the introduction of cimetidine. These so called cimetidine-resistant patients may represent a group with an unfavourable natural history and therefore more tendency towards recurrence.

In a small number of patients ischaemic necrosis of the lesser curve causes extensive ulceration, a catastrophe that can easily be diagnosed. However, a number of recurrences occur as gastric ulcers instead of a pre-operative location of the ulcer in the duodenum, or in the pre-pyloric antrum. The question arises whether such ulcers may be the result of operation, either through changes in motility or through interference with the blood circulation along the lesser curvature.

Recurrent ulcer may also be caused by new ulcer disease. Besides the gastric ulcer already mentioned, a gastrinoma producing a Zollinger-Ellison syndrome may become manifest after the operation. The diagnosis of gastrinoma can best be made by measuring gastrin levels after secretin stimulation. It is as yet unknown whether HSV is associated with long term increased incidence of gastric carcinoma.

Finally, exogenous factors may induce recurrent ulcers. Foremost among these are medication, especially acetylsalicylic acid and nonsteroidal anti-inflammatory drugs. A meticulous history of the use of such drugs should always be taken. Whether corticosteroids are ulcerogenic is still disputed. The effect of alcohol and smoking in the induction of ulcer recurrence is less clean cut. Alcohol can damage the gastric mucosa, while smoking is associated with increased incidence and recurrence of ulcer disease and impaired ulcer healing. However, as yet no systematic investigation of the influence of smoking on post-vagotomy ulcer recurrence has been done.

This compilation of the state of our ignorance suggests that the practical clinician will have to take a more pragmatic approach. After a diagnosis of recurrence he should check for the use of ulcerogenic drugs, excessive smoking and alcoholism. A gastrinoma should also be excluded. Although differentiation between technical failure and true recurrence may be of scientific importance it is probably of little significance in practice.

We now come to the heart of the question: how should the recurrent ulcer be treated?

In my opinion an attempt should always be made to restart medical management. At the moment maintenance treatment with a histamine H_2-receptor antagonist is probably most suitable. Comparative studies between vagotomy and cimetidine suggest that vagotomy is a stronger inhibitor of acid production than cimetidine. However, it is likely that more powerfull histamine H_2-receptor antagonists, or drugs like omeprazole may produce acid inhibition equal to, or better than, vagotomy.

Indications for re-operation, which always entails more mutilating surgery, are a failure of conservative treatment, or recurrent haemorrhage. Failure of conservative therapy is often due to unwillingness of the patient to accept medical maintenance treatment. The newer once daily regimens can result in better compliance and a decreased number of treatment failures. In practice, recurrent haemorrhage is uncommon during maintenance treatment with histamine H_2-receptor antagonists.

It is probably wise to avoid re-operation in patients who have already experienced post-operative sequelae such as diarrhea, or dumping after HSV. These patients may be even more prone to such complications after gastric resection and truncal vagotomy than the average patient. A statement made by dr Wormsley is pertinent at this point: 'If problems occur after surgery, they are irreversible, whereas as far as is known all the drug induced problems are reversible'.

Finally we are left with the question what role the physician can play in preventing ulcer recurrence after HSV. Selection of patients by pre-operative secretion studies is supported by a small minority of authors. Most studies do not show an increased risk of recurrence in hypersecretors. This means that the physician using this criterion to select patients for HSV or resection may well be condemning a number of patients to an unnecessarily mutilating operation. Peroperative tests for complete vagotomy have enjoyed a certain vogue and were discussed yesterday by professor Allgöwer. However, little has been published about the long term results of these procedures and they can probably only contribute to the prevention of technical failures. Most studies do seem to indicate that a physician would do well to send his patient to an experienced surgeon.

References

1. Poppen B, Andres D. Parietal cell vagotomy for duodenal and pyloric ulcers. Am J Surg 1981;141:323 – 329.
2. Jensen HE, Kjaergaard J, Meisner S. Ulcer recurrence two to twelve years after parietal cell vagotomy for duodenal ulcer. Surgery 1983;94:802 – 806.
3. Adami HO, Enander LK, Enskog L, Ingvar C, Rydberg B. Recurrences 1 to 10 years after Highly Selective Vagotomy in prepyloric and duodenal ulcer disease. Ann Surg 1984;199:393 – 399.
4. Joffe SN, Crocket A, Doyle D. Morphologic and functional evidence of reinnervation of the gastric parietal cell mass after parietal cell vagotomy. Am J Surg 1982;143:80 – 85.
5. Debas HT. Proximal gastric vagotomy interferes with a fundic inhibitory mechanism. Am J Surg, 1983;146:51 – 56.
6. Hansen JH, Knigge U. Failure of proximal gastric vagotomy for duodenal ulcer resistant to cimetidine. Lancet 1984;2:84 – 86.
7. Gledhill T, Clark CG. Vagotomy for cimetidine resistant ulcers. Lancet 1984,2:697.
8. Wormsley KG. In: Tijtgat GN (Ed). Ranitidine, the selective new H_2-receptor antagonist. Theracom, Guildford 1982:37 – 40.

28. Management of recurrent duodenal ulcer after treatment with histamine H$_2$-receptor antagonists and highly selective vagotomy

E. AMDRUP, P. FUNCH-JENSEN AND A. TØTTRUP

The organization of the Aarhus University Clinic of Surgical Gastro-enterology is somewhat unusual. While patients admitted as emergencies are surgical, the out-patient ward receives also large numbers for conservative treatment of gastroenterological disease. The department's endoscopy unit is central in the Country Hospital System. It has thus been possible to collect series of patients with the same disease treated surgically as well as by conservative means. This has been especially used in relation to peptic ulcer disease.

From 1972 to 1977 the department in co-operation with two other hospitals, performed a vagotomy trial on 900 patients. The aim was to compare hihgly selective vagotomy (HSV) without drainage with selective gastric vagotomy with a drainage (SGV), in the hands of well-trained surgeons not specially interested in vagotomy technique, but seeking some years of training in a specialized gastroenterological department. They assisted and were assisted by staff members, until they got a licence to work for themselves. The patients had a postoperative clinical follow-up every year. Endoscopy was not performed as a routine, but whenever even slight symptoms developed. Furthermore, patients were seen immediately whenever they developed recurrent symptoms. Thus it has been possible to collect precise information of the time of recurrence. A few years ago a recurrence meant a recurrence after surgical treatment, but today we have to recognize that it can also occur after medical treatment and even spontaneously.

Before surgery endoscopy with biopsy was always performed in patients with lesions at, or proximal to the pylorus, and in every case

346

where X-ray examination did not show a duodenal ulcer without any doubt. Thus a distinction between duodenal, pyloric and pre-pyloric ulcers could be made. In this series the location of ulcer was not taken into consideration for the randomization between operations. These studies were performed in co-operation with Daniel Anderson, Hans Høstrup and Finn Hanberg Sørensen.[1,2,3]

Later on a randomized trial between HSV with drainage and SGV with drainage for pyloric and pre-pyloric ulcer has been done in co-operation with Daniel Anderson and Finn Hanberg Sørensen. Results have not yet been published.

Cimetidine became available in 1977. In co-operation with the above surgeons, a randomized comparison between this drug and surgery was begun. Preliminary reports have been published.[4] The evaluation of the comparison has to be delayed until at least 5 years have passed after surgery. The series has, however, supplied us with information on results of cimetidine treatment in a considerable number of patients. It has to be stressed that the medically treated patients had exactly the same severity of ulcer disease, as those treated in the above vagotomy trial.

In our first cimetidine trial 145 patients were randomized to cimetidine 1 g/day for 8 weeks and then operation was advised in instances of no therapeutic effect or recurrence. 148 patients had the same treatment, but in instances of recurrence repeated courses of the drug were advised, until such time as the patients might opt for an operation. In the medically treated patients clinical evaluation was done every third months.

In a later cimetidine trial 260 patients had the same initial treatment as above. At recurrence half were randomized to surgery and half to long-time treatment with cimetidine 400 mg at night. The best gift of the physician to the surgeon was that we did not have to operate on recurrent ulcers in the old, the fat and those with severe concomitant disease. We can treat them for a life-time with histamine H_2-receptor antagonists and keep them symptom free.

During the years a number of patients with recurrent ulcer after HSV performed in this, or other departments have been admitted. Experiences with this group are not based on randomization. Before 1977 most patients were antrectomized, later on cimetidine was always the first choice.

Results

HSV versus SGV + D

The results are given in figure 1.

The number of recurrences is rising in time, at five years to 9% after SGV + D and 14% after PCV for duodenal ulcer. Following the same operations for pre-pyloric ulcer, the figures were 13% and 33%, respectively. Technical expertise is very important, because the highest rate of recurrence was in the first years. We had to learn to do the operation properly.

160 patients with pyloric and pre-pyloric ulcer were followed after either HSV with drainage, or SGV with drainage. At three years the cumulative recurrence rate was 8% after either operation. Can we bring down the recurrence rate for pre-pyloric ulcers? The pre-pyloric ulcer has an unacceptably high recurrence rate after HSV. After selective vagotomy and drainage the results are not much better. What might be the reason that the pre-pyloric ulcer is so difficult to treat with a vagal procedure? Acid secretion in these patients and controls was the same. Motility of the duodenum and antrum differs in patients with pre-pyloric ulcer compared with patients with duodenal ulcer and normals. The serum gastrin concentration did not differ very much, so further follow-up is needed.

Cimetidine treatment

When these patients with severe peptic ulcer disease stopped treatment after one course recurrence came very fast, the cumulative rate (fig. 1) being more than 60% after 6 months and more than 80% after 1 year. Ninety per cent of these patients had to choose between multiple courses of cimetidine and surgery. When full quote doses was continued directly into a low dose course, recurrence rate was considerably lower: 40% at three years.

Recurrence after HSV

The results are listed in Table I.

Before the cimetidine era 16 patients had an uncomplicated antrectomy. All had slight to moderate dumping, 14 being graded as Visick II. Two had a new recurrence, treated successfully with long term cimetidine.

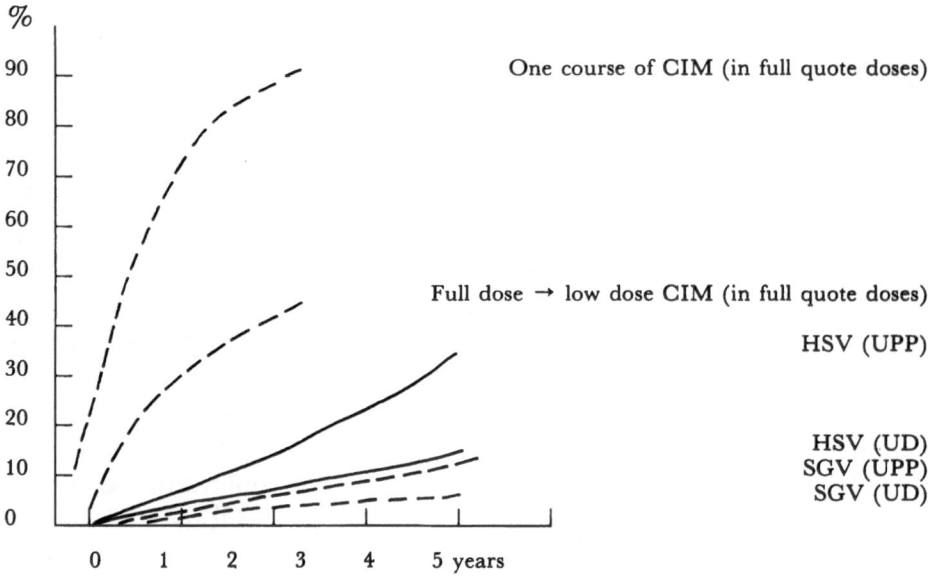

%

90 — One course of CIM (in full quote doses)

80 —

70 —

60 —

50 —

40 — Full dose → low dose CIM (in full quote doses)

30 — HSV (UPP)

20 —

10 — HSV (UD)
SGV (UPP)
SGV (UD)

0 —

0   1   2   3   4   5 years

UD   Duodenal ulcer
UPP Pre-pyloric ulcer
CIM Cimetidine

Figure 1. Cumulative recurrence rates (%) of duodenal and pre-pyloric ulcer after treatment with cimetidine (CIM), parietal cell vagotomy (CV) and selective gastric vagotomy (SGV).

After 1977 cimetidine treatment was the first choice. Eleven healed after 1 – 2 courses and have remained symptom-free for 2 – 4 years. Eight went through several courses before antrectomy had to be performed with uneventful courses. Eleven patients have been on long-term treatment from 1 – 6 years. Two have recurred, one treated with full dose cimetidine once again, the other being antrectomized. There were no deaths.

Table I. Treatment of recurrence after HSV (number of patients).

	Duodenal	Pre-pyloric	Total
Antrectomy	12	4	16
recurrence treated medically	2	0	2
CIM 1–2 courses	8	4	12
recurrence treated medically	0	1	1
CIM multiple courses	7	1	8
recurrence treated medically	7	1	8
CIM long-term	6	5	11
recurrence treated medically	1	0	1
antrectomy	1	0	1

Conclusions

The present conclusion is that every patient should have at least one formal course with histamine H_2-receptor antagonists, even if the history of ulcer is long and severe.

If contra-indications against surgery (old age, obesity, concomitant disease) exists conservative treatment should be continued indefinitely in appropriate dosage.

The young and fit chronic duodenal ulcer patient should make his own choice between long-term medical treatment and highly selective vagotomy, based on realistic information about advantage and disadvantage.

Patients with pre-pyloric ulcer remain a special problem, as the best surgical treatment would be vagotomy and antrectomy. Therefore
a more conservative course may be preferable.

In patients with recurrence after HSV, treatment with histamine H_2-receptor antagonists is the first choice. If it fails antrectomy is suggested.

References

1. Amdrup E, Andersen D, Høstrup H. The Aarhus County Vagotomy Trial I. World J Surg 1978;2:85–90.
2. Andersen D, Høstrup H, Amdrup E. The Aarhus County Vagotomy Trial II. World J Surg 1978;2:91–100.
3. Andersen D, Amdrup E, Høstrup H, Handberg Sørensen F. Trends in the problem of recurrent ulcer after parietal cell vagotomy with drainage. World J Surg 1982;6:86–92.
4. Andersen D, Amdrup E, Hanberg Sørensen F, Jensen KB. Surgery or cimetidine. World J Surg 1983;7:372–384.

29. A national inquiry into the diagnosis and treatment of peptic ulcers by Dutch physicians and gastroenterologists[1] in 1984

G.F. NELIS, M.D.

Department of Internal Medicine, Sophia Ziekenhuis Zwolle, The Netherlands

There is some intuitive feeling how peptic ulcers are diagnosed and treated at present in The Netherlands, but we don't know for certain what the real facts are. Therefore we decided to send a questionnaire to all Dutch consultant physicians and gastroenterologists appointed to general hospitals, in february 1984 and collected the data till august 1984.

People were addressed according to the Geneeskundig Adresboek voor Nederland, edited by H.W. Blok, Rotterdam edition 1983 – 984 (Medical Adress book for The Netherlands). For University hospitals the Head of the Department of Internal Medicine and of the Department of Gastroenterology were addressed and invited to respond on behalf of their Departments as a whole. If physicians responded and stated that the answer was on behalf of all the physicians in their hospital, all members of this group were counted as responders. Thus *all* percentages express the total number of responding physicians divided by the total number of consultant physicians appointed to general hospitals. This last number, calculated from the Geneeskundig Adresboek, was 625. Physicians who specifically restrict themselves to only a limited part of internal medicine (as *e.g.* haematology or haemodialysis in some cases) were disregarded.

The total number of responses from general hospitals represented the answers from 465 physicians, which made the overall response rate 76%.

The response rate was highest from the A-teaching hospitals (90%) and lowst from hospitals without teaching facilities (70), while the B-teaching hospitals were in between (77%).[2]

Analyzed by the number of beds, the larger hospitals reached higher response rates; with the total number of beds smaller than 200 the response rate was 55% and with the total number of beds more than 600 the response rate was 92%.

In most hospitals (81%) one physician from the group of physicians was specifically responsible for the care of gastroenterological patients.

Research on peptic ulcer (including drug trials) has been performed by 16% during their training in internal medicine and by 19% after completion of the training period. Of the physicians who later became appointed to A-teaching hospitals, 36% did research during training and 46% after training; for those appointed to B-teaching hospitals these figures were 19% and 28% respectively and for those appointed to hospital without training facilities 6 and 7% respectively.

Protocols for the management of peptic ulcer were extant in 56% of the hospitals within the group of physicians and protocols concerning the indications for surgery were available in 45%. Protocols were more frequently present in bigger, than in smaller hospitals. (Table I)

If patients with uncomplicated ulcer presented at the department of surgery, the patient was referred to the department of internal medicine for the supervision of conservative treatment in nearly all cases (86%). Only in university hospitals conservative treatment was supervised by the department of surgery in most of those cases (69%).

Table I. Protocols for treatment of peptic ulcer, divided by number of beds.

	Total	Number of beds		
		< 250	250 – 500	> 500
Physicians only, conservative management	56%	50%	64%	70%
Physicians and surgeons, indications for surgery	45%	19%	44%	56%

In general hospitals there appeared to be no standard diagnostic procedure[3] for the patient presenting with symptoms suggestive of peptic ulcer.

Endoscopy was performed as the primary procedure by 32% of the physicians, another 32% chose radiology as a primary procedure and 36% chose either procedure equally often. In this respect there were no differences between teaching and non-teaching hospitals. Only in university hospitals there was a 100% preference for endoscopy as the primary procedure. From the total data (Table II) it can be calculated that on average 75% of the patients with peptic ulcer undergo endoscopy and less than 50% radiology. The use of radiology increases in the following order: university hospitals, non-university teaching hospitals, non-teaching hospitals. The opposite is true for endoscopy.

Table II. Use of radiology and endoscopy in the diagnosis of peptic ulcer.

	Physicians primarily using	
	radiology	endoscopy
In less than 30% of patients	43%	10%
In 30–60% of patients	17%	11%
In 60–90% of patients	17%	34%
In more than 90% of patients	23%	45%

The number of upper gastrointestinal endoscopies per hospital showed immense variations, from 45 to 3500 per year, the median being 486. In more than ⅔ of the hospitals the total number of endoscopies was less than 700 per year. Endoscopy with forceps biopsies is performed as a standard procedure in nearly all patients with gastric ulcer (99%), but only in 52% the number of biopsies was large enough to differentiate reliably gastric ulcer from gastric carcinoma according to accepted standards (8 biopsies or more). (Table III)

Table III. Number of biopsies in gastric ulcer.

	1–4	5–8	>8
University hospitals	12%	15%	73%
General hospitals			
teaching	1%	34%	65%
non-teaching	7%	45%	48%

Emergency endoscopy was performed as a standard procedure in cases of upper gastrointestinal haemorrhage by 84%; in university hospitals this was 100%, in non-university teaching hospitals 90% and in non-teaching hospitals 75%. The time lag between admission and emergency endoscopy was shorter in teaching hospitals than in non-teaching hospitals. (Table IV)

General therapeutic measures such as bed rest, absence from work and a fixed dietary prescription were almost never advised: only in university hospitals and in the south of the country was absence from work advised regularly. Prescriptions for antacids were routinely given by 17%, frequently by 15% and infrequently, or never, by 68%.

Table IV. Time lag between admission and emergency endoscopy.

	<6 hr	6–12 hr	12–24 hr	>24 hr
Overall	15%	43%	36%	6%
Teaching hospitals	14%	56%	30%	0%
Non-teaching hospitals	17%	29%	43%	11%

The duration of drug treatment for uncomplicated ulcer is dependent on the frequency of ulcer recurrences in all university hospitals and in 78% of the general hospitals, while in the remaining 22% a standard course of treatment is given irrespective of whether ulcers recur frequently.

In university hospitals patients on life-long maintenance treatment are followed-up regularly. In general hospitals 20% of the physicians refer their patients back to the general practitioner, which probably means that 20% of the patients on life-long drug treatment take their medication practically uncontrolled.

In patients with infrequently recurrent uncomplicated peptic ulcer, despite a possibly great total number of recurrences during a prolonged period, intermittent medical therapy is favoured by all.

In patients with frequently recurrent uncomplicated peptic ulcer, intermittent medical treatment at the time of recurrence is preferred by 21% for younger patients and 22% for elderly patients, continuous medical treatment by 25% and 50% respectively and surgery by 49% and 21% respectively. In university hospitals there is more preference for continuous medical treatment for younger and older patients. (Table V)

Table V. Treatment preferences in frequently recurrent uncomplicated peptic ulcer in university hospitals (UH) and general hospitals (GH), analyzed by age.

	Younger patients		Older patients	
	UH	GH	UH	GH
Medical treatment				
intermittent	29%	20%	17%	23%
continuous	53%	23%	71%	48%
Surgery	6%	53%	0%	23%
No preference	12%	4%	12%	6%

In patients who have beld twice or more, 80% of the physicians consider some kind of definitive treatment indicated: either surgery, or continuous medical treatment. Medical treatment is preferred by 16% for younger patients and by 46% for older patients.

As to the choice of drugs: cimetidine was prescribed most frequently by 86% and ranitidine by 11%. If the prices of these two drugs would be the same the figures would be 55% and 37% respectively, 8% of the physicians having no preference. An overview of drug prescriptions is given in the Tables VI and VII.

Table VI. Prescriptions in gastric ulcer (Bis = bismuth subcitrate, Cim = cimetidine, Pir = pirenzepine, Ran = ranitidine, Suc = sucralfate).

	Bis	Cim	Pir	Ran	Suc
Never/infrequently	76%	18%	92%	58%	74%
Regularly	16%	17%	8%	25%	10%
Frequently	5%	36%	0%	9%	12%
First choice	2%	29%	0%	9%	4%

Table VI. Prescriptions in duodenal ulcer (Bis = bismuth subcitrate, Cim = cimetidine, Pir = pirenzepine, Ran = ranitidine, Suc = sucralfate).

	Bis	Cim	Pir	Ran	Suc
Never/infrequently	94%	5%	92%	46%	91%
Regularly	6%	9%	6%	33%	6%
Frequently	0%	30%	2%	7%	0%
First choice	0%	56%	0%	14%	3%

Notes

1. In the complete text physicians stands for: physicians and gastroenterologists.
2. A-teaching hospitals: complete training facilities for internal medicine (5 years).
   B-teaching hospitals: restricted training facilities for internal medicine (2 years).
3. As a standard procedure we defined only those procedures that will be performed in every patient, unless impossible due to technical failures, refusal or contra-indications.

30. The results of a national inquiry among Dutch surgeons on the present treatment of peptic ulcer disease

J. BOEVÉ, M.D.

Department of Surgery, Sophia Ziekenhuis Zwolle, The Netherlands

Introduction

After Billroth successfully performed his gastric resection in 1881 for cancer of the antrum, resection became the treatment of choice for peptic ulcer during the following 60 years.

During the Second World War truncal vagotomy with drainage (TVD) was introduced by Dragstedt, but this procedure did not find a great deal of support in Europe. Dragstedt was not the first surgeon who performed vagal surgery, Latarget, a French surgeon had already in 1922 done a vagotomy with gastroenterostomy on 24 patients. This operation did not find general acceptance either. But his anatomical investigation on the function of the vagal nerve must have been the foundation of all work on the vagus. The selective vagotomy with drainage, as described by Jackson and Frankson in 1948, found a little more response. In 1957 Griffith and Harkins described a surgical technique in which the acid producing part of the stomach is de nervated, but the motility is preserved. Holle performed this operation for the first time on patients, but he always did a pyloroplasty as well. Then in 1976 Amdrup and Johnston simultaneously introduced the highly selective vagotomy (HSV). Antral motility is intact sothat a drainage procedure is not necessary. From 1975 onwards an enormous decrease in the number of gastric resections for peptic ulcer can be detected.

A questionnaire was sent to all surgeons in Holland about their personal working conditions and the manner in which peptic ulcer is treated by them.

Results

The questionnaire was answered by 264 surgeons with training facilities and by 250 without these facilities: a response of 89%. The Dutch training system is divided into full training centres (university hospitals and A-hospitals), in which a complete programme for surgical training is given and B-hospitals, in which a partial programme is given. Their hospital units have about 60–172 surgical beds, while their gastroenterological departments have about 10–50 beds. Gastroenterology is a big field of interest among the surgeons. In some departments 14 surgeons are working on this subject. In 40% only one member of the surgical group is mainly responsible for this area. Research in gastroenterology was prosecuted in 30% of the centres mainly in the bigger hospitals during training, and in 80% a publication resulted.

Retrospective research on conservative treatment was hardly ever performed, but research was mainly conducted on the results of surgical therapy. The diagnosis of the uncomplicated peptic ulcer is established by the medical department in 70% of the patients. Endoscopic investigation is only performed by the surgeons in 10%, mostly in the larger hospitals. In almost all cases the medical department performes an endoscopic investigation, while radiological investigation is still performed in 70% of the departments.

During the endoscopic investigation of a gastric ulcer at least 8 biopsies are taken. Follow-up of the conservative treatment is in nearly 100% of the patients done by the medical department.

Short medical treatment for 6–12 months is favoured by the surgeons in the acute phase in 27%, the long-term treatment up to 2 years in the same percentage, also 27%. In 50% of the hospitals there is an arrangement between the medical and surgical department on the therapeutic approach and the kind of surgical therapy that must follow when and if indicated.

Uncomplicated peptic ulcer

Infrequently, recurrent peptic ulcer will be treated conservatively by 84% of the surgeons, whatever the age of the patient. Frequently recurrent peptic ulcer will be treated surgically by 80% of the surgeons, if the patient is younger than 45 years by 84%, and patients older than 65 years by 77% of the surgeons. The operation of choice for uncomplicated duodenal ulcer is as could be expected: 92% of the surgeons choose HSV, 3% will do a truncal vagotomy with a drainage procedure, and only 5% do a gastric resection.

Table I. Uncomplicated duodenal ulcer.

Operative treatment of choice	Percentage
HSV	92
Resection	5
TVD	3

When HSV is not possible for technical reasons in uncomplicated cases, 40% of the surgeons choose truncal vagotomy with drainage, and 69% a resection. The individual surgeons and B-hospitals prefer the Billroth II resection. In the university hospitals a truncal vagotomy with antral resection is the first, while the Billroth II is the second choice. A-hospitals prefer truncal vagotomy + drainage.

Table II. Operative treatment of duodenal ulcer (HSV not feasible).

Hospital	Operative treatment of choice
University hospitals	TV + antral resection
A-hospitals	TVD
B-hospitals	Resection
Non-training hospitals	Resection

In a small percentage lifelong conservative treatment is advised for patients above 65 years of age. Follow-up after surgery is by surgical and medical department equally, the mean time of surgical follow-up being one year. The recurrence rate is dependent on the time of follow-up and type of operation. The lowest recurrence is seen after truncal vagotomy with antral resection (between 1 and 2%), HSV has a recurrence varying from 5 to 18%. (Table III)

Table III. Recurrence rate.

Operative treatment	Percentage
TV + antral resection	1– 2
HSV	5–18

The treatment of choice for the first recurrence is equally divided between medical and surgical management. If surgery is chosen, resection is done in 67% and in 31% truncal vagotomy with antral resection. All training hospitals follow the same pattern.

Gastric ulcer

The surgical therapy for patients with an uncomplicated gastric ulcer is resection in 74% and vagotomy in 26%. This therapeutic approach is followed by all categories of surgeons. (Table IV)

Table IV. Uncomplicated gastric ulcer.

Operative treatment	Percentage
Resection	74
HSV	26

Complicated peptic ulcer disease

In 86% of the training hospitals there is an agreement with the medical department that the surgeon will see all the patients with upper gastrointestinal bleeding. In the non-teaching hospitals this only happens in 14% of the institutions. Endoscopy is performed in 90% of the cases. The diagnosis is reached within 12 hours in 80% of the cases. If there is a recurrence of bleeding within 24 hours, 87% of the surgeons will operate immediately, not only on the younger, but also on the older patients. A bleeding duodenal ulcer in a patient below 45 years will be treated by suture ligation of the ulcer and by HSV by 49% of the surgeons. 22% perform a gastric resection. In the university and A-hospitals the treatment of choice will be vagal surgery, while the B-hospitals and surgeons without training facilities prefer gastric resection. In the patient older than 65 years, the most favoured approach is suturing the ulcer and truncal vagotomy, with pyloroplasty done by 34% of the surgeons. The second choice is the Billroth II resection (28% of the surgeons). (Table V)

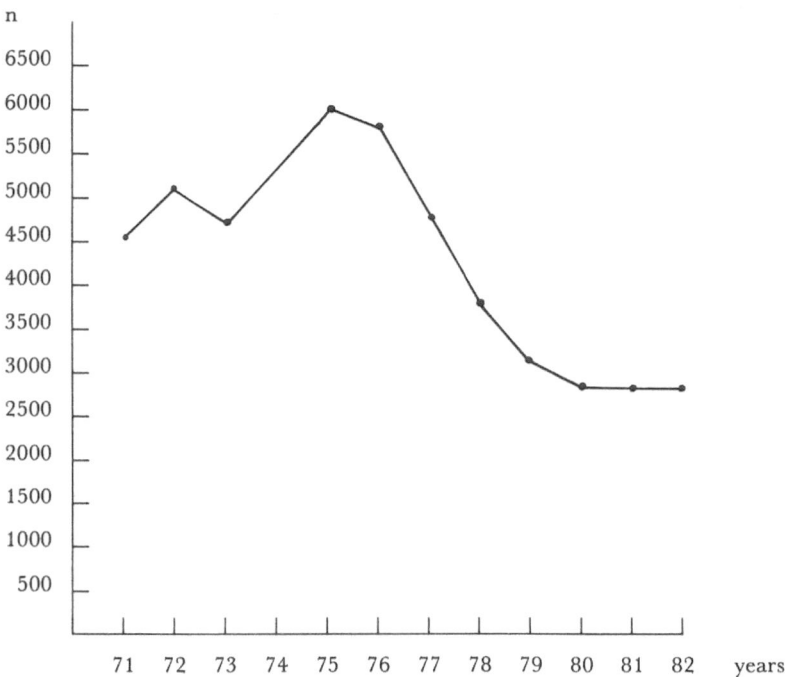

Figure 1. Number of operations for peptic ulcer in The Netherlands. Data from: Stichting Medische Registratie (SMR). Note: histamine H_2-receptor antagonists (cimetidine) was marketed in the Netherlands in 1977.

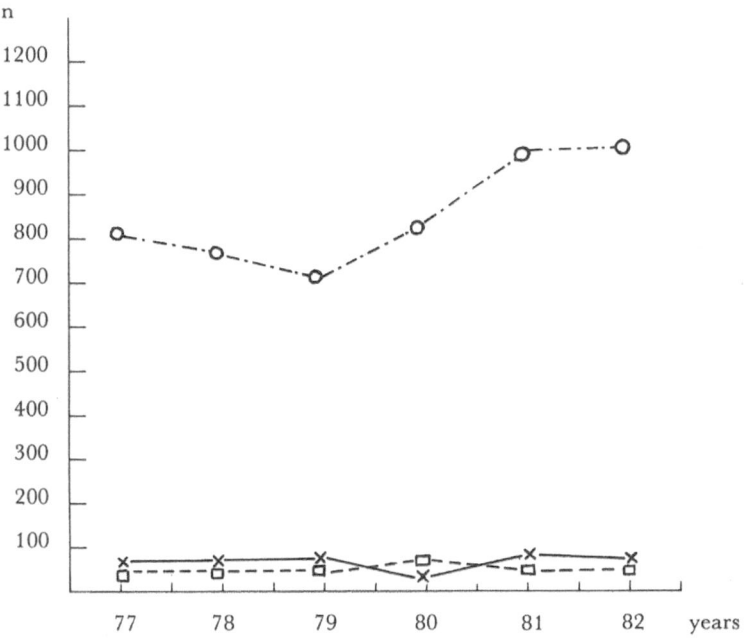

Figure 2. Duodenal ulcer in The Netherlands. Number of highly selective vagotomies (HSV) per year. Data from: Stichting Medische Registratie (SMR).

Table V. Bleeding duodenal ulcer (percentage).

	Suture + HSV	Resection
Under 45 yr	49	22
	Suture + TVD	Resection
Above 65 yr	34	28

Perforation of duodenal ulcer with a short history will be treated by suturing and histamine H_2-receptor antagonists (62% of the surgeons). In patients with a long history, the perforation will be sutured and HSV is performed by 43% of the surgeons, while 28% perform a resection. The university and A-hospitals prefer HSV and the surgeons without training facilities resection. (Table VI)

Table VI. Perforated duodenal ulcer.

Short history	62% suture + H_2-receptor antagonist	All hospitals
Long history	43% suture + HSV	University and A-hospitals
	28% resection	B-hospitals and non-training hospitals

In cases of a pyloric stenosis resection is done by 52% of the surgeons and HSV and dilatation only by 13%.

The number of gastric operations in The Netherlands has been obtained form the data of the SMR. This is a national organization, to which nearly all hospitals in Holland send data about all patients admitted to the hospital, classified according to the international code of disease. Results are shown in figures 1 and 2. It will be seen that the number of gastric operations diminished from 1975 onwards. In 1982 the decrease is nearly 40%. The precentage for duodenal and gastric ulcer is the same.

The answers to the questionnaire show the same trend regarding the decreased number of operations for duodenal ulcer and the change to HSV. As is well known, mortality after surgery for peptic ulcer disease has gone down after the introduction of vagal surgery, but the strongest decline came after the introduction of histamine H_2-receptor antagonists. Exact data from The Netherlands cannot be traced exactly but vary between 2–4%.

Conclusion

- Highly selective vagotomy is the operation of choice for uncomplicated duodenal ulcer.
- In complicated duodenal ulcer truncal vagotomy with antral resection, or Billroth II resection is performed.
- Recurrent peptic ulcer will be treated with surgery in all patients by 84% of the surgeons.
- Infrequently recurrent ulcer will be treated conservatively by 84% of the surgeons.
- Uncomplicated gastric ulcer will be treated with resection by 74% of the surgeons, and by 26% with highly selective vagotomy.

31. Discussion VII

Johnston:

Dr van Blankenstein, you stated that technical failures of HSV result in no decrease in pentagastrin-stimulated acid secretion. However, there are many incomplete vagotomies in which stimulated acid secretion is lowered though admittedly to a lesser extent than in complete vagotomy. Although neither intra-operative, nor post-operative testing is really reliable in predicting a relapse, the patients with a positive post-operative insulin test are four times as likely to get a recurrent ulcer than the negative patients. This does not mean that patients with negative insulin tests will be free of recurrences.

Kennedy:

There is a group of patients with inappropriately high levels of gastric acidity and serum gastrin without having a gastrinoma, or antral G-cell hyperplasia. Probably these patients have G-cell hyperactivity. The recurrence rate after HSV in these patients is very high.

Festen:

Dr Lamers from Nijmegen described a similar patient. The diagnosis can be made by determination of meal-stimulated, or bombesin-stimulated serum gastrin. Bombesin infusion is the most specific test as it only stimulates gastrin of antral origin. The treatment should be antrectomy.

Amdrup:

We had 3 patients with recurrent prepyloric ulcer after selective vagotomy and drainage, who had high serum gastrin levels and a considerable meal-stimulated increase. these patients were cured by antrectomy and post-operatively basal and meal-stimulated serum gastrin returned to normal. Antral G-cell hyperplasia was documented in the operation specimens, with the G-cells in multiple layers.

Van Rooijen:

Are you looking for these multiple layers of G-cells in antral biopsies?

Amdrup:

It cannot be seen in biopsies, it can only be seen in resection specimens.

Kennedy:

I agree. The G-cells are not evenly distributed in the antral mucosa, so biopsies give sampling errors. Moreover, you have to have a very devoted pathologist.

Tijtgat:

Antral G-cell hyperfunction does exist, but I would not advise an antrectomy just because of a high serum gastrin, or an abnormal rise after a meal. We followed two of such patients on conservative treatment and their serum gastrin returned to near-normal levels spontaneously with time. I would advise antrectomy only if the ulcer cannot be successfully treated medically.

Busman (Leeuwarden):

We studied fasting serum gastrin concentrations before and after HSV and found no relation to ulcer recurrence, neither was there any relation established between the decrease in acid output and the rise in serum gastrin. It has been speculated that denervation of the proximal stomach results in the 'removal' of a gastrin inhibiting factor from the fundic mucosa.

Johnston:

Serum gastrin levels and the possible relation to the outcome of HSV are of scientific interest. But this should have no impact on clinical decisions as these matters have not adequately been solved. On the basis of the low mortality and moribidity rates, patients should still be treated by HSV until further research on acid output and gastrin warrants a change in this policy.

Van Blankenstein:

This discussion is merely indicating our lack of knowledge. If an operation fails for non-technical reasons, we probably are dealing with the natural history of disease, which does not respond to inhibition of acid but should be dealt with an alternative approach, such as chelating agents.

Johnson:
There is a irreducible limited percentage of recurrences. Despite an ideal surgical technique, 3 or 4% will recur, for example because of anomalous vagal nerve fibres. Even the patients with recurrent ulcer after HSV could profit from the operation, as the response to medical treatment can be better after HSV, than before. Moreover, we should not view the recurrence rate as an ever increasing figure, but we should take into account the interval rate of the absence of recurrence.

Bilsky (Haarlem):
Is there any place left for selective vagotomy with drainage?

Amdrup:
Either truncal vagotomy and antrectomy because the recurrence rate is low, or HSV because the mortality and morbidity rates are low, but nothing in between.

Spencer:
According to the Dutch national inquiry on diagnosis and treatment of ulcers, physicians almost exclusively make use of histamine H_2-receptor antagonists. But mucosa protective agents are as effective as and cheaper than histamine H_2-receptor antagonists.

Nelis:
In part this prescribing attitude will be determined by historical grounds. If one is going to manage a patient with continuous medical treatment, it seems logical to choose the same drug for the acute and the maintenance period and this will mostly be an histamine H_2-receptor antagonist. Of the chelating agents bismuth compounds are not advised for maintenance treatment because of the possible toxic effects of bismuth accumulation and there is only limited experience in maintenance treatment with sucralfate. However, if one selects acute treatment only, there are many arguments in favour of a chelating agent. Among these are cost-effectiveness and also a lower recurrence rate has been claimed by some authors.

Van Blankenstein:

The histamine H_2-receptor antagonists were first on the scene. Given the effectiveness and safety profile there are not many arguments to change. Moreover, (Dutch) physicians are mostly not aware of the price of the drugs they prescribe.

Tijtgat:

In which proportion of the patients with recurrent ulcer after HSV is the recurrence due to incompleteness of the vagotomy?

Amdrup:

It is hard to say. In my opinion, with complete HSV the recurrence rate will not be less than 5% at 10 years.

Johnston:

All tests on completeness are of limited value as they only predict that the chance of a recurrence is more or less, but they do not predict whether an ulcer is indeed going to recur or not.

Busman (Leeuwarden):

Possibly stress factors have an influence in this matter. Poppen demonstrated on biopsy material that even after an ideal HSV 25% of the patients still had some innervation left. So perhaps 25% of the procedures is incomplete by definition.

Johnson:

Why should we assume that every ulcer heals with complete vagotomy. Not all ulcers heal with histamine H_2-receptor antagonists either. If there is a technical failure with HSV many ulcers will stay unhealed or recur. If the HSV is done properly some ulcers will stay unhealed or recur.